GROSS PATHOLOGY

A COLOUR ATLAS

BY R·C·CURRAN

& E·L·JONES

GROSS PATHOLOGY

A COLOR ATLAS

BY R·C·CURRAN MD·FRCP(Lond)·FRS(Edin)·FRC Path

Leith Professor of Pathology, University of Birmingham
Consultant Pathologist, United Birmingham Hospitals
and Birmingham Regional Hospital Board
Chairman, Division of Pathological Studies

& E·L·JONES MD·MRCS(Eng)·LRCP(Lond)·MRC Path

Senior Lecturer, Department of Pathology, University of Birmingham
Consultant Pathologist, United Birmingham Hospitals

FOREWORD BY PROFESSOR SIR THEO CRAWFORD

with 762 illustrations in full color

OXFORD UNIVERSITY PRESS—NEW YORK

All rights including translations reserved by
Harvey Miller · 20 Marryat Road · London SW19 5BD · England

Published in the USA and Canada by
Oxford University Press, 200 Madison Avenue, New York NY 10016, USA

First Edition 1974, Reprinted 1975

Library of Congress Card Number 74-77295

A Harvey and Elly Miller Production

Text composed by Art Reprographic (London) Ltd.
Colour origination by Schwitter AG Basel · Switzerland
Printed by de Lange/van Leer · Deventer · Holland
Bound by van Rijmenam · The Hague · Holland
Manufactured in Holland

CONTENTS

FOREWORD

THE INCREASING AMOUNT of knowledge that the young doctor must acquire during his training has inevitably led to attempts to prune some of the older subjects of the classical medical curriculum. As every gardener knows, pruning is a process which, if properly conducted, leads to tidier, better organised and more fruitful growth: but if the process is crudely or ruthlessly performed the plant may wither and become unproductive. Amongst subjects of the medical curriculum that have suffered in this way Gross—or Anatomical—Pathology comes high on the list.

Those of us who were undergraduates between the wars were sated with descriptive gross pathology. We learned by rote the text book descriptions and culinary metaphors applied to a host of morbid anatomical states, for we knew—or thought we knew—that survival through a testing examination depended on this knowledge. Which of us dared to enter such an examination without being on familiar terms with such delicacies as nutmeg liver, hard-bake spleen, or bread-and-butter pericardium—or a host of other irrelevancies acquired by hours spent in the post-mortem room, at tutorials, or with the text books? It is right that much of this preoccupation with the details of gross anatomical change as a result of disease has been pruned away to find time for a more functional approach to pathological processes; but, as so often happens, there is danger of the pruning being too radical and producing a generation of medical graduates who carry in their mind's eye no mental picture of the altered anatomy of the diseased organs whose abnormality they detect by their increasingly sophisticated diagnostic tests. Such doctors are clearly at a disadvantage in acquiring a full understanding of their patients and the impact of their disease upon them. The dilemma, therefore, is to retain time for an updated version of the classical morbid anatomy and simultaneously to find time for the countless new facets of knowledge in the field of pathology with which the student now has to be acquainted.

Gross pathology is a visual subject, and like all visual subjects it is to be learned only by frequent exposure to the visual patterns involved—and, furthermore, if it is to be remembered, periodic re-exposure is essential. Traditionally these exposures have involved long hours spent in the post-mortem room and in the museum, with resort to reference books for rather indifferent black-and-white illustrations for home study or when less common conditions are being considered.

This Atlas of Gross Pathology is a serious, and—in my view—successful attempt to solve these problems. It brings together in a single volume no less than 762 technically-superb illustrations in colour of all the common and very many of the rarer pathological disturbances of anatomy found in the operating theatre and post-mortem room. These pictures have great advantages over the specimens in most museums: they look 'alive' rather than preserved, and in many instances the important features are emphasised by 'close-up' viewing. Furthermore, the clear and concise text which accompanies the illustrations gives just the amount of commentary that is needed for what is essentially a visual exercise.

Professor R. C. Curran is the natural author for such a book. His origins in Glasgow ensure a proper appreciation of the value of morphological detail in the understanding of disease: and this, tempered by his sojourns in Sheffield, London (at St. Thomas's) and Birmingham, and by his personal research in inflammation and repair, further ensures that the details of gross pathology are appropriately related to the histological features which formed the subject of Professor Curran's earlier Atlas.

Professor Curran has been fortunate and wise to enlist the aid of Dr. E. L. Jones as his co-author for this Atlas. Dr. Jones is a Senior Lecturer in Professor Curran's department in

Birmingham but, still in his early thirties, he is young enough to know by experience the pressures on the contemporary student population and on our young pathologists in training. Between them Professor Curran and Dr. Jones have solved enormously difficult problems. The technical quality of the photography is superb and is matched by the skilful selection and preparation of specimens. The result is a collection of pictures which are superior in educational value to many of the fixed specimens to be found in pathological museums. No-one would suggest that direct experience of pathological material in the laboratory and post-mortem room could ever be replaced by illustrations in the training of our future pathologists. But for the undergraduate it makes sense to short-circuit the learning process in this way: and the trainee pathologists too will find it an invaluable adjunct to the more rapid acquisition of their essential stock-in-trade of visual memory.

T.C.

AUTHORS' PREFACE

From the late 18th century, when Morgagni published his great classic, *De Sedibus*, advances in medicine were generally based on the principle of correlating the clinical and pathological features of a disease. This was done by determining the structural changes present in the tissues and then considering how these changes might lead to disordered function and in turn to the symptoms and signs characteristic of that disease. This approach is still valid, and modern analytical techniques have extended it from the macroscopic to the subcellular and molecular levels. We believe that a sound knowledge of the macroscopic changes in the tissues is still the firmest foundation on which to build an understanding of disease and its clinical manifestations. Students are quick to recognise this. However the pressures of a crowded curriculum have tended to reduce the time available to them for studying tissues at first hand, either in the form of surgical specimens or through attendance at post-mortem examinations. It is hoped that this Atlas will help to remedy this deficiency, by presenting a balanced and comprehensive coverage of the structural derangements found in most of the diseases likely to be encountered in clinical practice.

The 'visual' content of tissue pathology is high, and to convey this in the most effective way, unfixed or lightly fixed tissues have been used wherever possible. They are shown in considerable detail, often in close-up in a way normally experienced only by the pathologist handling tissues in the laboratory or post-mortem room. Correlation of the macroscopic and microscopic abnormalities is aided by occasional brief descriptions of the main histological features. As a rule scales have been omitted from the illustrations. Instead we have included a sufficient amount of the affected organ, or shown its architecture in such detail by means of 'close-ups', as to make it easy to estimate the size of the lesion. Where more precision is required, the measurements are given in the text. The colour balance of the pictures has been carefully adjusted so as to be satisfactory for most forms of lighting, but for viewing them artificial (tungsten) light is better than daylight or light from gas discharge (fluorescent) tubes.

The concise text allows the essential features of each lesion to be readily grasped, the intention being that the student should complement this knowledge by reading the fuller descriptions available in the standard textbooks of pathology. On the other hand the Index is comprehensive to make it easy to locate a particular lesion or a macroscopic appearance. The Atlas has been planned primarily for undergraduate students but it is hoped that it will prove of interest and value not only to postgraduate students in pathology but also to those training in other branches of medicine.

ACKNOWLEDGEMENTS

We wish to express our sincere thanks to past and present colleagues in this Department, and especially to Professor W. Thomas Smith, for providing many of the lesions for photography; and one of us (R.C.C.) also wishes to acknowledge with gratitude the help given in this respect by former colleagues in St. Thomas's Hospital Medical School, London. We are also particularly indebted to Dr. H. Thompson and the late Dr. C. W. Taylor for allowing us access to their personal collections of photographs. The same privilege was granted by a number of pathologists and clinicians in this Medical Centre and in other centres; and several pathologists allowed us to photograph specimens in their Museums. In this way it was possible to extend the range of the Atlas considerably and to all these individuals, whose contributions are listed below, we are deeply grateful.

Our thanks are due also to Miss Mary Domone FIMLT and Mr. Allan Cooper FIMLT, who took many of the photographs; to Mrs. J. E. Collar B.Sc. and Mrs. A. D. Simmons AIMLT for technical help; and to Mrs. B. S. Richardson for secretarial assistance.

The colour reproduction has been carried out by Schwitter A.G. Basel and the printing by de Lange-van Leer, Deventer with great care and skill under the guidance of Harvey and Elly Miller. To all of them we express our thanks.

Professor J. R. Anderson, Department of Pathology, Western Infirmary, Glasgow.   13.34.

Mr. G. H. Baines, Consultant Surgeon, Department of Urology, Queen Elizabeth Hospital, Birmingham. 10.59; 10.60.

Dr. D. R. Barry, Birmingham and Midland Eye Hospital, Birmingham.   9.87; 9.89; 9.90.

Professor W. A. J. Crane, Department of Pathology, University of Sheffield.   5.10; 5.39; 6.32; 6.33; 6.44; 7.25; 7.26; 7.50; 10.25; 10.66; 11.9; 13.62; 13.64; 14.22.

Professor G. Cunningham, *M.B.E.*, formerly Sir William Collins Professor of Pathology and Conservator of Pathological Collection, Royal College of Surgeons, London.   4.32; 4.34; 6.9; 7.11; 7.40; 9.18; 10.53; 12.50; 13.1; 13.12; 13.27; 13.37; 13.38; 13.45; 13.48; 13.51; 13.53.

Mr. T. F. Dee, Chief Medical Photographer, Department of Medical Illustration, Queen Elizabeth Medical Centre, Birmingham.   1.3; 1.16; 12.11; 14.1; 14.2; 14.3; 14.4; 14.5; 14.7; 14.8; 14.9; 14.10; 14.12; 14.13; 14.14; 14.18; 14.21; 14.23; 14.24; 14.25; 14.27; 14.28; 14.31.
We are grateful to the following consultants for allowing us to reproduce the above photographs of patients in their clinical care:
Professor J. M. Bishop, Mr. W. H. Bond, Mr. V. S. Brookes, Mr. G. W. Dalton, Mr. P. E. Dawson-Edwards, Dr. E. A. Fairburn, Mr. A. Gourevitch, Dr. C. F. Hawkins, Dr. G. M. Holme, Mr. O. T. Mansfield, Professor G. Slaney.

Professor J. L. Emery, Department of Pathology, Children's Hospital, Sheffield.   3.4; 8.14; 9.7; 9.22; 9.23; 9.33; 9.82; 14.36.

Professor T. Gibson, Director, Plastic and Oral Surgery Service, Canniesburn Hospital, Glasgow.   1.12.

Dr. C. Giles, Department of Pathology, North Staffordshire Royal Infirmary, Stoke-on-Trent.   9.28.

Professor R. B. Goudie, Department of Pathology, Royal Infirmary, Glasgow.   4.64; 8.27; 9.37; 9.50; 10.24; 11.30.

Professor J. Gough, 22 Park Road, Whitchurch, Cardiff.   7.22; 7.23; 7.24.

Professor N. F. C. Gowing, Department of Histopathology, Royal Marsden Hospital, London.   2.15; 3.12; 3.13; 3.15; 7.9; 8.25; 8.35; 10.26; 12.7; 13.14; 13.70; 13.71; 13.82; 13.84; 13.85; 14.20; 14.29; 14.30; 14.34.

Dr. C. H. W. Horne, Department of Pathology, University of Aberdeen. 4.6.

Dr. C. R. Knappett, Department of Pathology, North Staffordshire Royal Infirmary, Stoke-on-Trent. 4.57.

Dr. F. Kurrein, Department of Pathology, Worcester Royal Infirmary, Worcester. 7.47.

Dr. A. J. McCall, Department of Pathology, North Staffordshire Royal Infirmary, Stoke-on-Trent. 1.15; 2.21; 4.5; 4.18; 4.63; 5.4; 5.13; 5.25; 6.4; 6.5; 6.11; 6.45; 6.72; 6.78; 7.16; 8.3; 9.34; 9.39; 11.12; 13.55; 13.81; 13.90.

Dr. A. M. MacDonald and Dr. A. A. M. Gibson, Department of Pathology, Royal Hospital for Sick Children, Glasgow. 4.10; 4.55; 5.16; 5.24; 5.38; 6.1; 6.2; 6.8; 8.12; 8.13; 9.24; 9.88; 10.2; 10.3; 11.27; 13.3; 13.59; 13.80; 13.89.

Dr. P. Mackay, Department of Pathology, University of Aberdeen. 1.25.

Dr. J. S. McKinnell, Department of Pathology, Selly Oak Hospital, Birmingham. 13.25; 13.52; 13.68; 13.69.

Dr. A. G. Marshall and Dr. Shirley P. Ward, Department of Pathology, The Royal Hospital, Wolverhampton. 1.22; 5.18; 8.15; 11.11; 13.67.

Professor A. Munro Neville, Division of Pathology, Chester Beatty Research Institute, London. 8.22; 11.29; 12.68.

Dr. R. G. F. Parker, Department of Pathology, East Birmingham Hospital, Birmingham. 4.4; 4.24; 6.54; 7.33; 7.37; 10.54; 11.3; 11.19; 13.20; 13.27.

Dr. D. I. Rushton, Department of Pathology, Birmingham Maternity Hospital, Birmingham. 12.47; 12.48; 12.54.

Dr. R. M. E. Seal, Department of Pathology, Sully Hospital, Sully, Glam. 7.29.

Dr. S. Sevitt, Department of Pathology, Birmingham Accident Hospital and Rehabilitation Centre, Birmingham. 6.19; 6.29; 6.34; 9.19; 13.28; 13.29; 13.30; 13.33.

Dr. W. R. Shortland-Webb, Department of Pathology, Dudley Road Hospital, Birmingham. 3.5.

Professor H. A. Sissons, Department of Morbid Anatomy, Royal National Orthopaedic Hospital, London (Wellcome Museum of Orthopaedics). 9.57; 13.2; 13.4; 13.21; 13.24; 13.63.

Professor A. L. Stalker, Department of Pathology, University of Aberdeen. 4.3; 4.6; 6.73; 6.74; 8.29; 9.9; 11.8; 13.22; 13.36.

The late **Dr. C. W. Taylor,** Department of Pathology, University of Birmingham. 9.79; 12.19; 12.20; 12.21; 12.22; 12.25; 12.27; 12.31; 12.33; 12.34; 12.35; 12.36; 12.38; 12.39; 12.42; 12.43; 12.44; 12.45; 12.46; 12.51; 12.55; 12.56; 12.58; 12.59; 12.60; 12.61; 12.65; 12.70; 12.71; 13.86.

Professor O. L. Wade, Department of Clinical Pharmacology, University of Birmingham. 7.31.

Dr. T. Wade-Evans, Department of Pathology, Birmingham and Midland Hospital for Women, Birmingham. 12.26; 12.28; 12.29; 12.30; 12.63; 12.69.

Professor D. H. Wright, Department of Morbid Anatomy and Experimental Pathology, University of Southampton. 1.2; 2.18; 2.26; 2.30; 3.14; 4.8; 4.27; 5.23; 5.40; 6.16; 6.18; 9.15; 12.72.

Injury to tissue initiates a series of events which tend to destroy or limit the spread or effect of the injurious agent. These events constitute inflammation. The earliest responses are mainly vascular and the later phases of repair and healing of the injured tissue may be regarded as parts of the same defensive process. The agents that injure tissues and thereby evoke an inflammatory response include bacteria and other types of microorganisms, and non-living agents such as trauma, heat, cold, radiant and electrical energy, and chemicals. The diversity of the aetiological factors is the principal reason for inflammation being one of the commonest and most important conditions in pathology. There are also immunological mechanisms which are defensive in nature but which may in some circumstances prove harmful to the host. This chapter illustrates some aspects of the inflammatory response; and examples of lesions produced by a wide variety of agents or by mechanisms of an infective, physical and immunological nature are given.

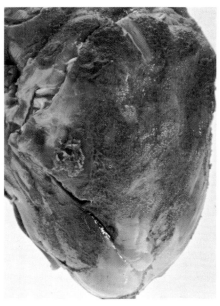

1.1 Acute fibrinous pericarditis

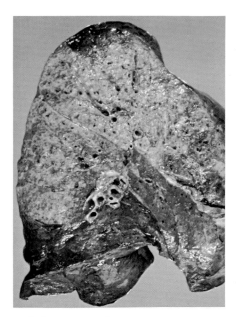

1.2 Lobar pneumonia

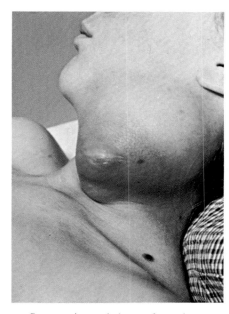

1.3 Suppuration and abscess formation: branchial cyst

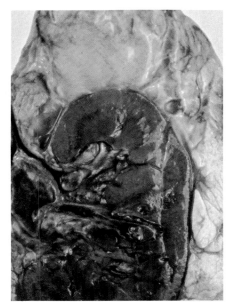

1.4 Perinephric abscess

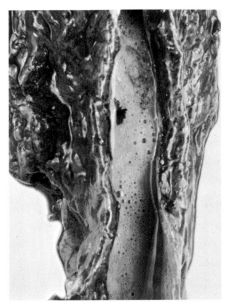

1.5 Acute tracheobronchitis

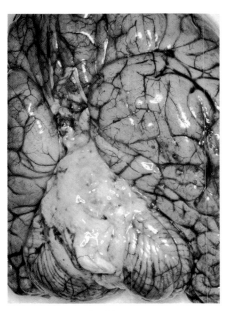

1.6 Purulent meningitis

1.1 Acute fibrinous pericarditis. Fibrinous inflammation frequently involves serous membranes and the meninges. This shows the epicardial surface of the heart covered with a fibrinous exudate which is slightly blood-stained in places. A protein-rich fluid was also present in the pericardial sac. Fibrinous pericarditis may be caused by a pneumococcal infection but the most extreme forms are found in acute rheumatic fever. Fibrinous inflammation is also often seen on the pleura overlying a pneumonic process. **1.2 Lobar pneumonia.** In lobar pneumonia, a fibrin-rich inflammatory exudate fills the pulmonary alveoli in such a way as to cause one or more lobes to become solid (consolidation) and liver-like (hepatisation). This is the left lung and there is extensive consolidation of the whole of the upper lobe and apical segments of the lower lobe. The consolidated lung is pale grey, a stage of consolidation referred to as grey hepatisation. It is preceded by red hepatisation and generally occurs four to eight days after the onset of the acute illness. The cut surface of the affected lung is dry, granular and airless, and the firm consistence is shown in the way that the cut surface retains sharp straight edges. Lobar pneumonia is most often caused by a pneumococcal infection and the classical appearances of red and grey hepatisation are seen much less frequently than previously. **1.3 Suppuration and abscess formation: branchial cyst.** Two of the signs of acute inflammation are evident, viz. redness and swelling. The redness is caused by vasodilatation and the swelling mainly through the accumulation of exudate. The underlying lesion is a branchial cyst on the side of the neck

of a young girl. The cyst has become infected and acutely inflamed and pus has formed within it to produce an acute abscess. **1.4 Perinephric abscess.** Infection in the tissues around the upper pole of the kidney has caused acute inflammation which has gone on to the formation of an abundant thick green exudate of pus (purulent or suppurative inflammation). Pus contains large numbers of neutrophil polymorph leucocytes as well as necrotic cells and tissue. Initially thick and creamy, it often becomes thinner in consistence following the release of proteolytic enzymes from dying and dead polymorphs. Perinephric abscess usually complicates acute pyelonephritis, following rupture of renal abscesses into the perinephric tissues. **1.5 Acute tracheobronchitis.** Catarrhal inflammation affects mucous membranes and is characterised by copious secretion of mucus, by formation of an exudate which is at first serous and later mucopurulent, and sometimes by desquamation of the mucosal epithelium. The changes are typically confined to the superficial tissues. In this case, the mucosa of the trachea and bronchi were affected and the trachea is filled with frothy greenish mucopurulent secretion. For many years the patient had chronic bronchitis, a condition which is liable to be complicated by episodes of acute inflammation. **1.6 Purulent meningitis.** The undersurface of the brain is shown. A thick green purulent exudate fills the subarachnoid space over the brain-stem and cerebellum. The patient was treated for leukaemia and subsequently developed acute meningitis. The causative organism was *Staphylococcus aureus*.

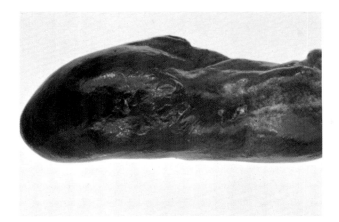

1.7 Acute cholecystitis and empyema

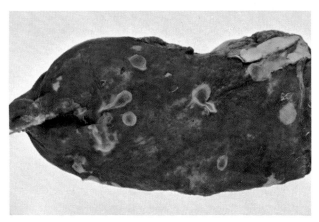

1.8 Acute gangrenous cholecystitis

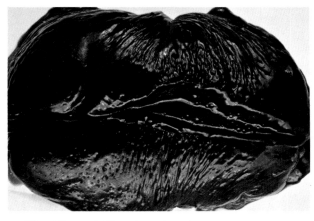

1.9 *Clostridium welchii* septicaemia: spleen

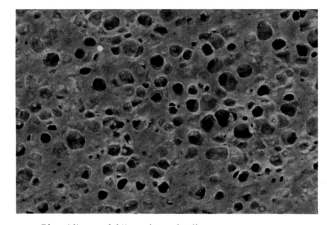

1.10 *Clostridium welchii* septicaemia: liver

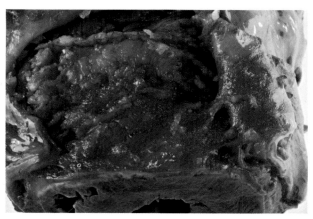

1.11 Organising fibrinous pericarditis

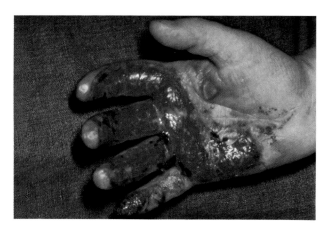

1.12 Granulating burn

1.7 Acute cholecystitis and empyema. An empyema is a collection of pus within a natural sac. This shows a gall-bladder which is enlarged, firm and a dark reddish-brown colour. The wall is increased in thickness, from the presence within it of an inflammatory exudate and extravasated blood. The lumen was distended with a mixture of bile, pus and blood, but gall-stones were not present. Acute cholecystitis may be caused by streptococci, staphylococci or enteric microorganisms. **1.8 Acute gangrenous cholecystitis**. In some forms of acute cholecystitis (generally suppurative), vascular obstruction may occur, causing haemorrhagic infarction and gangrene of the gall-bladder. In this example, the wall of the gall-bladder is a dusky-brown colour, because of the underlying infarction, and multiple round yellowish-green abscesses are present over the serosal surface. These abscesses tend to rupture and produce fatal acute diffuse peritonitis. **1.9 and 1.10 *Clostridium welchii* septicaemia**. The clostridia are strictly anaerobic gram-positive bacilli and they include the organisms responsible for gas-gangrene. In the terminal stages of gas-gangrene, the organisms invade the bloodstream and are widely distributed to all tissues. If the necropsy is delayed a few hours, gas formation is evident in most organs. **1.9**. This is the spleen from a fatal case of *Clostridium welchii* septicaemia. The organ is enlarged and the capsule is very wrinkled. The pulp is dark red, almost black, and

semi-fluid. Gas bubbles can be seen exuding from the cut surface. Apart from the gas bubbles, a similar change in the spleen can be seen in many acute systemic infections, a condition termed acute reactive hyperplasia or 'septic splenitis'. In some instances the follicles are enlarged and prominent as grey dots. **1.10**. This is the cut surface of the liver from the same case. The large numbers of gas bubbles present give the organ a honeycomb appearance. **1.11 Organising fibrinous pericarditis**. This is an example of repair by organisation. The pericardial sac has been opened with some difficulty, the two layers being firmly adherent to each other, to show numerous thick strands of fibrin covering the surface of the heart and causing it to adhere to the parietal pericardium. The fibrin has been partly organised, the process of organisation leading to the formation of fibrous tissue. The appearances of this stage of fibrinous pericarditis should be compared with those shown in 1.1. **1.12 Granulating burn**. This shows a 3-week-old deep burn of the palmar surface of the hand of a child. Where the epithelial tissues have been destroyed, the surface is covered with bright red granulation tissue. The granulation tissue would eventually form considerable amounts of fibrous tissue. For this reason skin grafts are used to cover severe burns, after resection of necrotic tissue. In this way formation of granulation tissue and scar tissue is greatly reduced and severe deformities are avoided.

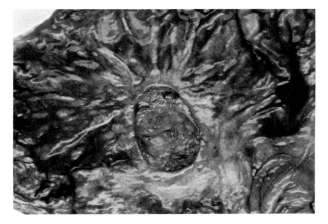

1.13 Chronic peptic ulcer: stomach

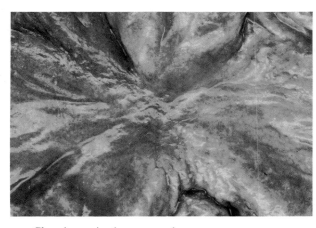

1.14 Chronic peptic ulcer: stomach

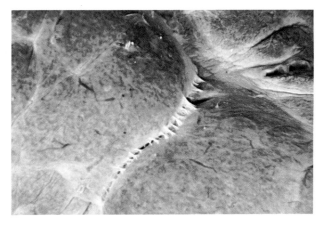

1.15 Tertiary syphilis: liver

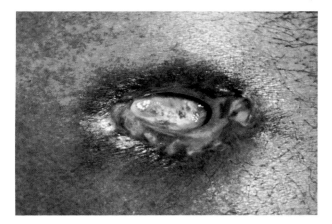

1.16 Gummatous ulcer: skin

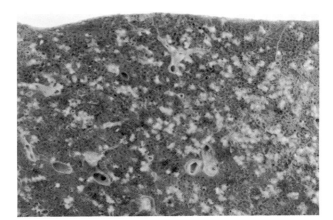

1.17 Miliary tuberculosis: lung

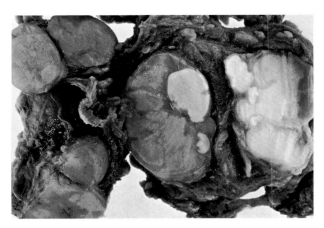

1.18 Caseous tuberculosis: lymph nodes

1.13 and 1.14 Chronic peptic ulcer: stomach. Ulceration means a circumscribed loss of substance from the surface of an organ, usually accompanied by inflammation of the adjacent tissues. **1.13** The stomach and first part of the duodenum are frequent sites of ulceration and this shows a large gastric ulcer situated in the body of the stomach. The artery visible in the ulcer crater had been eroded by the deepening ulcer and the patient died from haematemesis. **1.14** A shallow healed ulcer is present on the lesser curve, with mucosal folds radiating out from the central epithelialised crater. Microscopy showed the epithelium covering the tissue occupying the ulcer to be flat and lacking specialised secretory elements. Contraction of the fibrous tissue in and around the ulcer has produced an hour-glass deformity of the stomach. Contraction may also produce pyloric stenosis. **1.15 and 1.16 Tertiary syphilis.** In tertiary syphilis, fibrosis and necrosis affect many tissues, and a gumma is a large area of necrosis. Gummas appear 8 to 25 years after the initial infection. They may be solitary or multiple and vary from microscopic size to 10 cm or more in diameter. Common sites of occurrence are the skin, liver, bone and testes. Absorption of the necrotic tissue in the gumma is followed by

reparative fibrosis of unusual severity. The scar tissue tends to produce considerable distortion, particularly in the liver. **1.15** In this example, destruction of the hepatic tissue followed by fibrous repair has produced a grossly distorted liver with the formation of large lobes (hepar lobatum). Several lobes are joined by dense fibrous adhesions. **1.16** A large gummatous ulcer of the abdominal wall is shown. It is deep and the base is covered by a necrotic slough. The surrounding skin is undermined. **1.17 Miliary tuberculosis: lung.** In this condition, numerous small white nodules (miliary tubercles), 1 mm or more in diameter, are found in many organs, including the lung, as shown here. Miliary tuberculosis results from dissemination of large numbers of tubercle bacilli by the bloodstream. Each tubercle is a small granuloma composed of epithelioid cells and giant cells. The name miliary is derived from the fact that the tubercle resembles a millet seed. **1.18 Caseous tuberculosis: lymph nodes.** Several enlarged discrete lymph nodes are present within fat and fibrous tissue. The two largest nodes contain white areas of caseation necrosis.

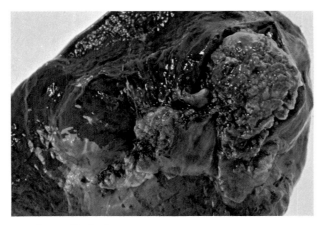

1.19 Aspergillosis: lung

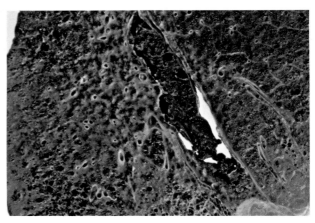

1.20 Silicosis: lung

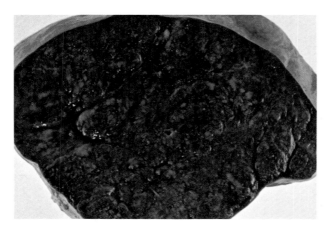

1.21 Sarcoidosis: spleen

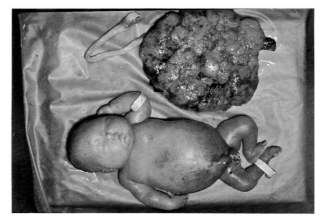

1.22 Hydrops fetalis (erythroblastosis fetalis)

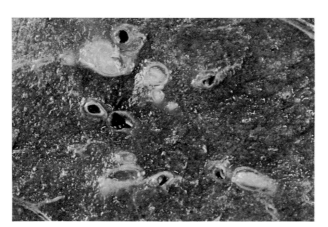

1.23 Bronchial asthma

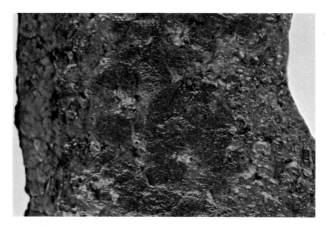

1.24 Honeycomb lung

1.19 Aspergillosis: lung. Aspergillosis is a mycotic infection produced by organisms usually regarded as non-pathogenic which invade under conditions of lowered resistance of the body. Thus it is usually an 'opportunistic' infection, secondary to some predisposing disease, disturbed metabolic state, or therapeutic regime. Where there is a pre-existing cavity, 'fungus balls' may form within them, as in this case. The lung is from a woman aged 32 with Fallot's tetrad, and a large aspergillotic 'ball' is visible in the apex of the upper lobe. **1.20 Silicosis: lung.** The patient was a foundry worker. The right middle lobe is collapsed but extensive areas of silicotic scarring are visible as pale nodules throughout the other lobes. The lung also shows diffuse focal dust emphysema and patchy centrilobular emphysema. The blackening is due to the presence of carbon pigment, more severe peripherally. Inhaled silica particles are phagocytosed by pulmonary macrophages and provoke formation of nodules of dense hyaline collagenous tissue. This nodularity gives silicosis its unique appearance among the pneumoconioses. The tendency to tuberculosis is much enhanced in silicosis. **1.21 Sarcoidosis: spleen.** Sarcoidosis is characterised by the presence of granulomas composed of epithelioid cells and giant cells arranged in follicles similar to those seen in tuberculosis. The aetiological agent is however unknown. The spleen is enlarged but grey-white sarcoid tissue has replaced most of the splenic tissue. Rarely the splenic involvement is so severe in proportion to lesions in other organs as to appear the 'primary' lesion. **1.22-1.30** illustrate a variety of conditions in which the pathogenetic mechanism is either known or suspected to be immunologically-mediated. **1.22 Hydrops fetalis (erythroblastosis fetalis).** The placenta (top) is swollen and yellow, in contrast to the deep red of the normal full-term placenta. The fetus is grossly oedematous (hydrops fetalis). Erythroblastosis fetalis arises when a rhesus-negative mother carries a rhesus-positive fetus. Fetal antigen induces antibody formation in the mother, and her antibodies cross the placenta to cause severe haemolysis in the fetus. In severe cases the anaemia may be so marked as to cause generalised oedema of the fetus, as here. **1.23 Bronchial asthma.** Bronchial asthma is an example of an immediate (Type I) hypersensitivity reaction mediated in atopic individuals by various antigens reacting with tissue cells passively sensitised by antibody produced elsewhere and leading to the release of pharmacologically-active substances. In the acute stages the lungs are pale and distended and the medium and small bronchi are plugged by thick viscid mucus which contains numerous eosinophils and desquamated epithelial cells. The plugging of the medium and small bronchi by mucus plugs is clearly seen in this case. The adjacent branches of the pulmonary arteries also are thick-walled and unduly prominent. **1.24 Honeycomb lung.** In some non-atopic individuals inhalation of organic dusts such as fungal spores or bird secretions gives rise not to an immediate (Type I) reaction but to a Type III reaction. The result is gradual destruction of the alveolar structure and formation of larger cystic spaces—honeycomb lung. The lung on the right shows these changes of diffuse fibrosis with the formation of multiple small thick-walled cysts, and the pleural surface (left) appears nodular. In addition, the central portion is red-brown, with large areas of bronchopneumonic consolidation.

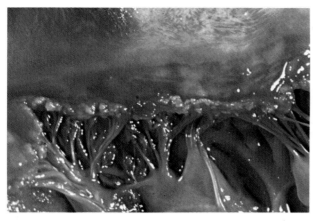

1.25 Acute rheumatic endocarditis: mitral valve

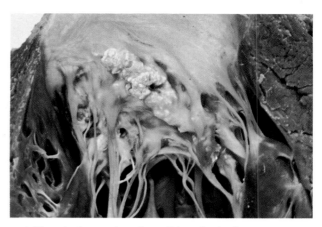

1.26 Chronic rheumatic endocarditis: mitral valve

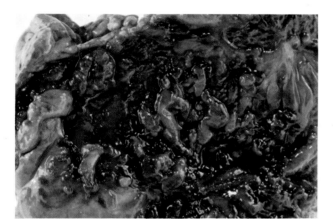

1.27 Ulcerative colitis

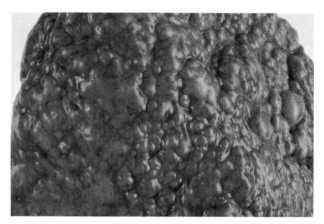

1.28 Macronodular cirrhosis

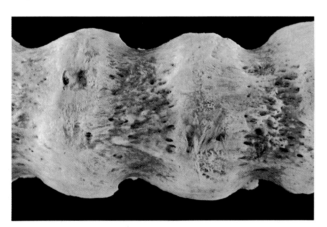

1.29 Ankylosing spondylitis

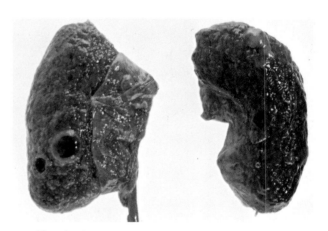

1.30 Chronic glomerulonephritis

1.25 and 1.26 Acute and chronic rheumatic endocarditis. Acute rheumatism causes acute inflammation of the heart and especially of the valves on the left side. Fibrotic lesions develop in the heart as a result of repeated attacks. The condition is probably mediated by a disordered immunological response to streptococcal infections, usually of the nasopharynx. **1.25** This is an acutely inflamed mitral valve. The valve leaflets are swollen and oedematous, with loss of translucency. Along the line of contact of the atrial surfaces of the cusps there are many tiny grey wart-like vegetations, each 1-3 mm in diameter. Their small size is characteristic. Acute rheumatic valvulitis most commonly affects the mitral valve, but vegetations are also often found on other valves and they sometimes extend to the endocardium of the left atrium (McCallum's patch). The patient was a child of 7 who developed acute rheumatism following a streptococcal throat infection. **1.26** The vegetations are organised and after several attacks there is considerable scarring of the valves, sometimes with dystrophic calcification. The undersurface of an affected mitral valve is shown, with part of the left ventricle and left atrium. The mitral valve cusps are fused and distorted due to severe fibrous contraction and nodular calcification. The chordae tendineae are also considerably thickened and shortened. These changes caused severe stenosis of the valve orifice and this led to cardiac failure. **1.27 Ulcerative colitis.** This is an example of a fulminating acute inflammatory process, affecting the mucous membrane of the colon, which has led to ulceration and haemorrhage. The surviving areas of mucosa, by attempting to regenerate and repair the areas of ulceration, have formed raised polypoid

masses which are sometimes referred to as pseudopolyps. **1.28 Macronodular cirrhosis.** This is the capsular surface of the liver. It has a coarse 'hob-nail' appearance, from the presence within it of large nodules of regenerating liver cells, combined with marked fibrosis. The regeneration nodules range from 0.5 to 1.5 cm in diameter. The liver usually weighs between 700 and 1000 g. **1.29 Ankylosing spondylitis.** This is another example of a chronic fibrosing condition with the additional feature, because of the involvement of osteogenic tissue, of considerable formation of new bone. The thoraco-lumbar spine has been macerated to remove the soft tissues and then dried. The most notable feature is the formation of new bone between the vertebral bodies, obscuring the articulations, spinal ligaments and intervertebral discs, and fusing the bodies into a solid bony column. In ankylosing spondylitis, there is chronic inflammation of the posterior intervertebral, costovertebral and sacroiliac joints. The disease mainly occurs in males and is closely related to rheumatoid arthritis. **1.30 Chronic glomerulonephritis.** This condition also may be regarded as a chronic inflammatory process, immunologically-mediated, which ends in severe fibrosis and destruction of normal structure and function. Both kidneys are shrunken, characteristically to an equal extent. The surface of each organ is pitted and diffusely granular, due to the underlying fibrosis. A few small 'retention' cysts (left) are present. Small contracted kidneys can be caused by a number of conditions other then glomerulonephritis and it may be difficult to identify *post mortem* which one was responsible.

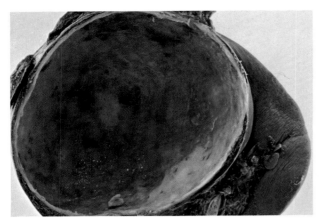

2.1 Simple (non-parasitic) cyst: spleen

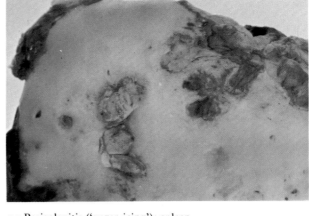

2.2 Perisplenitis ('sugar-icing'): spleen

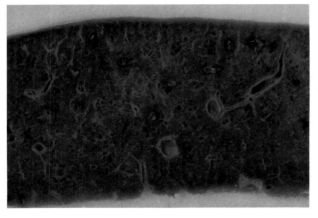

2.3 Chronic venous congestion: spleen

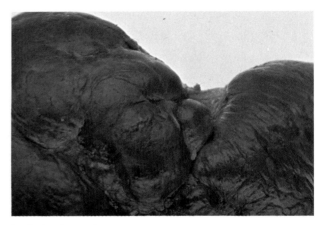

2.4 Infarction: spleen

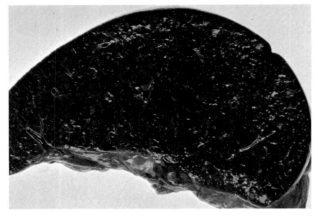

2.5 Portal hypertension and congestion: spleen

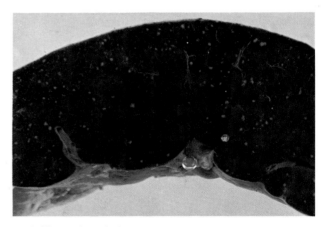

2.6 Miliary tuberculosis: spleen

2.1 Simple (non-parasitic) cyst: spleen. The cyst is large (23 cm diameter) and roughly spherical, with a thick wall which consisted of heavily calcified fibrous tissue. Its inner surface contains deposits of necrotic yellow material. Histological examination revealed no specific features, e.g. of a dermoid cyst. Cysts of the spleen are rare. They may be parasitic, hydatid cyst being the commonest; neoplastic, including cystic lymphangiomas and dermoids; or 'pseudocysts' resulting from degeneration in an area of haemorrhage and infarction. **2.2 .Perisplenitis ('sugar-icing'): spleen.** The spleen, which was small and atrophic, is encased in dense fibrous tissue, with some portions of fatty tissue adherent. This change in the splenic capsule may be seen in senile atrophy, and in some enlarged spleens the surface is patchily affected. In long-standing cases the fibrous tissue may undergo calcification. Milder forms of the condition are often observed at necropsy. **2.3 Chronic venous congestion: spleen.** Chronic passive congestion is caused by interference with the venous return from the spleen. The increase in venous pressure may be confined to the portal circulation or it may be part of the generalised increase in systemic venous pressure found in cardiac decompensation. The spleen was moderately enlarged, weighing 225 g, and very firm. The increase in consistence is shown in the way the cut edges remain 'sharp'. The cut surface is dark red and 'dry' and the trabecular markings are prominent. **2.4 Infarction: spleen.** Several broad depressed areas distort the external surface of the spleen. They represent old infarcts which have undergone organisation and fibrosis, with subsequent contraction of the fibrous tissue. Most splenic infarcts are caused by emboli from the heart, and this patient had subacute bacterial endocarditis affecting the aortic valve, the valve having been rendered stenotic and incompetent by chronic rheumatic heart disease. **2.5 Portal hypertension and congestion: spleen.** The spleen was moderately enlarged. The splenic tissue appears dark brown and pale grey trabeculae are prominent. A number of red-brown siderotic nodules (Gamna-Gandi bodies) are present, centred on dilated blood vessels. Siderotic nodules are the result of haemorrhages within the pulp, with subsequent repair by organisation and fibrosis. Calcium and iron salts impregnate the connective tissue fibres. This patient had cirrhosis of the liver and ascites. **2.6 Miliary tuberculosis: spleen.** Miliary tubercles, appearing as small white nodules, are visible throughout the organ, which was not enlarged. The spleen is usually involved in miliary tuberculosis and tubercles may be few or numerous. They rarely show central caseation, even microscopically. In a child, miliary tuberculosis may complicate a primary focus of infection, e.g. in a primary complex in lung and hilar nodes, whereas in older people miliary spread may be a terminal event in a chronic infection.

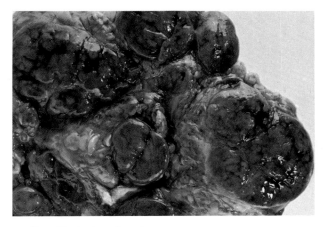

2.7 Sarcoidosis: lymph nodes

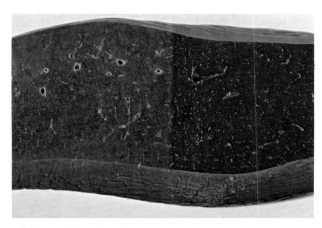

2.8 Haemosiderosis: spleen

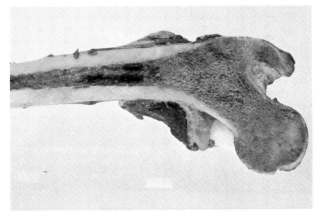

2.9 Primary haemochromatosis: vertebral bodies and femur

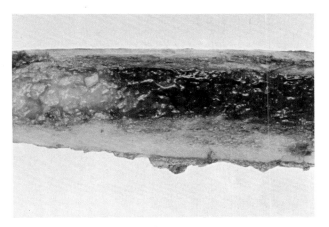

2.10 Aplastic anaemia: vertebrae

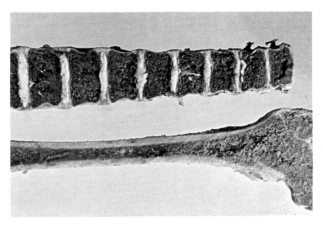

2.11 Aplastic anaemia: femur

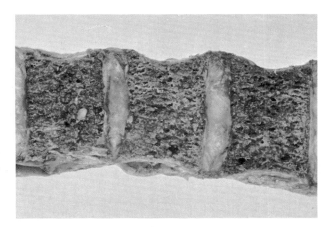

2.12 Hyperplasia of marrow: femur

2.7 Sarcoidosis: lymph nodes. A mass of enlarged lymph nodes is surrounded by fat and fibrous tissue. The nodes are enlarged (the largest at the top left is 6 cm in diameter) and the cut surface is a fleshy pink colour, with clear grey 'follicular' areas formed by fusion of many sarcroid follicles. Characteristically the lesions are granulomatous and non-caseous in the earlier stages and fibrotic in the later stages. **2.8 Haemo-siderosis: spleen.** The patient suffered from histiocytic lymphoma (reticulum cell sarcoma) complicated by auto-immune haemolytic anaemia. The iron released from the excessive haemolysis of red cells has been stored as haemosiderin in the reticuloendothelial system in amounts sufficient to give the splenic tissue on the left a dark rusty-brown colour. The splenic tissue on the right has been immersed in hydrochloric acid—potassium ferrocyanide solution (Perls' reaction) and the deep blue colour (Prussian blue) confirms the presence of the iron-containing pigment. **2.9 Primary haemochromatosis: vertebral bodies and femur.** In haemochromatosis there is a defect in the control of iron absorption and the excess iron taken in is stored as haemosiderin within the reticulo-endothelial system. One femur and the vertebral column from such a case are shown in section. The cut surface of each is a dark rusty-brown, from the presence of large amounts of haemosiderin within the marrow. **2.10 and 2.11 Aplastic anaemia.** The term aplastic anaemia should refer specifically to the anaemia which is secondary to bone marrow

depression, but it is sometimes used loosely for the state of pancytopenia which follows suppression of all haemopoietic elements in the marrow. **2.10** Three thoracic vertebral bodies are shown in hemi-section. The normal red marrow has been replaced by pale yellow marrow which microscopy confirmed to be markedly deficient in cells of both the erythropoietic and granulopoietic series. **2.11** In this longitudinal section of the upper femoral shaft, the marrow which extends down to the lower part of the femoral shaft, apart from a few red areas, is comparatively pale, because of a marked reduction in the normal erythropoietic tissue and an increase in fat. The red areas represent residual foci of haemopoietic activity, complete aplasia of the bone marrow being rare, and it is not uncommon to find areas of hyperplasia associated with aplasia. **2.12 Hyperplasia of marrow: femur.** Hyperplasia may be generalised, affecting all types of stem cell; or it may be selective, with hyperplasia confined to one type of cell, as e.g., the erythroid hyperplasia found in anaemia. This is a longitudinal section of the middle of the shaft of the femur from a patient who died from myelofibrosis (myelosclerosis). The hyperplastic red marrow on the right filled the proximal two-thirds of the medullary cavity and the pale fatty marrow (left) filled the distal third. In the normal adult, red marrow is found only in the head and proximal part of the femoral shaft.

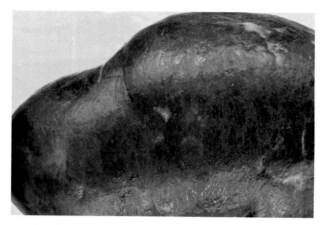

2.13 Myelofibrosis (myelosclerosis): spleen

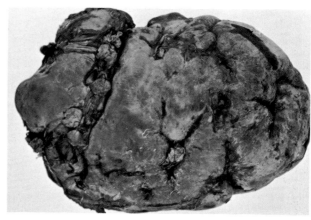

2.14 Myelofibrosis (myelosclerosis): spleen

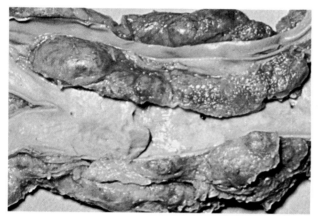

2.15 Myelofibrosis (myelosclerosis): lymph nodes

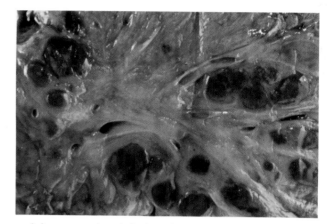

2.16 Acute granulocytic leukaemia: lymph nodes

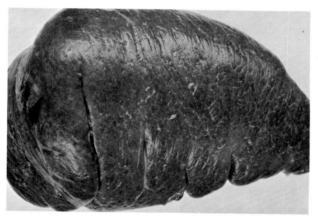

2.17 Acute monocytic leukaemia: spleen

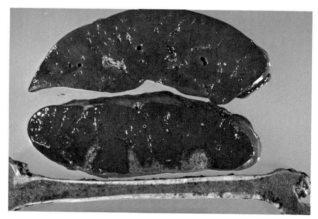

2.18 Chronic granulocytic leukaemia: spleen and femur

2.13-2.15 Myelofibrosis (myelosclerosis). This condition is regarded as a myeloproliferative disorder which may affect the precursors of the red cells, granulocytes or platelets, and the blood may show elevation of any of these three cell lines. There is increasing fibrosis of the marrow, suggesting some type of primary marrow failure, with resumption of blood formation in the various fetal sites (myeloid metaplasia). However the state of the marrow is variable, and it may be of normal cellularity or even hypercellular. The extramedullary haemopoiesis may therefore be a basic component of the disease and not a secondary development. **2.13** The spleen was massive, weighing 5 kg, and haemopoietic elements formed the bulk of the tissue. The capsular surface is shown. The irregular greyish-white areas are recent infarcts. The same tendency to infarction is found in the enlarged spleen of chronic granulocytic (myeloid) leukaemia. **2.14** This spleen also is very big. The capsular surface is irregularly scarred and notched due to the underlying scarring and contraction of numerous old infarcts. It also shows pale yellowish areas of recent infarction associated with the old scarred areas. The pale colour of the spleen is also partly due to the presence of considerable haemopoietic tissue. The spleen is generally the main site of extramedullary haemopoiesis. **2.15** This shows uniformly enlarged para-aortic lymph nodes. Histology confirmed that the enlargement was due to the presence of haemopoietic tissue. The lymph nodes are not usually involved in myelofibrosis. **2.16 Acute granulocytic leukaemia: lymph nodes.** Many enlarged

but discrete reddish-brown lymph nodes are present in the fatty tissues of the mesentery. The cut surface of the nodes has a 'meaty' appearance, and the normal structure has been replaced by leukaemic tissue. Lymph node enlargement is uncommon in acute granulocytic leukaemia. **2.17 Acute monocytic leukaemia: spleen.** This shows the surface of the spleen which weighed 800 g and had a homogeneous rubbery consistence at necropsy. The surface is wrinkled and the capsule appears to bulge. Histology showed an intense infiltrate of leukaemic cells of the monocyte series. Monocytic leukaemia is closely related to acute granulocytic leukaemia. The neoplastic monocytes are thought to be derived from a marrow precursor cell which can also give rise to the granulocyte series of cells, and mixed forms of leukaemia are occasionally seen in which both monocytes and granulocytes are present. **2.18 Chronic granulocytic leukaemia: spleen and femur.** Both halves of the much-enlarged spleen (33 cm long) are shown. The cut surface has a uniform dark red ('meaty') appearance, and extensive yellowish-white areas of infarction are visible beneath the capsule in the lower half. The enlargement is caused by the presence of vast numbers of granulocytes. The medullary cavity of the femur is filled with pinkish-red leukaemic tissue. In a normal subject of the same age, the distal part of the medullary cavity of the femur would contain fat, with red haemopoietic tissue confined to the proximal third of the shaft.

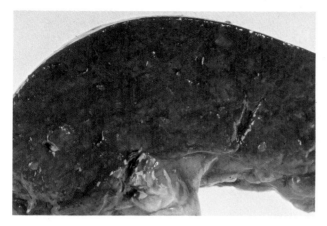

2.19 Myelomatosis: spleen

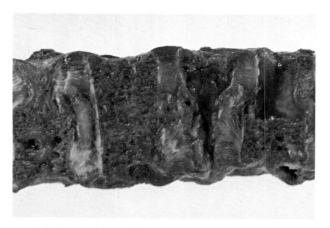

2.20 Myelomatosis: vertebrae

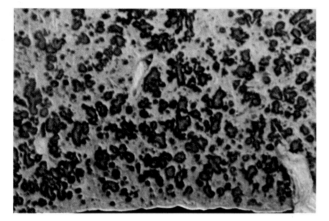

2.21 Amyloidosis: spleen

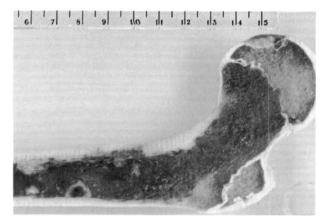

2.22 Hodgkin's disease: femur

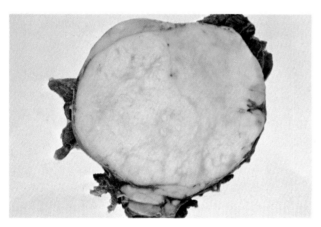

2.23 Hodgkin's disease: lymph node

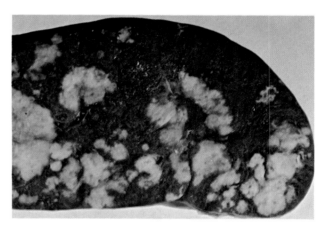

2.24 Hodgkin's disease: spleen

2.19 and 2.20 Myelomatosis. This is a malignant neoplasm of plasma cells. It may present as a solitary tumour (myeloma) or it may be a widespread lesion involving the bone marrow and other organs (myelomatosis or multiple myeloma). **2.19** Splenomegaly occurs in about 10% of cases of myelomatosis and this spleen was enlarged. The cut surface has an irregular nodular pattern due to pale areas of infiltration by myeloma cells. **2.20** The first four lumbar vertebral bodies are shown in section. Three are largely destroyed by myelomatous tissue, and the two on the right have collapsed. The intervertebral discs are also eroded. Characteristically, the neoplastic plasma cells are osteolytic and radiological evidence of bone destruction can generally be found in patients with myelomatosis, the bones most commonly involved being the ribs, sternum and vertebral bodies. Pain, swelling, deformity or pathological fracture result. **2.21 Amyloidosis: spleen.** Amyloidosis may be a complication of myelomatosis. In systemic amyloidosis the spleen is the organ most frequently involved. This spleen was sectioned and the cut surface immersed in Lugol's iodine, which stains the amyloid a dark mahogany-brown colour. In this close-up of the cut surface, the brown deposits of amyloid, which before staining may be compared with sago grains, stand

out as distinct nodules against the pale yellow-brown red pulp. The deposits of amyloid are centred on the Malpighian bodies. In the diffuse form the amyloid is deposited in close association with the fine connective tissue fibrils throughout the organ. Only in the more advanced stages of the disease is the spleen enlarged. **2.22-2.24 Hodgkin's disease.** This is the commonest type of malignant lymphoma. **2.22** The head and upper third of femur of a 13-year-old girl who died from disseminated Hodgkin's disease are shown. The marrow is infiltrated by fairly well-demarcated greyish-white deposits of Hodgkin's tissue. The lesions are confined to the medullary cavity. **2.23** The disease frequently begins in the mediastinal group of lymph nodes, and this shows a greatly enlarged (8 cm diameter) mediastinal lymph node. The cut surface is cream-coloured, with occasional paler areas of necrosis. Nodes affected by Hodgkin's disease feel firm and rubbery and not uncommonly several enlarged nodes are matted together into a large firm mass. **2.24** This is the spleen. It is greatly enlarged, weighing 1353 g. Many large whitish deposits of Hodgkin's tissue are present, along with smaller satellite nodules. The splenic involvement in Hodgkin's disease may be nodular, as here, or more diffuse.

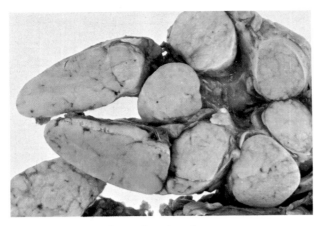

2.25 Follicular lymphoma: lymph nodes

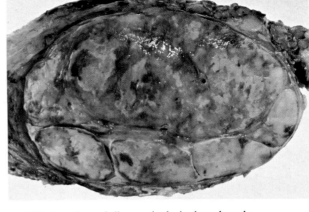

2.26 Histiocytic medullary reticulosis: lymph node

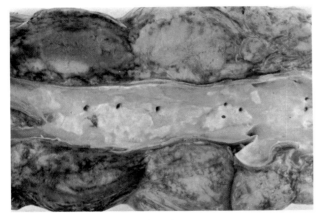

2.27 Lymphosarcoma: lymph nodes

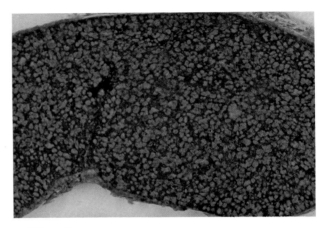

2.28 Lymphosarcoma: spleen

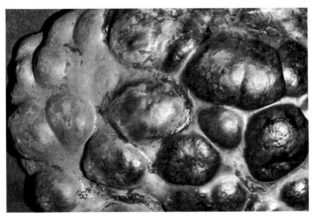

2.30 Burkitt's (African) lymphoma: spleen

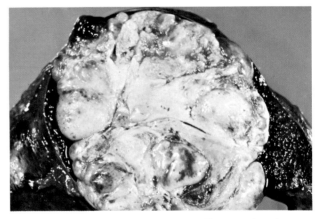

2.29 Histiocytic lymphoma (reticulum cell sarcoma): spleen

2.25 Follicular lymphoma: lymph nodes. The lymph nodes are enlarged (the largest measuring 6 cm in its long axis) and replaced by lymphomatous tissue. The cut surface is creamy-white. Some of the nodes are discrete but others are matted together as a result of pericapsular infiltration. A follicular pattern can be distinguished histologically in this type of lymphoma. Clinically the nodes felt firm and rubbery. **2.26 Histiocytic medullary reticulosis: lymph node.** Histiocytic medullary reticulosis is a rare type of lymphoma. This affected lymph node is greatly enlarged (14 cm in its long axis) and surrounded by a thickened capsule. The cut surface shows coarse nodularity and is pinkish-yellow from extensive necrosis and underlying haemorrhage. **2.27 and 2.28 Lymphosarcoma. 2.27** The para-aortic lymph nodes are enlarged and matted together. Some have been bisected to show the pale pinkish-grey lymphomatous tissue, in which there are extensive areas of necrosis. The matting together of the lymph nodes in lymphomas is due to pericapsular infiltration by neoplastic cells. Incidentally the intima of the opened abdominal aorta is atherosclerotic. **2.28** This shows a greatly enlarged spleen (23 cm in its long axis). Large numbers of small nodules of lymphosarcomatous tissue (each 3 or 4 mm diameter) are visible, distributed evenly throughout the organ. The pattern of splenic involvement in lymphosarcoma may also be diffuse. **2.29 Histiocytic lymphoma (reticulum cell sarcoma): spleen.** The capsular surface of the spleen is bosselated from the presence within the organ of large rounded deposits of histiocytic lymphoma. Many of the nodules are red and haemorrhagic, and some have a central depressed area (umbilication), the result of necrosis and cavitation. **2.30 Burkitt's (African) lymphoma: spleen.** The organ is expanded by a large, lobulated white mass (9 cm diameter) in which there are areas of recent haemorrhage and central yellow areas of necrosis. Burkitt's lymphoma is a malignant, poorly differentiated lymphosarcoma, mainly of children, with a predilection for the jaw and facial bones. In some patients, however, involvement of facial bones is slight and they present with abdominal tumours affecting e.g. both ovaries or kidneys. Involvement of peripheral lymph nodes and spleen is not a usual feature.

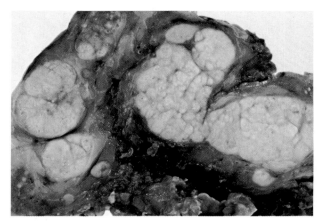

2.31 Secondary carcinoma: lymph nodes

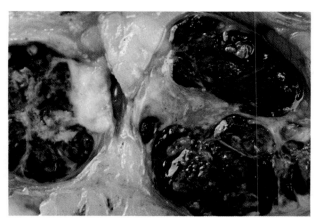

2.32 Secondary melanoma: lymph nodes

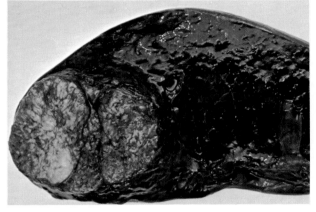

2.33 Secondary carcinoma: spleen

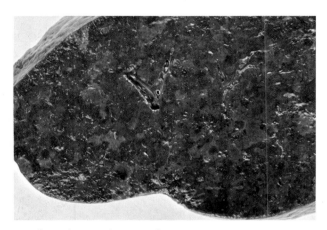

2.34 Secondary carcinoma: spleen

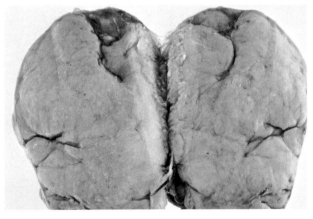

2.35 Thymoma

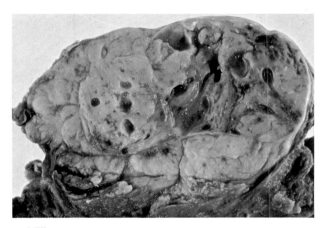

2.36 Thymoma

2.31 Secondary carcinoma: lymph nodes. The mesenteric tissues contain several enlarged lymph nodes, the largest being 4 cm in diameter. The enlargement is caused by the presence of greyish-white deposits of secondary carcinoma. The primary tumour was in the rectum. **2.32 Secondary melanoma: lymph nodes.** The lymph nodes lying in fatty tissue are enlarged and largely replaced by melanin-laden secondary deposits of malignant melanoma. **2.33 and 2.34 Secondary carcinoma: spleen.** Invasion of the spleen by malignant cells may take place either directly from the primary growth or from deposits in the splenic lymph nodes. The tumour usually enters the spleen at its hilum and spreads mainly along the trabeculae. **2.33** This spleen is only slightly enlarged and contains a rounded solitary metastasis in one pole of the organ (left). The primary tumour was a bronchial carcinoma. The reported frequency of involvement of the spleen by metastatic tumour varies widely, from rare to as high as 50%. The lesions may be either nodular or diffuse. Most probably result from haematogenous spread from the primary. Splenic involvement occurs late in the course of the disease and is usually not found in the absence of metastases to other organs. The primary tumour is generally in lung, breast, prostate, colon or stomach. **2.34** Invasion of the main trabecular veins by the tumour may cause infarction. This spleen weighed 1400 g. The cut surface is reddish-brown, with numerous pale

white areas of infarction. Histological examination of the spleen revealed extensive invasion by carcinoma. Rarely, fatal haemorrhage from an affected spleen may occur. **2.35 and 2.36 Thymoma.** The term thymoma is generally taken to include all intrinsic tumours of the thymus. Thymoma is an uncommon tumour and it is rare in subjects under twenty years of age. Most are situated in the upper anterior mediastinum, where they grow expansively. The majority are lobulated or multinodular and appear well-encapsulated, although some are non-encapsulated and extend by local invasion. There is considerable variation in size and they range from 1 to 20 cm in diameter. Histologically four types are recognised based on the cell type: lymphoid, spindle-cell, epithelial and rosette-forming. The lymphoid type is the most common. **2.35** This bisected specimen is a compact firm tumour with the characteristic lobulation and a well-demarcated fibrous capsule. It appears to involve the whole gland. The colour is a pale yellowish-grey. **2.36** In this case the patient suffered from myasthenia gravis, as do one third of all patients with thymoma. Part of the normal thymus is shown along with an oval tumour mass measuring 8 cm in length. The neoplasm weighed 70 g. Its cut surface shows the characteristic bosselated appearance, with fibrous trabeculae dividing the growth into lobules. Numerous small cystic areas are present and also areas of haemorrhage.

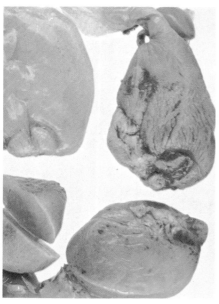

3.1 Nasal polyps

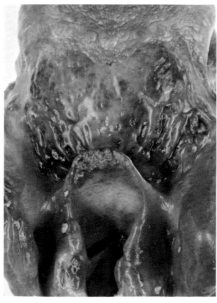

3.2 Ulceration: tongue and larynx

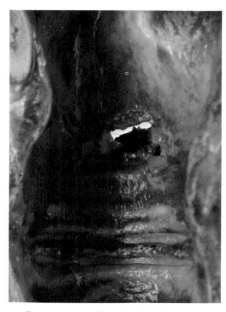

3.3 Pressure necrosis and ulceration: trachea

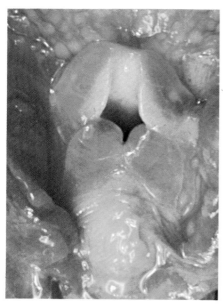

3.4 Oedema: glottis

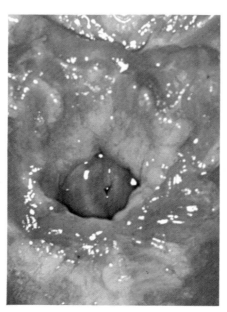

3.5 Acute epiglottitis

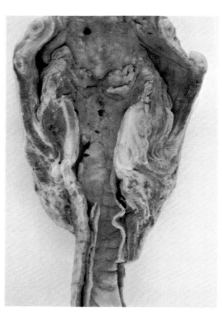

3.6 Diphtheria: larynx

3.1 Nasal polyps. The polyps are smooth shiny semi-translucent and bluish-grey, with many fine blood vessels traversing their surface. Histologically they consisted of oedematous fibrous tissue, with a sparse inflammatory cell infiltrate in which eosinophils were conspicuous. Nasal polyps most probably result from inflammatory oedema and hypertrophy of the nasal mucosa in chronic sinusitis, associated at times with allergic rhinitis. They are common lesions, occurring mainly in adults and are most often found in the ethmoidal region. They may fill the nasal cavity and cause obstruction. **3.2 Ulceration: tongue and larynx.** Shallow irregular areas of ulceration are present around the base of the tongue, epiglottis and larynx. The base of each ulcer is covered with necrotic fibrin-rich exudate. The ulcers probably resulted from an overwhelming secondary infection by organisms within the oral cavity, made possible by the reduction of the normal cellular defence mechanisms which would accompany the aplastic anaemia and pancytopenia from which the patient died. **3.3 Pressure necrosis and ulceration: trachea.** The patient sustained a head injury which required endotracheal intubation and intermittent positive-pressure respiration; a tracheostomy had been performed two weeks earlier. The trachea has been opened to display the internal aspect of the tracheostomy stoma. The tracheal cartilages are visible. Beneath the stoma there is a horizontal ulcer which resulted from pressure necrosis caused by the cuffed endotracheal tube. The patient died from ulcerative tracheobronchitis and bronchopneumonia. **3.4 Oedema: glottis.** Oedema fluid has collected in the soft areolar tissues

of the glottis and surrounding tissues, rendering them swollen and translucent. Oedema generally first involves the arytenoid cartilage and the ary-epiglottic folds, and spreads into the epiglottis and vestibular folds to cause obstruction of the air passage. The causes of the oedema are various. Angioneurotic oedema sometimes involves the tissues of the larynx as a manifestation of allergic hypersensitivity to some particular food or drug; bee or wasp stings may, on the same basis, prove fatal; but the most dangerous causes are diphtheria and streptococcal infection and the acute inflammation that accompanies inhalation of steam or irritant gases. **3.5 Acute epiglottitis.** The acutely inflamed epiglottis is grossly swollen from inflammatory oedema but no ulceration is visible. Histologically the changes were those of a non-specific acute inflammation. Acute epiglottitis is a rare but important illness of early childhood. The illness often develops with startling rapidity, the child dying within a few hours of onset. It is caused by *Haemophilus influenzae* type B. **3.6 Diphtheria: larynx.** In diphtheria the bacteria generally infect the pharynx and posterior nares but occasionally spread downwards and cause acute tracheitis and bronchitis. However this type of specimen is or should be largely of historical interest. It shows an extensive pale yellowish-white diphtheritic pseudomembrane involving the larynx and trachea. The membrane is typically insecurely attached and can be readily desquamated and dislodged, to cause death from asphyxia through impaction in the larynx during a paroxysm of coughing.

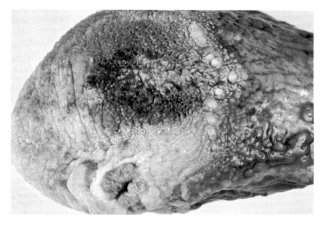

3.7 Squamous carcinoma: tongue

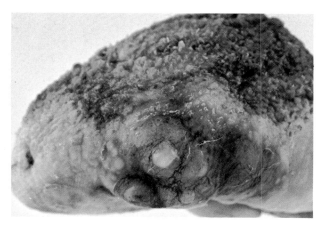

3.8 Adenoid cystic carcinoma: tongue

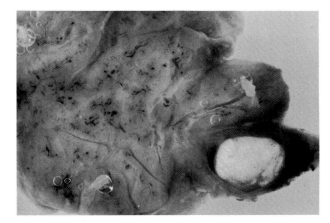

3.9 Calculus: submandibular salivary gland

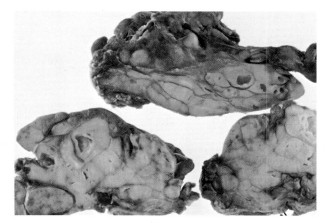

3.10 Benign lymphoepithelial lesion: parotid

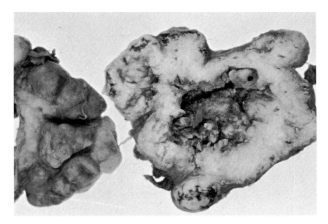

3.11 Pleomorphic adenoma: parotid

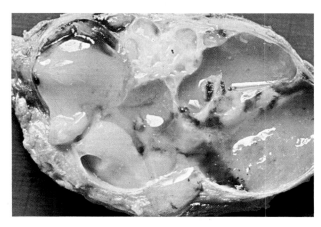

3.12 Adenolymphoma: parotid

3.7 Squamous carcinoma: tongue. The anterior surface of the dorsum of the tongue is covered by opaque white patches of leukoplakia (lower centre) and the centre of the tongue is covered by a dark brown ('hairy') plaque due to a fungal infection. There is also a small nodular squamous carcinoma on the lateral margin of the anterior two-thirds (bottom). Leukoplakia of the tongue, which is a precancerous condition, is common in heavy smokers and patients with tertiary syphilis, and affects men more often than women. **3.8 Adenoid cystic carcinoma: tongue.** The dorsal surface of the tongue is brownish-black from fungal infection. There is an irregular ulcerated tumour on the lateral margin of the anterior two-thirds of the tongue which extends on to the ventral surface. The tumour is an adenoid cystic carcinoma, a rare type of neoplasm which arises from one of the minor sublingual salivary glands around the tongue or more commonly in the hard palate. The lesion tends to be locally malignant and invasive. It does not appear to be associated with previous chronic irritation and leukoplakia. **3.9 Calculus: submandibular salivary gland.** A yellow calculus is impacted in the dilated main duct of the gland. The adjacent glandular tissue is pinkish-white, due to atrophy of the normal parenchyma and replacement by fibrous tissue and fat as a result of the chronic obstruction of the duct. Recurrent attacks of acute inflammation may also complicate sialolithiasis. Salivary calculi consist chiefly of calcium carbonate with small quantities of other salts. **3.10 Benign lymphoepithelial lesion: parotid.** The condition presented clinically as a painless enlargement of the parotid glands. The normal lobular pattern has been replaced by a much coarser pattern, and the tissue is paler and 'fleshier' than normal glandular tissue. Histologically the gland was infiltrated by mature lymphocytes surrounding islands of epithelial cells. The lesion may be mistaken for a lymphoma but although occasionally a lymphoma has developed many years later, it usually pursues a benign course. The aetiology is unknown but in some cases it may be a manifestation of auto-immunisation comparable to auto-immune thyroiditis. **3.11 Pleomorphic adenoma: parotid.** The external surface of the tumour is smooth and nodular (left) and the cut surface (right) shows a homogeneous greyish-white tissue with areas of softening, cyst formation and occasionally haemorrhage. This type of adenoma is very much commoner in the parotid than in the submandibular and sublingual salivary glands. It is generally fairly well-encapsulated but failure to remove the peripheral nodules at operation not infrequently leads to recurrence. Histologically myxomatous and pseudocartilaginous tissue is usually present along with the epithelial component which itself varies considerably in its pattern. **3.12 Adenolymphoma: parotid.** This rare benign slow-growing neoplasm of salivary duct origin generally presents as a soft lobulated mass. The cut surface of this specimen shows the presence of numerous cysts filled with a mucinous fluid which was rich in cholesterol crystals. The histological appearance is very distinctive, consisting of irregular papillae lined by epithelium consisting of two cell layers; and the abundant stroma consists of lymphoid tissue, often with well-formed follicles with germinal centres.

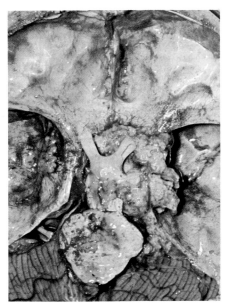

3.13 Nasopharyngeal carcinoma: skull

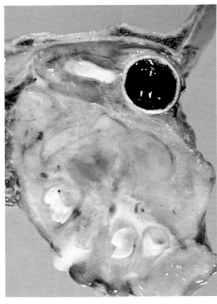

3.14 Burkitt's (African) lymphoma: maxilla

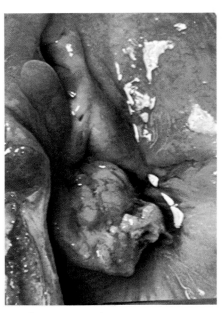

3.15 Squamous carcinoma: larynx

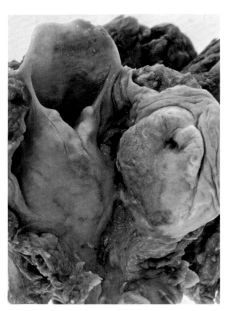

3.16 Squamous carcinoma: pharynx

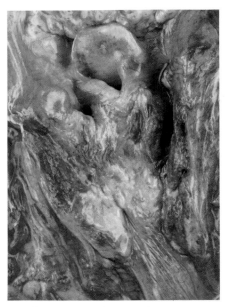

3.17 Squamous carcinoma: pharynx

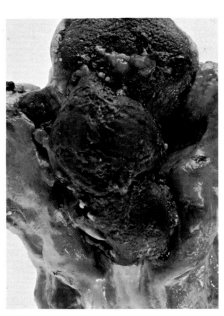

3.18 Sarcoma: pharynx

3.13 Nasopharyngeal carcinoma: skull. The tumour, a carcinoma arising from the sphenoid or ethmoid sinuses, has penetrated the base of the skull. Pinkish-white tumour is infiltrating the middle cranial fossae widely and encircling the optic chiasma and sella turcica. It extends laterally into both middle fossae and posteriorly over the basi-sphenoid and basi-occiput to approach the pons. **3.14 Burkitt's (African) lymphoma: maxilla.** This hemi-maxillectomy specimen shows the face in sagittal section. An eye (top right) and several teeth can be identified. A mass of pink fleshy tumour fills the maxilla and invades the surrounding tissues extensively. The jaw is a common site of origin of Burkitt's lymphoma. **3.15 Squamous carcinoma: larynx.** A polypoid subglottic carcinoma arising from the left vocal cord has extended into the anterior commissure. About 98% of malignant tumours of the larynx are squamous carcinomas and they fall into three groups: those arising from the vocal fold or anterior or posterior commissure, referred to as glottic carcinomas, are the commonest and have the best prognosis; those arising from the supraglottic tissues; and those arising from the subglottic space, which carry a poor prognosis. About two-thirds of all carcinomas of the larynx arise from the true vocal cords. **3.16 and 3.17 Squamous**

carcinoma: pharynx. 3.16 A large oval tumour mass is located in the right post-cricoid region of the hypopharynx. A small area of ulceration is present on its surface. Post-cricoid hypopharyngeal carcinoma is almost exclusively a disease of women and is preceded in many cases by the Plummer-Vinson syndrome. **3.17** Post-cricoid carcinoma frequently spreads to encircle the lower pharynx and upper oesophagus and cause a marked degree of stenosis and obstruction. The greyish-white tumour has invaded widely, with extension into the upper oesophagus, larynx and fossa of Rosenmuller. A poor degree of differentiation, aggressive local spread, and rapid metastasis to the regional nodes are the main characteristics of carcinomas arising in the nasopharynx and hypopharynx. **3.18 Sarcoma: pharynx.** A large brownish-black polypoid mass fills the hypopharynx, causing severe obstruction. The brownish-black colour of the tumour and tongue is due to fungal infection. Histologically the tumour was an undifferentiated sarcoma, probably synovial in origin. The patient was a 25-year-old woman who had undergone radiotherapy for this tumour previously. Sarcoma of the hypopharynx is a rare tumour. Occasionally a squamous carcinoma assumes a spindle-cell pattern which mimics sarcoma histologically (pseudosarcoma).

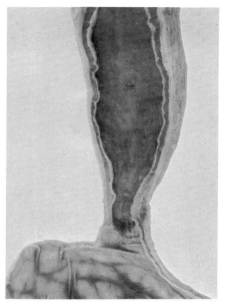

4.1 Achalasia of cardia (cardiospasm):
oesophagus

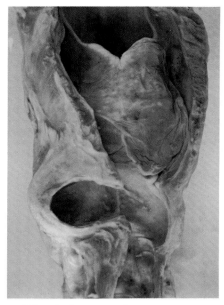

4.2 Diverticulum: oesophagus

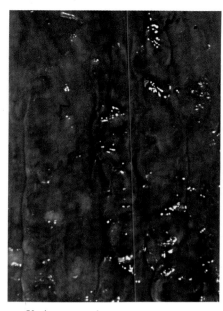

4.3 Varices: oesophagus

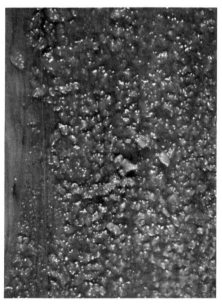

4.4 Candidiasis: oesophagus

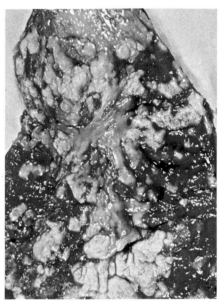

4.5 Achalasia, leukoplakia and squamous
carcinoma: oesophagus

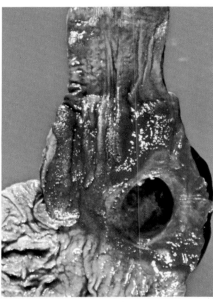

4.6 Hiatus hernia, oesophagitis and peptic
ulcer: oesophagus

4.1 Achalasia of cardia (cardiospasm): oesophagus. There is marked dilatation and hypertrophy of the oesophagus except for a short segment adjoining the stomach. Ganglion cells of the myenteric plexus were reduced in number or absent from this short segment, and as a result the 'sphincter' at the cardia failed to relax and the oesophagus proximal to the obstruction lost its normal peristaltic rhythm. Achalasia affects women predominantly. **4.2 Diverticulum: oesophagus.** Most diverticula are acquired and are usually 'false'; that is, they are formed by herniation of the mucous membrane and muscularis mucosae through weakened areas or defects in the muscularis externa. True diverticula consists of all layers of the oesophageal wall. Acquired diverticula may be pulsion diverticula and caused by raised intra-luminal pressure, or traction diverticula formed by distorting effects of a chronic inflammatory process outside the oesophagus. The posterior aspect of pharynx and oesophagus is shown. A small posterior pulsion diverticulum is present at the junction of the oesophagus and pharynx where the cricopharyngeal muscle is attached. This type of lesion mostly affects males. **4.3 Varices: oesophagus.** The venous drainage of the oesophagus includes a submucosal venous plexus and a serosal plexus. Both drain partly into the portal and partly into the systemic venous system. In portal hypertension the longitudinally-running submucosal plexuses dilate to form enormously-dilated channels beneath the mucosa. This patient had portal hypertension and 'varices' in the form of bluish-black tortuous veins are

clearly visible. Such 'varices' are prone to rupture and give rise to serious gastrointestinal haemorrhage. **4.4 Candidiasis: oesophagus.** The mucosal surface is covered with small raised yellowish 'mucoid' patches which consist of colonies of *Candida albicans*. Suppression of the normal bacterial flora in patients treated with immunosuppressants, cytotoxic drugs, antibiotics or steroids predisposes to fungal infection. **4.5 Achalasia, leukoplakia and squamous carcinoma: oesophagus.** In achalasia, stagnation of oesophageal contents results in chronic inflammatory changes in the mucosa with subsequent development of leukoplakia. This oesophagus is dilated and the mucosal surface covered with raised irregular warty white plaques of leukoplakia. Achalasia, especially when leukoplakia is present, predisposes to the development of squamous carcinoma in the dilated segment, and an early squamous carcinoma was found in this specimen. **4.6 Hiatus hernia, oesophagitis and peptic ulcer: oesophagus.** The distal oesophagus and proximal part of the stomach are visible. They are dilated and formed a sliding hiatus hernia. The mucosa is bright red, due to acute congestion and ulceration (peptic oesophagitis) and there is a penetrating peptic ulcer at the cardio-oesophageal junction. In the sliding type of hiatus hernia, the lower oesophagus and stomach herniate through the oesophageal diaphragmatic hiatus, thus predisposing to reflux of gastric juices and digestion oesophagitis and ulceration.

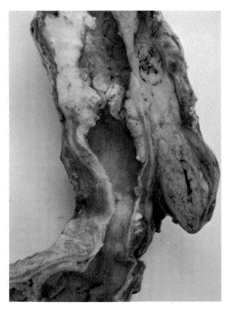

4.7 Squamous carcinoma: oesophagus

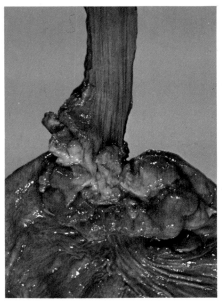

4.8 Carcinoma of the cardia

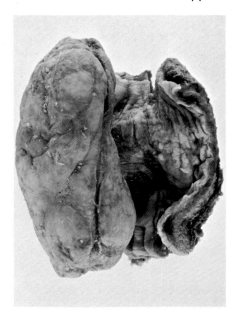

4.9 Pseudosarcoma: oesophagus

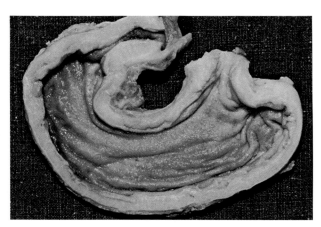

4.10 Congenital pyloric stenosis: stomach

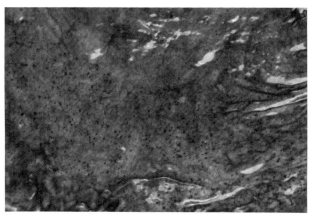

4.11 'Anoxic' haemorrhages: stomach

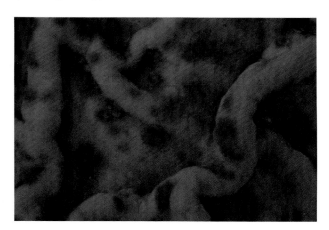

4.12 Mucosal haemorrhages: stomach

4.7 Squamous carcinoma: oesophagus. The middle and lower thirds of the oesophagus are almost encircled by an annular constricting growth. Extension of tumour through the wall has occurred, with infiltration of the serosa and two adjacent lymph nodes on the right. Direct spread to involve adjacent mediastinal structures is common. In men the lesion is rare in the upper third, most common in the middle third, and less frequent in the lower third of the oesophagus. There is some evidence that tumours of all types are more common opposite anatomical sites of narrowing of the oesophagus. **4.8 Carcinoma of the cardia.** Carcinomas at the cardio-oesophageal junction can be classified as intra-oesophageal, junctional or (largely) intragastric. This example of the junctional type is a large fleshy polypoid tumour with an ulcerated surface projecting into the cardia. About 75% of tumours of the cardia are adenocarcinomas, the remainder being squamous or mixed tumours. **4.9 Pseudosarcoma: oesophagus.** A large oval polypid tumour fills the lumen of the oesophagus. Pseudosarcoma is a rare tumour, usually seen in elderly patients and often located at the upper third. Histologically the lesion should be regarded not as a sarcoma but as a squamous carcinoma in which the neoplastic cells assume a spindle-cell form and evoke a marked stromal fibrous response. **4.10 Congenital pyloric stenosis: stomach.** This is the stomach of a neonate. There is marked concentric thickening of the pylorus which terminates abruptly at the first part of the duodenum and narrows the pyloric canal. Congenital pyloric stenosis is commoner in first-born male children and may be due to a recessive gene. It frequently presents between the second and fourth weeks of life. The circular muscle coat hypertrophies to between twice and four times its normal thickness. The primary defect is probably degeneration and/or diminution of myenteric ganglion cells. **4.11 'Anoxic' haemorrhages: stomach.** The mucosa of the stomach is intensely congested and multiple pin-point asphyxia-type petechiae are present. The patient had severe aortic stenosis and following insertion of an aortic valve prosthesis on cardio-pulmonary by-pass he suffered from generalised anoxia due to low aortic perfusion. **4.12 Mucosal haemorrhages: stomach.** This close-up view of the gastric rugae shows small mucosal haemorrhages. The patient had acute leukaemia and a bleeding diathesis is common in the later stages of this condition, as a result of deficiency of platelets. Haemorrhage tends to occur from the gums and mucosa of the gastrointestinal tract.

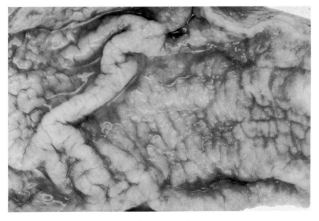

4.13 Granulomatous gastritis: stomach

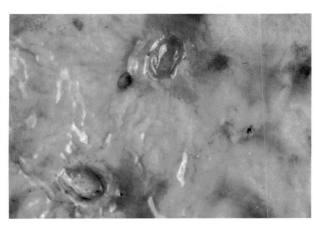

4.14 Acute 'stress' ulcers: stomach

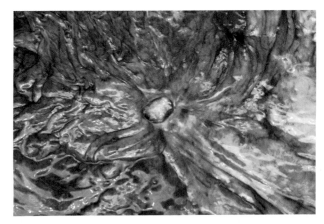

4.15 Chronic peptic ulcer: stomach

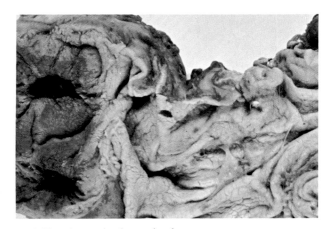

4.16 Chronic peptic ulcers: duodenum

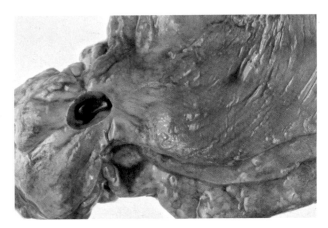

4.17 Perforated chronic peptic ulcer: duodenum

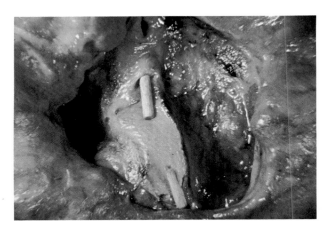

4.18 Chronic peptic ulcer: duodenum

4.13 Granulomatous gastritis: stomach. The normal mucosal pattern is lost, with flattening of the rugae and a regular 'cobblestone' pattern to the mucosa. Some cases of granulomatous gastritis may represent Crohn's disease of the stomach. The pyloric region is usually affected and the presenting clinical symptoms are generally dyspepsia and weight loss and of pyloric stenosis. There may be clinical evidence of disease in the small intestine. **4.14 Acute 'stress' ulcers: stomach.** Two acute ulcers which were situated in the fundus of the stomach are shown. The larger has punched-out edges. The patient, a young man, sustained a severe head injury 10 days prior to death. There is a recognised relation between acute peptic ulceration and lesions in the region of the hypothalamus and vagal nuclei, suggesting a neurogenic factor in their origin (Cushing's ulcers). Organic lesions elsewhere, such as cutaneous burns (Curling's ulcer), abdominal injuries, and surgical operations may be followed by acute peptic ulcers. **4.15-4.18 Chronic peptic ulcers.** Perforation, haemorrhage and obstruction are the principal complications of chronic peptic ulceration. Duodenal ulcers are especially prone to perforation. **4.15** A chronic peptic ulcer is present on the lesser curve of the stomach. The ulcer crater is oval and the base is covered with a greenish-yellow slough consisting of necrotic granulation tissue. The ulcer is healing by fibrosis, as shown by the folds of mucosa radiating from the ulcer. The adjacent mucosa is atrophic. In general gastric ulcers tend to be single, round or oval, less than 2 cm in diameter and situated on the lesser curve. The edges are clear-cut but not raised or rolled, and overhang to produce a flask-shaped appearance. Chronic ulcers penetrate the muscle and the ensuing fibrosis may lead to distortion and constriction. **4.16** Immediately distal to the pylorus are two chronic deeply-penetrating duodenal ulcers. The base of one contains a recent blood clot, and the patient died from a massive haemorrhage due to penetration of the gastro-duodenal artery by the ulcer. Posterior duodenal ulcers are particularly prone to penetration and haemorrhage. **4.17** The patient, a 78-year-old woman died from peritonitis following perforation of an unsuspected anterior duodenal ulcer. This shows the serosal aspect of the pyloric end of stomach and duodenum. The large orifice of the perforated ulcer is clearly visible. **4.18** This large ulcer has penetrated posteriorly into the common bile duct, the ends of which are identified by stick markers. Such a complication would result in a biliary peritonitis. An ulcer like this may also erode the pancreas or perforate into the lesser sac.

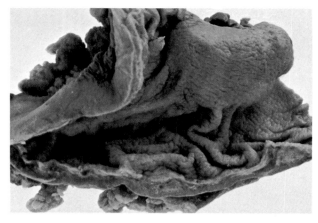

4.19 Leiomyoma: stomach

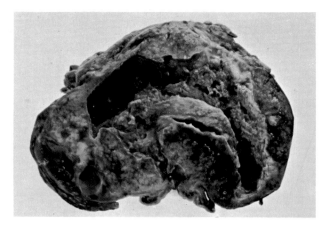

4.20 Neurolemmoma: stomach

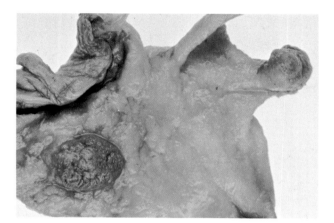

4.21 Papillary adenoma: stomach

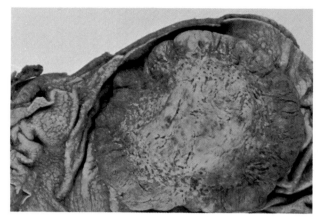

4.22 Carcinoma: stomach

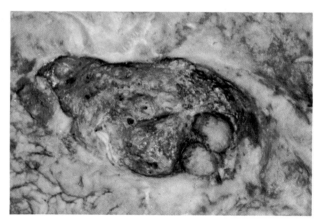

4.23 Carcinoma: stomach

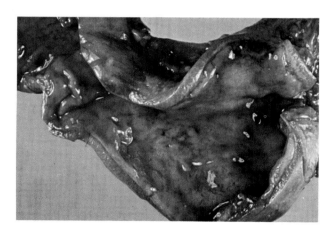

4.24 Carcinoma: stomach

4.19 Leiomyoma: stomach. The tumour is a smooth pinkish-grey mass projecting into the lumen of the stomach. Smooth-muscle tumours are not rare in the alimentary tract, and the stomach is the commonest site. They arise from the muscle coat and when small remain intramural. Microscopically they usually consist of clearly recognisable smooth-muscle cells. However there are well-recognised variants occurring mainly in old patients, which although generally benign and with the same macroscopic features show considerable cellular pleomorphism—the bizarre smooth-muscle tumours or leiomyoblastomas. **4.20 Neuro-lemmoma: stomach.** The tumour is large (15 cm diameter) and ovoid. The cut surface shows areas of necrosis, cystic degeneration and haemorrhage. Neurolemmomas account for 5-10% of all benign gastric neoplasms. Like this one, they are usually single, originate in the submucosa on the lesser curve, and grow into the lumen. Occasionally they may undergo sarcomatous change. **4.21 Papillary adenoma: stomach.** Two pedunculated papillary adenomas have arisen in the antrum and prepyloric region of the stomach. Their mucosal surface is lobulated. Benign epithelial tumours and polyps represent about 5% of all gastric epithelial tumours. They are usually single and tend to arise in the pyloric antrum. **4.22-4.24 Carcinoma: stomach.** The prognosis for gastric carcinoma is generally poor, the 5-year survival rate being less than 20%. Lymphatic spread readily occurs, along with metastasis to the liver. **4.22** The tumour is a large flat polypoid (fungating) mass arising from the body of the stomach. **4.23** This shows a large ulcerating type of growth: the edges are raised and the surrounding tissue is thickened, nodular and infiltrated. A large eroded artery is visible in the base of the ulcer. Ulcerated carcinomas usually present as shallow ulcers readily distinguished from the deeper flask-shaped peptic ulcers with their overhanging edges and comparatively normal surrounding mucosa. **4.24** This is a scirrhous growth. The stomach wall is diffusely thickened and the stomach contracted due to widely infiltrating carcinoma. The tumour cells have excited extensive fibrosis in the submucosa and muscularis externa and so produced the so-called leather-bottle stomach (linitis plastica).

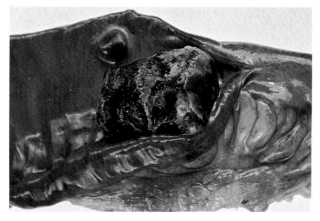

4.25 Acute obstruction: ileum

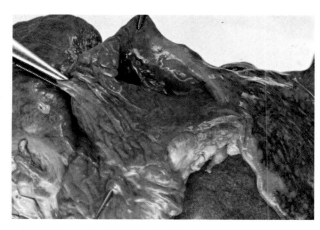

4.26 Cholecystoduodenal fistula: duodenum

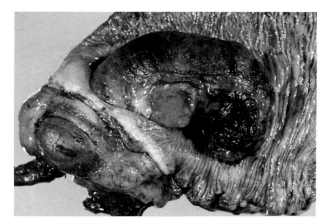

4.27 Intussusception: colon

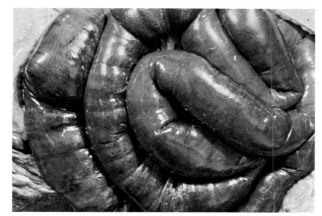

4.28 Volvulus: small intestine

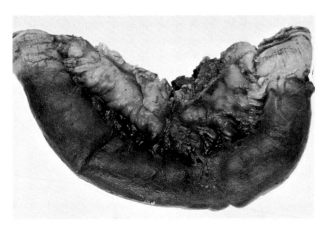

4.29 Strangulated hernia: small intestine

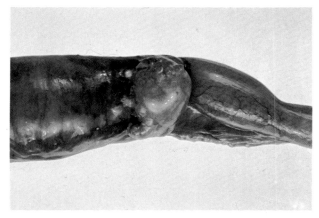

4.30 Ischaemic stricture: ileum

4.25 Acute obstruction: ileum. A large gall-stone is impacted in the terminal ileum. The proximal segment of the gut is dilated and the distal portion collapsed. The intestinal wall is red-brown and infarcted. Gall-stone obstruction (gall-stone ileus) usually affects the small intestine. **4.26 Cholecystoduodenal fistula: duodenum.** This shows the source of the gall-stone causing the lesion in 4.25. The undersurface of the liver is displayed with the duodenal loop laid open. A probe is present in the ampulla of Vater, and the pylorus and part of the gastric antrum are on the right. At the top, between the forceps, a large fistulous connection is visible between the first part of the duodenum and the gall-bladder which is closely adherent to the posterior wall of the duodenum. **4.27 Intus-susception: colon.** Intussusception is the invagination of a segment of the intestinal tract (intussusceptum) into the adjacent intestine (intus-suscipiens). Here the terminal ileum has intussuscepted into the ascending colon, the caecum and appendix being visible to the left. The intus-susceptum forms a red tumour-like mass with a granular surface. The swelling and discolouration are signs of oedema and early haemorrhagic infarction. Intussusception is primarily a disorder of children and young adults, in whom it tends to affect the region of the ileocaecal valve. In adults it may be initiated by a polypoid intraluminal tumour. **4.28**

Volvulus: small intestine. The coils of small intestine are greatly distended and blue-black, as a result of gangrenous infarction. Volvulus is the twisting of a loop (or loops) of intestine upon itself through 180° or more, a process which obstructs the intestine and interferes with its blood supply. The condition, which predominates in males, often affects the sigmoid colon. Predisposing factors include a long mesenteric attachment and congenital or acquired bands. **4.29 Strangulated hernia: small intestine.** This short segment of small intestine was incarcerated in an inguinal hernial sac. Obstruction of the passage of intestinal contents was followed by strangulation, i.e. obstruction to the venous return in the mesentery produced congestion and oedema culminating in arterial obstruction and haemorrhagic infarction. **4.30 Ischaemic stricture: ileum.** A localised ischaemic stricture is present (right of centre). The ileum beyond the stricture is collapsed but viable. The ileum proximal to the stricture is distended and the wall greenish-brown following infarction. A recent perforation has occurred, with prolapse of the mucous membrane through the necrotic wall of the ileum. The lesion was caused by partial blockage of the origin of the superior mesenteric artery by a thrombus on an atherosclerotic plaque.

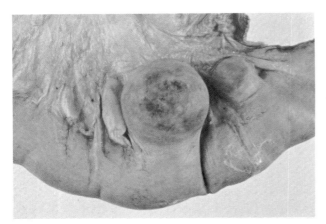

4.31 Diverticula: jejunum

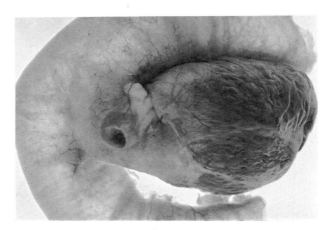

4.32 Meckel's diverticulum: ileum

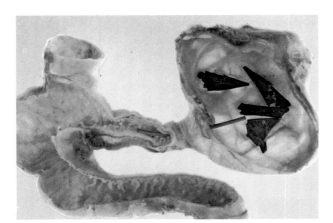

4.33 Meckel's diverticulum: ileum

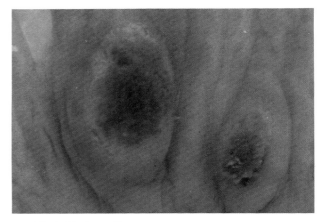

4.34 Typhoid ulcers: ileum

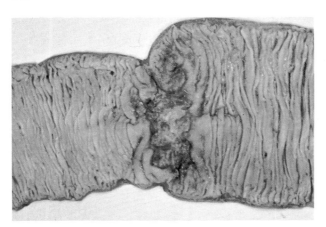

4.35 Tuberculous ulcers and stricture: ileum

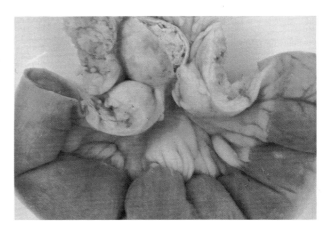

4.36 Calcified tuberculous lymph nodes: mesentery

4.31 Diverticula: jejunum. Two wide-mouthed diverticula are present on the mesenteric border of the lower jejunum. Diverticula of the small intestine are usually multiple, occurring along the mesenteric attachment and herniating through the gaps by which the blood vessels and nerves penetrate the muscle. They are usually wide-mouthed sacs and are rarely the cause of clinical disease. **4.32 and 4.33 Meckel's diverticulum: ileum.** Meckel's diverticulum is the persisting proximal portion of the vitello-intestinal duct and is the only common congenital diverticulum of the gastrointestinal tract, being found in 1-4% of individuals. It is situated on the antimesenteric aspect of the terminal ileum, 30-90 cm proximal to the ileocaecal valve. **4.32** About 25% of Meckel's diverticula contain heterotopic gastric mucosa, and peptic ulceration with haemorrhage and/or perforation tend to occur. The diverticulum in this case is a wide sac. There is a recent perforation on the neck of the sac. The perforation may not be in the diverticulum, as here, but in the adjacent ileum. **4.33** Any portion of the vitello-intestinal duct may persist as such or as a fibrous cord, or as a fistulous communication between Meckel's diverticulum and a vitelline cyst, or between Meckel's diverticulum and the umbilicus. This shows an opened Meckel's diverticulum (centre) communicating with a patent persistent vitello-intestinal duct which in turn communicates with a thin-walled vitelline cyst containing tomato skins. A vitelline cyst may contain enteroliths. The presence of a fibrous cord or a persistent vitello-intestinal duct may lead to volvulus or intussusception. **4.34 Typhoid ulcers: ileum.** This is the mucosa of the terminal ileum. It is ulcerated over two swollen masses of lymphoid tissue and the floor of each ulcer is necrotic. Typhoid ulcers have the same configuration as the lymphoid aggregates and are therefore elongated, with the long axis longitudinal. Typically, the ulcers have elevated margins, formed of surviving hyperplastic lymphoid tissue. The most serious complications are haemorrhage and perforation. **4.35 Tuberculous ulcers and stricture: ileum.** Tuberculous ulcers are usually situated in the ileocaecal region, with the long axis running circumferentially. Contracting scar tissue may produce a localised stricture, usually with partial rather than complete intestinal obstruction. In this example the lesion consists of an irregular transverse ulcer and a fibrous stricture which has caused dilatation of the ileum proximal to the stricture. **4.36 Calcified tuberculous lymph nodes: mesentery.** A portion of terminal ileum and its mesentery is shown. The mesentery shows fibrous scarring and there are two large calcified lymph nodes, representing old healed tuberculous lymphadenitis. In intestinal tuberculosis involvement of the mesenteric lymph nodes is very common, and calcified ileocaecal nodes are often encountered *post mortem*.

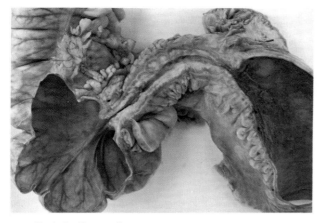

4.37 Crohn's disease: ileum

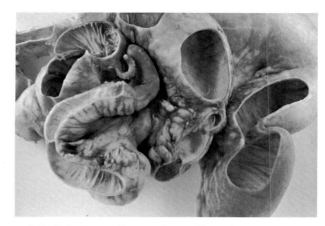

4.38 Crohn's disease: ileum and ascending colon

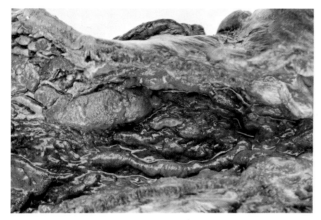

4.39 Crohn's disease: ileum

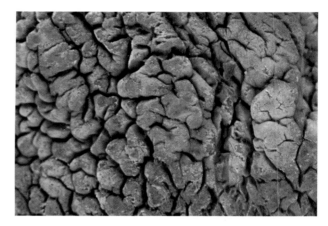

4.40 Crohn's disease: caecum

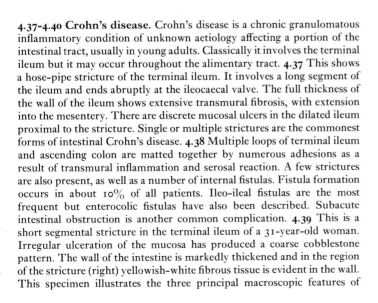

4.41 Carcinoma of ampulla of Vater: duodenum

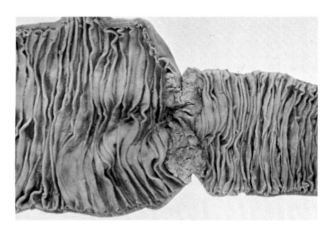

4.42 Carcinoma: jejunum

4.37-4.40 Crohn's disease. Crohn's disease is a chronic granulomatous inflammatory condition of unknown aetiology affecting a portion of the intestinal tract, usually in young adults. Classically it involves the terminal ileum but it may occur throughout the alimentary tract. **4.37** This shows a hose-pipe stricture of the terminal ileum. It involves a long segment of the ileum and ends abruptly at the ileocaecal valve. The full thickness of the wall of the ileum shows extensive transmural fibrosis, with extension into the mesentery. There are discrete mucosal ulcers in the dilated ileum proximal to the stricture. Single or multiple strictures are the commonest forms of intestinal Crohn's disease. **4.38** Multiple loops of terminal ileum and ascending colon are matted together by numerous adhesions as a result of transmural inflammation and serosal reaction. A few strictures are also present, as well as a number of internal fistulas. Fistula formation occurs in about 10% of all patients. Ileo-ileal fistulas are the most frequent but enterocolic fistulas have also been described. Subacute intestinal obstruction is another common complication. **4.39** This is a short segmental stricture in the terminal ileum of a 31-year-old woman. Irregular ulceration of the mucosa has produced a coarse cobblestone pattern. The wall of the intestine is markedly thickened and in the region of the stricture (right) yellowish-white fibrous tissue is evident in the wall. This specimen illustrates the three principal macroscopic features of

Crohn's disease: ulceration, stricture formation, and cobblestone appearance of the mucosa. **4.40** The classic cobblestone appearance is seen in about 25% of cases of Crohn's disease, and this view of the mucosa of the caecum depicts cobblestoning in detail. The cobblestones are formed by intercommunicating crevices and fissures surrounding islands of mucous membranes which are raised by underlying inflammation and oedema. This patient, a 33-year-old man, also had Hodgkin's disease affecting the colon. Carcinoma of the colon sometimes complicates Crohn's disease but a link between Crohn's disease and lymphoma remains to be established. **4.41 Carcinoma of the ampulla of Vater: duodenum.** The tumour is a small polypoid mass with an ulcerated surface. Ampullary carcinomas are often diagnosed early since they cause obstructive jaundice. They also have a tendency to bleed. They are typically polypoid. Histologically they are papillary adenocarcinomas and tend to resemble bile-duct carcinoma. **4.42 Carcinoma: jejunum.** The tumour has encircled the intestine to form an annular stricture. The proximal jejunum is hypertrophied and the distal portion collapsed and atrophic. Primary carcinomas of the small intestine form less than 1% of all intestinal carcinomas. They are distributed equally between the duodenum, upper jejunum and the lower ileum. An association with a gluten-sensitive enteropathy is sometimes found, as in this case.

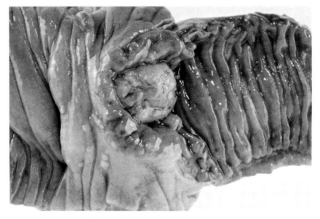

4.43 Carcinoid tumour (argentaffinoma): ileum

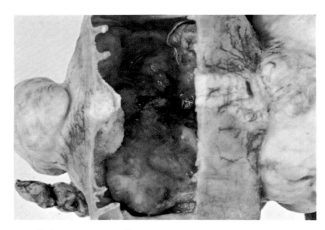

4.44 Leiomyosarcoma: ileum

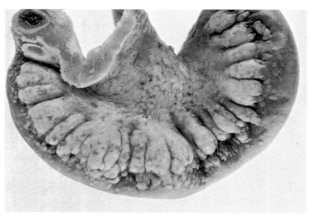

4.45 Histiocytic lymphoma: small intestine

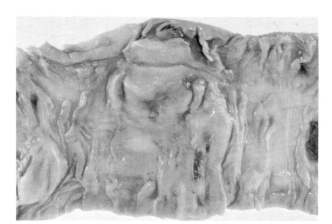

4.46 Lymphosarcoma: ileum

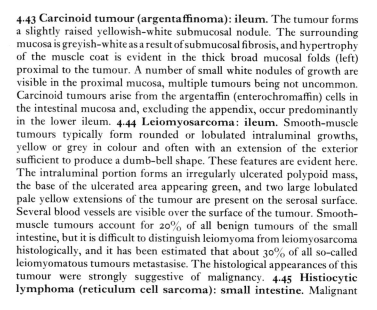

4.47 Secondary carcinoma: ileum

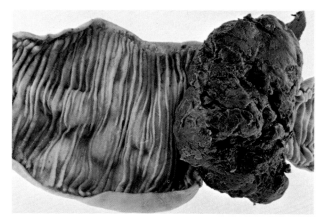

4.48 Secondary melanoma: small intestine

4.43 Carcinoid tumour (argentaffinoma): ileum. The tumour forms a slightly raised yellowish-white submucosal nodule. The surrounding mucosa is greyish-white as a result of submucosal fibrosis, and hypertrophy of the muscle coat is evident in the thick broad mucosal folds (left) proximal to the tumour. A number of small white nodules of growth are visible in the proximal mucosa, multiple tumours being not uncommon. Carcinoid tumours arise from the argentaffin (enterochromaffin) cells in the intestinal mucosa and, excluding the appendix, occur predominantly in the lower ileum. **4.44 Leiomyosarcoma: ileum.** Smooth-muscle tumours typically form rounded or lobulated intraluminal growths, yellow or grey in colour and often with an extension of the exterior sufficient to produce a dumb-bell shape. These features are evident here. The intraluminal portion forms an irregularly ulcerated polypoid mass, the base of the ulcerated area appearing green, and two large lobulated pale yellow extensions of the tumour are present on the serosal surface. Several blood vessels are visible over the surface of the tumour. Smooth-muscle tumours account for 20% of all benign tumours of the small intestine, but it is difficult to distinguish leiomyoma from leiomyosarcoma histologically, and it has been estimated that about 30% of all so-called leiomyomatous tumours metastasise. The histological appearances of this tumour were strongly suggestive of malignancy. **4.45 Histiocytic lymphoma (reticulum cell sarcoma): small intestine.** Malignant lymphoma of the gastrointestinal tract characteristically presents as multiple infiltrative annular or plateau-like elevations of the mucosa, and this one consists of multiple raised plaque-like masses, cream-coloured but with discrete greenish areas of ulceration. A lymphoma may arise as a primary lesion in the gastrointestinal tract or be a manifestation of generalised disease. **4.46 Lymphosarcoma: ileum.** Multiple small greyish-white polypoid tumours project into the lumen of the terminal ileum, a pattern known as multiple lymphomatous polyposis and found most often in the large intestine. The mesenteric lymph node shown in section is enlarged and replaced by lymphoma. Most patients with malignant lymphoma of the gastrointestinal tract rarely survive more than two years after diagnosis. Lymphosarcoma has a better prognosis than histiocytic lymphoma (reticulum cell sarcoma). **4.47 Secondary carcinoma: ileum.** The serosal surface of this loop of ileum is covered with tiny (miliary) white deposits of secondary carcinoma. The mesentery is heavily infiltrated and confluent deposits of white tumour have replaced the normal fat. There is also a well-marked mesenteric fibrosis. The primary tumour in this case was in the stomach. **4.48 Secondary melanoma: small intestine.** A solitary deposit of malignant melanoma forms a large black deeply-pigmented irregular polypoid tumour filling the lumen of the small intestine. It had caused subacute obstruction.

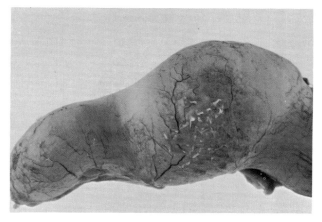

4.49 Mucocele: appendix

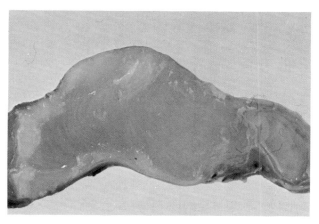

4.50 Mucocele: appendix

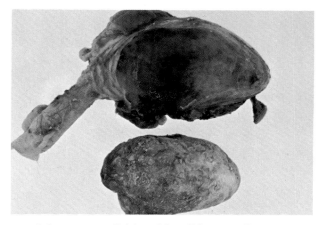

4.51 Subacute appendicitis and faecolith: appendix

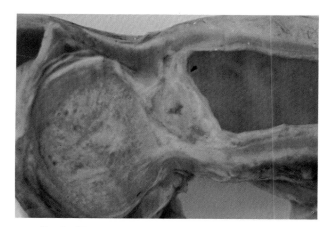

4.52 Carcinoid tumour: appendix

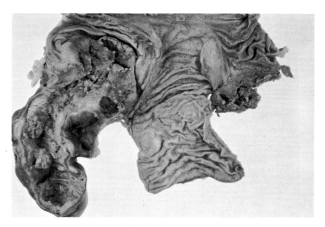

4.53 Carcinoma: appendix

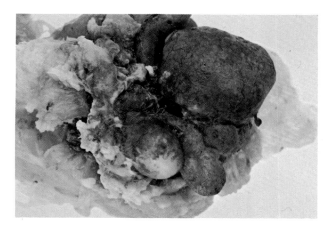

4.54 Carcinoma: appendix

4.49 and 4.50 Mucocele: appendix. A mucocele is a cystic dilatation distal to a complete obstruction, usually the result of cicatricial stricture following inflammation. **4.49** The appendix is greatly distended and its base is scarred. The serosa is not inflamed, however, being pale pink and with delicate branching vessels visible. **4.50** The appendix shown in 4.49 has been sectioned longitudinally and is full of thick glairy pale yellow mucus. The wall is thinned. Occasionally a mucocele ruptures and discharges mucin and epithelial cells into the peritoneal cavity, giving rise eventually to myxoma peritonei. **4.51 Subacute appendicitis and faecolith: appendix.** The appendix (top) has been sectioned longitudinally to display considerable dilatation of the distal half of the lumen. The wall is thickened and white, suggestive of underlying fibrosis. The mucosal surface shows superficial haemorrhagic ulceration and an irregular perforation is present on the inferior aspect. Below the appendix there is an oval faecolith with a projecting spur. About 60% of inflamed appendices contain faecoliths. **4.52 Carcinoid tumour: appendix.** This is the tip of the appendix. It contains a small round apparently-encapsulated yellow tumour. Carcinoids form 85% of all tumours of the

appendix and are found in about 0.1% of all resected appendices. The tumour often infiltrates muscle and spreads locally onto the peritoneal surface but metastasis occurs in less than 1% of cases. **4.53 and 4.54 Carcinoma: appendix.** Carcinoma of the appendix is a rare tumour, being found in approximately 0.01% of all resected appendices. It is usually situated at the base and may infiltrate the appendix and project into the lumen. The organ may not show any external evidence of disease. **4.53** This specimen consists of the opened terminal ileum, caecum and first part of the ascending colon. The appendix (left) is largely filled with an irregular polypoid tumour, maximal at the base. Histologically the tumour was an adenocarcinoma of colonic pattern, a type which readily invades the caecum, mesoappendix and regional lymphatics. **4.54** Some appendiceal carcinomas are mucus-secreting (colloid) carcinomas, a type of growth which often shows evidence of extension through the wall of the appendix with peritoneal dissemination and the development of a myxoma peritonei—a lesion sometimes referred to as a 'malignant mucocele'. In this instance a grossly distorted and kinked appendix, largely replaced by tumour, is surrounded by thick gelatinous mucus.

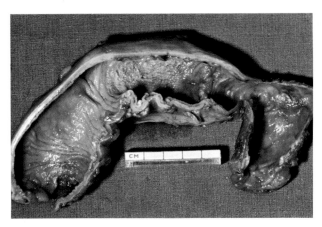

4.55 Congenital aganglionic megacolon
(Hirschsprung's disease)

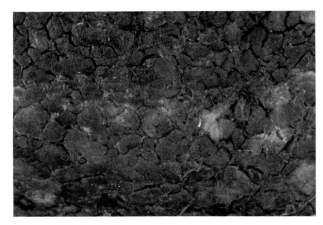

4.56 Ischaemic colitis

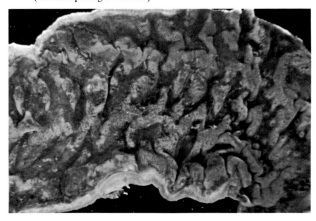

4.57 Pseudomembranous enterocolitis: colon

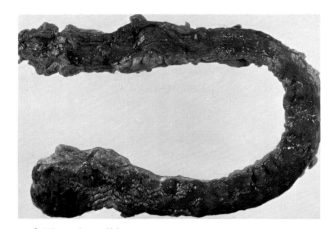

4.58 Ulcerative colitis

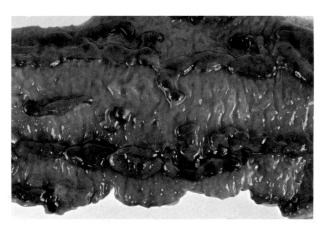

4.59 Ulcerative colitis

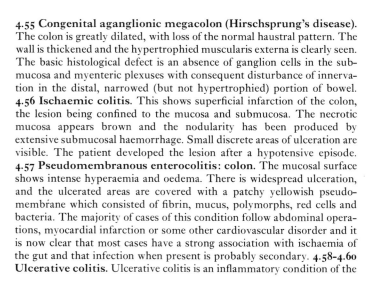

4.60 Ulcerative colitis

4.55 Congenital aganglionic megacolon (Hirschsprung's disease). The colon is greatly dilated, with loss of the normal haustral pattern. The wall is thickened and the hypertrophied muscularis externa is clearly seen. The basic histological defect is an absence of ganglion cells in the submucosa and myenteric plexuses with consequent disturbance of innervation in the distal, narrowed (but not hypertrophied) portion of bowel. **4.56 Ischaemic colitis.** This shows superficial infarction of the colon, the lesion being confined to the mucosa and submucosa. The necrotic mucosa appears brown and the nodularity has been produced by extensive submucosal haemorrhage. Small discrete areas of ulceration are visible. The patient developed the lesion after a hypotensive episode. **4.57 Pseudomembranous enterocolitis: colon.** The mucosal surface shows intense hyperaemia and oedema. There is widespread ulceration, and the ulcerated areas are covered with a patchy yellowish pseudomembrane which consisted of fibrin, mucus, polymorphs, red cells and bacteria. The majority of cases of this condition follow abdominal operations, myocardial infarction or some other cardiovascular disorder and it is now clear that most cases have a strong association with ischaemia of the gut and that infection when present is probably secondary. **4.58-4.60 Ulcerative colitis.** Ulcerative colitis is an inflammatory condition of the colonic mucosa of unknown aetiology. **4.58** This is a total colectomy specimen from a patient with an acute exacerbation of the disease opened to display the mucosal surface. The mucosa is granular, velvety and plum-red, and ulceration is very extensive. The colour is due to the intense vascularity. The disease is most severe in the left colon (bottom left) where patchy yellow-white exudates are visible. There is loss of the normal haustral pattern due to muscular contraction and the length of the colon and rectum is reduced. **4.59** The earliest form of ulceration consists of superficial erosion of the mucous membrane. Later there is full-thickness ulceration. The ulcers are sometimes linear and this pattern of linear ulceration is very pronounced in this colon. Full-thickness mucosal ulceration followed by undermining of adjacent intact mucosa tend to cause the surviving mucosa to project into the lumen as pseudopolyps ('inflammatory polyps' or 'mucosal tags'). In this case the pseudopolyps formed by the longitudinally-running ridges of congested mucosa contrast with the pale areas denuded of mucosa. **4.60** Pseudopolyps may be present in large numbers and assume bizarre shapes. They may also fuse together to form irregular mucosal bridges. Such a development, termed colitis polyposa, is shown here. Discrete punched-out superficial ulcers are present on some of the broad ridges and folds.

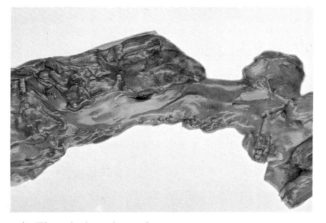

4.61 Thoracic duct obstruction

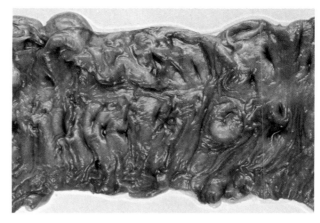

4.62 Diverticular disease: colon

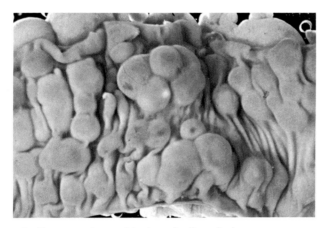

4.63 Pneumatosis cystoides intestinalis: colon

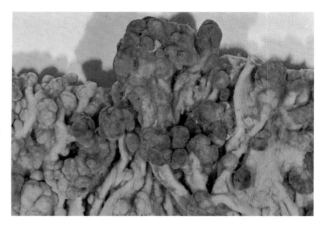

4.64 Familial adenomatous polyposis: colon

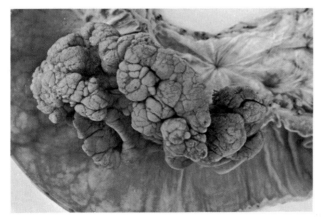

4.65 Papillary adenoma: colon

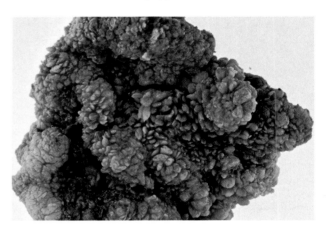

4.66 Villous papilloma: rectum

4.61 Thoracic duct obstruction. This shows a greatly dilated thoracic duct encased in dense fibrous tissue, the result of retroperitoneal fibrosis which in turn was due to a diffusely infiltrating retroperitoneal lymphosarcoma. The patient had chylous ascites, the ascitic fluid appearing milky from its high fat content. **4.62 Diverticular disease: colon.** Diverticula of the colon are the commonest type of diverticula of the gastrointestinal tract. They are found throughout the colon but are commonest in the descending and sigmoid colon. They are frequently multiple and are more common in men. They occur on the convexity of the intestine opposite the mesenteric attachment and between the longitudinal muscle bands (taenia coli). This shows the mucosa of the sigmoid colon. The orifices of the diverticula are seen in two parallel rows. Note the prominence of the mucosal folds owing to the underlying muscular thickening. Diverticula of colon are important clinically because in approximately 10-15% of cases inflammatory complications develop. **4.63 Pneumatosis cystoides intestinalis: colon.** The mucosa has a coarse cobblestone appearance from the presence of many submucosal gas-filled cysts. Cystic penumatosis is a rare condition, and the small intestine is more often affected than the colon. About 50% of the cases are associated with gastric or duodenal ulcers, and a strong link with respiratory disease, notably asthma, has also been observed. **4.64 Familial adenomatous polyposis: colon.** The mucosa of this part of an affected colon is covered with sessile polypoid adenomas of various sizes. The large pedunculated polyp (top centre) has undergone carcinomatous change. Familial polyposis is transmitted as an autosomal dominant trait and the lesion usually becomes manifest in childhood or adolescence. The premalignant character of the lesion is well-established, about 60% of patients presenting in adult life with carcinoma which is often multicentric. **4.65 Papillary adenoma: colon.** Neoplastic polyps of the colon fall into two main types, adenomatous polyps and villous papillomas, the adenomatous type of growth being much more common than the villous. This shows in close-up a large adenomatous polyp (papillary adenoma) of the sigmoid colon. The smooth lobulated surface is traversed by intercommunicating clefts and fissures. Some papillary adenomas are transitional in pattern and have areas of villous type. **4.66 Villous papilloma: rectum.** A large sessile villous papilloma of the rectum is shown. The surface is shaggy and made up of numerous thin finger-like processes. Villous papillomas may secrete large quantities of mucus and are more likely to undergo malignant change than adenomatous polyps. Villous and papillary tumours are found throughout the large bowel but are more common in the rectum.

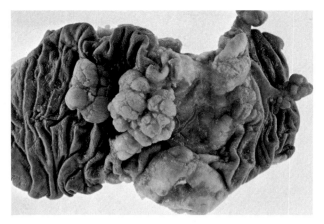

4.67 Carcinoma and papillary adenoma: colon

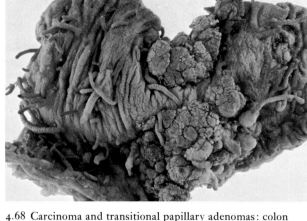

4.68 Carcinoma and transitional papillary adenomas: colon

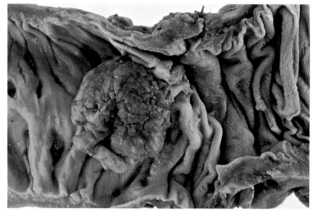

4.69 Carcinoma: colon

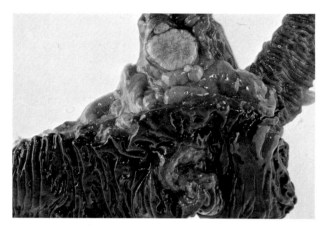

4.70 Carcinoma: colon

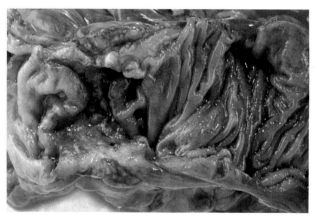

4.71 Carcinoma: colon

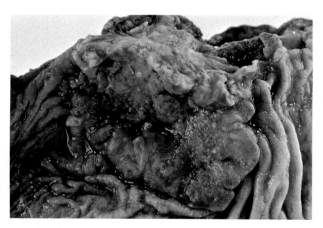

4.72 Carcinoma: rectum

4.67 Carcinoma and papillary adenoma: colon. The dark-brown colour of the colonic mucosa is due to melanosis coli. An ulcerated carcinoma is present (right of centre). There are also two sessile papillary adenomas in continuity with the carcinoma to its left, as well as two small pedunculated polypoid adenomas (right and above right). **4.68 Carcinoma and transitional papillary adenomas: colon.** A large sessile polypoid growth, combining the superficial features of a transitional or mixed papillary adenoma and a villous papilloma, encircles the colonic wall, causing a partial stricture. Histology showed carcinomatous change with invasion of the bowel wall. Multiple unusually thin (filiform) polyps are also present. **4.69-4.71 Carcinoma: colon.** Carcinoma of colon may be classified into three types depending on the macroscopic appearance; the polypoid, the annular stenosing, and the raised flat ulcer. **4.69** This red-brown growth is an example of the polypoid or protruberant type of lesion. Polypoid carcinomas are usually small and tend to bleed readily. They are often situated in the caecum and right colon but this one was situated on the sigmoid colon. The orifice of a diverticulum can be seen

to the left of the tumour. **4.70** The specimen consists of the terminal portion of ileum, caecum, and part of the ascending colon, with a portion of the attached mesentery. The mucosa of the colon is very dark from melanosis coli. The tumour takes the form of a small irregular ulcerated mass. An ileocaecal lymph node is infiltrated by secondary carcinoma (top). **4.71** The annular stenosing variety is the commonest type. It grows slowly, spreading circumferentially around the wall. A considerable fibrous tissue stroma develops, which subsequently contracts and narrows the lumen. These features are evident in this ulcerated constricting tumour of the descending colon. The margins of the growth are everted and the base covered by a greenish necrotic slough. The stromal fibrosis is visible on the cut surface of the tumour and adjacent serosa (top centre). **4.72 Carcinoma: rectum.** Carcinomas of the rectum do not have a characteristic gross pattern; many are bulky ulcerated growths but some are flatter with raised everted edges. In this case the tumour is large, flat, and slightly raised. The centre is necrotic and ulcerated and the edge is elevated and everted.

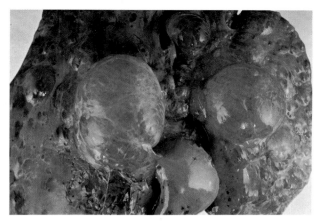

5.1 Polycystic disease: liver

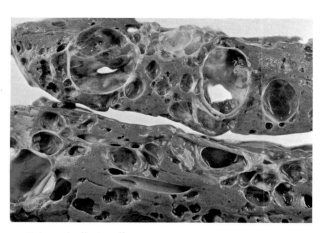

5.2 Polycystic disease: liver

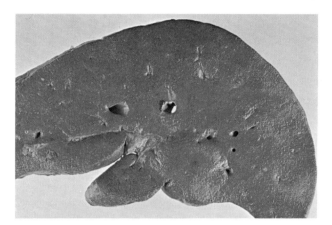

5.3 Haemosiderosis: liver

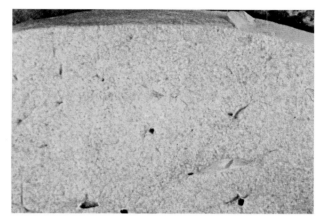

5.4 Fatty change: liver

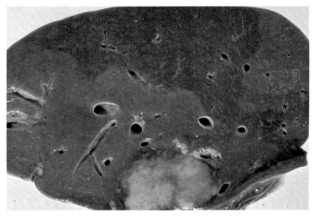

5.5 Zahn's infarct: liver

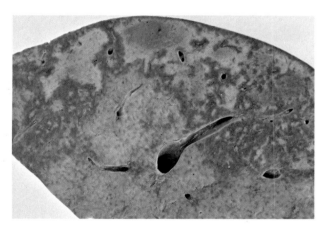

5.6 Infarction: liver

5.1 and 5.2 Polycystic disease: liver. This is a congenital lesion of unknown pathogenesis. **5.1** This is part of the surface of the liver. Cysts are present throughout the organ. Some are large and project from the surface but most are small. The diameter varies from one to five cm. Sometimes the cysts may be of microscopic size, appearing as small greyish dots throughout the liver. **5.2** This is a section of the same liver, showing the smooth lining of the cysts, many of which are multilocular. Some cysts contain yellowish fluid. The liver tissue shows fatty change. The patient also had polycystic kidneys. **5.3 Haemosiderosis: liver.** The liver is a dull brick-red colour instead of the usual rich brown. The patient had received many hundreds of pints of blood by transfusion and massive amounts of haemosiderin were present in macrophages and in the Kupffer cells. There was also increase in fibrous tissue in the portal tracts but this had not advanced to the stage of cirrhosis. **5.4 Fatty change: liver.** This is a section of the right lobe of the liver. The hepatic tissue is a uniform yellow colour, from the presence of large quantities of neutral fat within the liver cells, and the normal lobular pattern is obscured. The patient was an alcoholic and the commonest cause of diffuse fatty change

is chronic alcoholism. Fatty change may also be found in association with obesity, malnutrition, wasting diseases and kwashiorkor. **5.5 Zahn's infarct: liver.** This is a section of the right lobe of the liver. The upper portion shows a well-demarcated roughly triangular dusky-brown zone which measured about 8×4 cm. It is a Zahn-type infarct, in which the liver cells become atrophic but not necrotic. Zahn's infarcts usually result from intrahepatic obstruction of the portal vein or one of its tributaries. They may follow severe congestive failure or, more usually, neoplastic infiltration of the portal vein; and in this case a secondary deposit of carcinoma (bottom centre) has infiltrated the portal vein. The cut surface of the liver also shows a fine mottling, due to fatty change from passive congestion. The nutmeg change is more obvious in the infarcted tissue. **5.6 Infarction: liver.** There is a recent subcapsular infarct. The necrotic parenchyma is pale yellow and is bounded by a deep brown haemorrhagic border. The non-infarcted liver is bile-stained and light green. True infarction of the liver is rare and is usually due to obstruction of the hepatic artery or one of its branches.

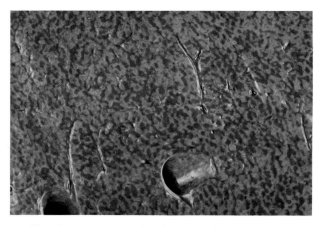

5.7 Chronic venous congestion (nut-meg change): liver

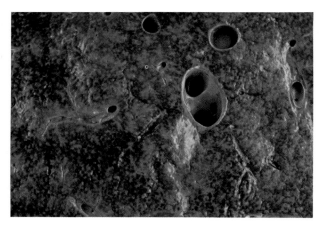

5.8 Cardiac cirrhosis: liver

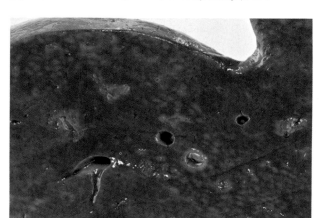

5.9 Waldenström's macroglobulinaemia: liver

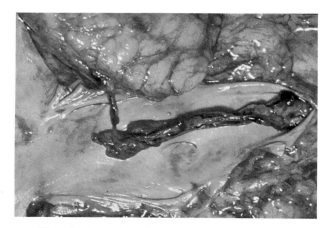

5.10 Thrombosis: portal vein

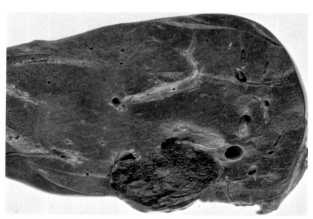

5.11 Haemangioma: liver

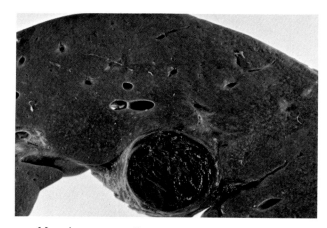

5.12 Mycotic aneurysm: liver

5.7 Chronic venous congestion (nut-meg change): liver. This shows the cut surface of the liver. The yellow colour of the fatty change, which is mainly around the central lobular veins, contrasts with the darker brown colour of the relatively unaffected peripheral parts of the lobules. **5.8 Cardiac cirrhosis: liver.** True cardiac cirrhosis with nodular regeneration is a rare complication of congestive cardiac failure and this example is only moderately severe. The cut surface of the liver is finely nodular, with a typical variegated light yellow and dark brown colour (nut-meg appearance). The hepatic veins are dilated. The portal tracts are unduly prominent, with increased amounts of fibrous tissue. The patient had long-standing congestive cardiac failure secondary to ischaemic heart disease. **5.9 Waldenström's macroglobulinaemia: liver.** The cut surface is paler than normal and there are many small greyish-white nodules which histology showed to consist of periportal collections of lymphocytes and plasmacytoid cells. Two main branches of the portal vein are filled with antemortem thrombus. **5.10 Thrombosis: portal vein.** The portal vein contains a pale coiled thrombus. The liver is pale yellow and shows coarse macronodular cirrhosis. Cirrhosis of

the liver with portal hypertension predisposes to extrahepatic thrombosis of the portal vein. The orifices of the superior mesenteric and splenic veins where they enter the portal vein are just visible on the left. **5.11 Haemangioma: liver.** The lesion is a red haemorrhagic mass approximately 4 cm in diameter on the undersurface of an otherwise normal liver. Cavernous haemangiomas are common. They are usually an incidental finding at necropsy, varying from a few mm to several cm in diameter. They are usually subcapsular but may be deep within the organ. Microscopically the large blood-filled spaces are lined by a single layer of endothelium and separated by fibrous tissue septa. A number undergo fibrosis and calcification. **5.12 Mycotic aneurysm: liver.** There is a spherical aneurysmal sac approximately 5 cm in diameter and full of dark red thrombus on the inferior surface of the liver. Its wall consists of fibrous tissue and compressed liver tissue. The patient suffered from bacterial endocarditis and fragments of vegetation had carried micro-organisms *(Streptococcus viridans)* into a branch of the hepatic artery where they proliferated and caused the wall of the artery to weaken and bulge.

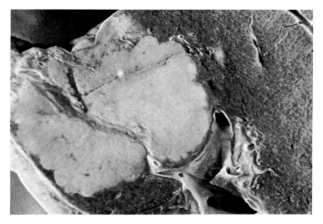

5.13 Gumma: liver

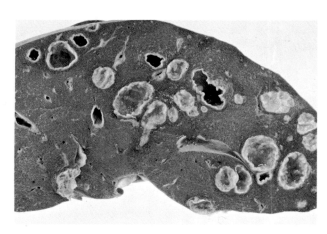

5.14 Multiple abscesses (Aspergillosis): liver

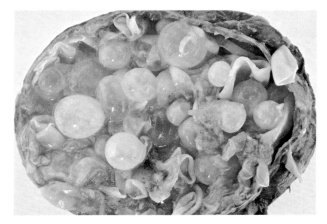

5.15 Hydatid cyst: liver

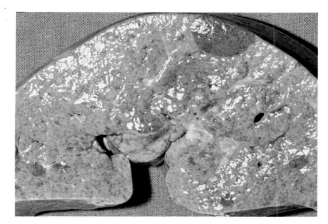

5.16 Neonatal (giant-cell) hepatitis: liver

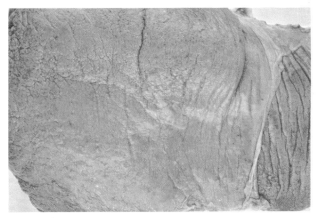

5.17 Acute diffuse necrosis: liver

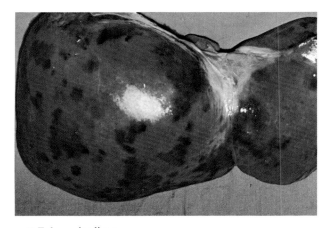

5.18 Eclampsia: liver

5.13 Gumma: liver. A large gumma is visible in this section of liver. Its centre is necrotic and a dull yellow-white colour. The gumma is typically irregular in shape and clearly delineated from the surrounding liver by granulation tissue and fibrous tissue. About 15% of patients with acquired syphilis are likely to develop gummas of the liver in the tertiary stage. They may be solitary or multiple, and several may coalesce to form a large mass. **5.14 Multiple abscesses (Aspergillosis): liver.** Multiple abscess cavities are scattered throughout the organ. They have a thick fibrous wall and are lined by greenish tissue. The contents of the abscesses were found to consist of necrotic liver and colonies of *Aspergillus flavus*. Infection had reached the liver by the systemic circulation. The patient was receiving immunosuppressive therapy. **5.15 Hydatid cyst: liver.** The main cyst (13 cm diameter) has been opened to show large numbers of daughter cysts. The average diameter of these was 1.5 cm. Most of them are thin-walled and translucent and filled with clear yellowish fluid but a few appear opaque. Some have ruptured. Each small cyst contained large numbers of scolices. **5.16 Neonatal (giant-cell) hepatitis: liver.** The patient was a five-month-old male infant. The cut surface of the liver is pale green, from bile stasis. A fine nodularity is present, with diffuse increase of fibrous tissue. The fibrosis also evident in the portal areas suggests progression to cirrhosis. Histologically

there was bile stasis, formation of giant multinucleated hepatocytes, and intralobular fibrosis. Neonatal or giant-cell hepatitis commonly develops in the first or second week of life and the condition may be seen in such diverse diseases as cytomegalovirus inclusion disease and galactosaemia. In a proportion of cases there is no known aetiology. The majority of patients recover with no permanent damage, but a few die in the acute stage and a few progress to cirrhosis. **5.17 Acute diffuse necrosis: liver.** This shows the diaphragmatic surface of the right lobe and part of the left lobe. The deep brown colour of the normal organ has been replaced by a much lighter reddish-brown colour. The capsule is also very wrinkled, particularly over the left lobe (left), as a result of shrinkage of the liver tissue. The organ weighed only 445 g and microscopy showed that almost all the remaining liver cells were necrotic. The patient died after an operation in which halothane was the anaesthetic. **5.18 Eclampsia: liver.** Liver disease is rare in eclampsia, but in patients who die of eclampsia the liver frequently shows haemorrhagic zones alternating with paler areas of necrosis. The capsular surface of this liver is blotchy and discoloured from the presence of large and small subcapsular haemorrhages. Microscopically the periportal and peripheral zones of the lobules were found to be necrotic. The sinusoids frequently contain fibrin thrombi in eclampsia.

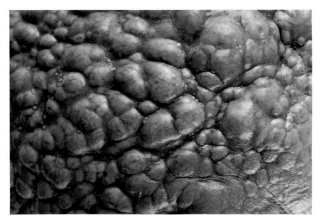

5.19 Macronodular cirrhosis: liver

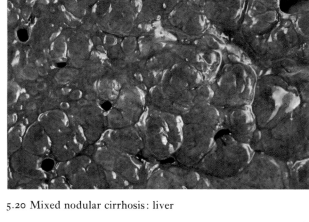

5.20 Mixed nodular cirrhosis: liver

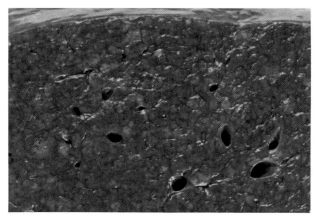

5.21 Micronodular cirrhosis: liver

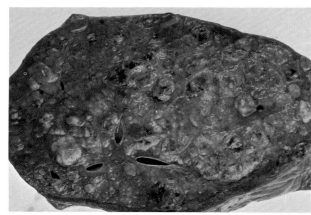

5.22 Macronodular cirrhosis and hepatocellular
carcinoma: liver

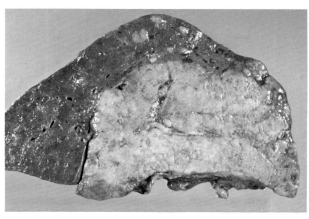

5.23 Hepatocellular carcinoma: liver

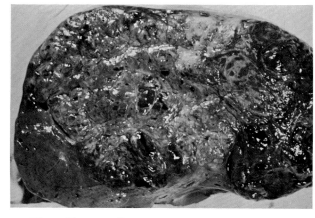

5.24 Hepatoblastoma: liver

5.19 Macronodular cirrhosis: liver. This is a close-up of the capsular aspect of the organ. Large (0.5-2 cm diameter) nodules of hyperplastic liver cells are separated by fibrous trabeculae. **5.20 Mixed nodular cirrhosis: liver.** The cut surface of the liver, which was moderately enlarged, is yellowish-brown. The organ consists of nodules of regenerating liver cells of very variable size. Some are only 1 or 2 mm in diameter whereas others measure 2.5 cm or more. The pattern therefore is a mixed micronodular and macronodular one. The central veins are prominent and thickened. The fibrous tissue septa between the regenerating nodules are prominent. **5.21 Micronodular cirrhosis: liver.** The liver, which was moderately enlarged, is a pale yellow-brown colour. The capsular surface is fairly smooth but in places shallow depressed scarred areas are visible. The cut surface shows the organ to be made up of more or less uniform nodules of regenerating liver cells 1-3 mm in diameter. Some of the nodules are pale. The patient was a middle-aged man who died from chronic bronchitis and the changes in the liver were an unexpected finding. No aetiological factor was found (cryptogenic cirrhosis). **5.22 Macronodular cirrhosis and hepatocellular carcinoma: liver.** There is a very advanced macronodular cirrhosis with destruction of the normal architecture. The brown regeneration nodules are relatively large and can be seen most clearly at the bottom. In addition, however, there are many large nodules of carcinomatous tissue, some pale,

some haemorrhagic and dark in colour, some greenish and bile-stained. Histology showed that the tumour was a hepatocellular carcinoma which developed on top of the cirrhotic process. **5.23 Hepatocellular carcinoma: liver.** In contrast to the multicentric lesion in 5.22, this neoplasm is a single large mass replacing most of the right lobe of the liver. There are also several small satellite nodules in the surrounding liver. The hepatic tissue appears paler than normal but is not cirrhotic. Hepatocellular carcinoma comprises 75-80% of primary liver cancers. It shows a striking difference in frequency in various parts of the world. In Europe and the United States, this varies from 0.1% to 0.7% of all necropsies, whereas in parts of Africa the figure rises to 10 to 20%. This patient lived in Uganda. There is a strong association with cirrhosis, most marked in Africa, where approximately 60% of cirrhotic males develop liver cancer. **5.24 Hepatoblastoma: liver.** Most hepatocellular carcinomas in infants and children are large multinodular lesions that usually arise in non-cirrhotic livers. Some of these tumours contain sarcomatous elements and the name mixed hepatoblastoma is applied to them. Hepatoblastomas are highly malignant. This liver has been almost completely replaced by the tumour. The neoplastic tissue is pale but there are many areas of necrosis and haemorrhage. A small portion of surviving liver is visible at the bottom left corner.

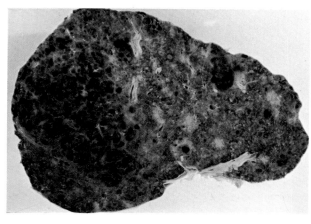

5.25 Haemangioendothelial sarcoma: liver

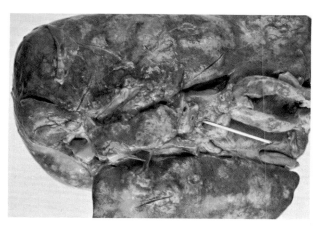

5.26 Secondary carcinoma: liver

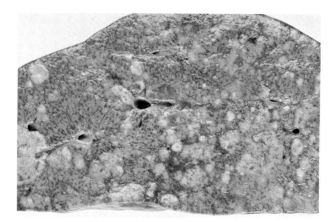

5.27 Secondary carcinoma: liver

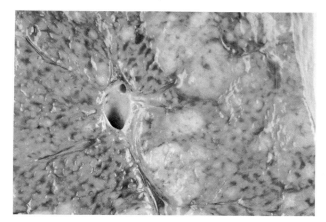

5.28 Secondary carcinoma: liver

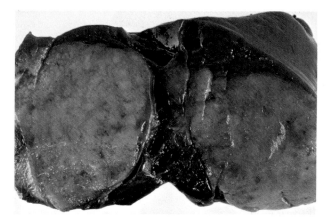

5.29 Secondary carcinoid tumour: liver

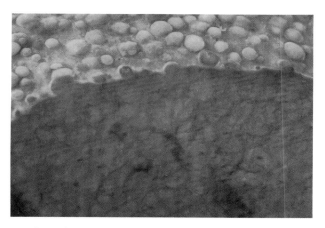

5.30 Lymphosarcoma: liver

5.25 Haemangioendothelial sarcoma: liver. The liver is diffusely infiltrated by tumour. Most of the tumour appears haemorrhagic but yellowish-white nodules of solid tumour are also present and there are areas of cystic degeneration (left). The surviving liver tissue is stained bright green by retained bile (centre). The patient had received thorotrast more than 20 years prior to his death in the course of diagnostic radiology. Thorotrast is deposited in the reticuloendothelial system in the liver, spleen and bone marrow. The carcinogenic factor in it is thorium[228] which gives off alpha and beta particles and gamma rays. Haemangio-endothelial sarcoma of the liver was the first tumour to be associated with thorotrast. **5.26-5.28 Secondary carcinoma: liver.** Metastatic carcinoma may reach the liver via the portal vein, hepatic artery, hilar lymphatics or by direct extension. The tumour often grows within sinusoids. **5.26** This shows the undersurface of the liver. The organ is a dark green colour from bile stasis and it is studded with subcapsular deposits of secondary carcinoma. The deposits vary greatly in size and their appearance is also variegated, with areas of yellowish tumour and red haemorrhage. Some deposits have undergone central necrosis and this has produced a central depressed area on the surface of the deposits—'umbilication' (lower centre). Extensive spread is also seen in the porta hepatis, in lymph nodes and around the gall-bladder (right). The common

bile duct was compressed by these metastases (note the probe in the cut end of the common duct) and the patient presented with signs of obstructive jaundice. The primary was in the stomach. **5.27** The liver is pale, from fatty change, and large numbers of pinkish-white deposits of secondary carcinoma are scattered throughout the organ. The tumour nodules vary in diameter from 4 cm down to 1 or 2 mm. The patient had had a carcinoma of breast removed previously. **5.28** This is a close-up view of the lesions shown in 5.27. The carcinomatous tissue is paler than the brownish liver tissue. There are, however, haemorrhagic foci throughout the deposits, which are not well-demarcated from the hepatic tissue. On the left, very small whitish deposits of tumour can be seen infiltrating the sinusoids among the liver trabeculae. **5.29 Secondary carcinoid tumour: liver.** A single deposit of carcinoid tumour has been bisected to show the cut surface. It is yellowish-brown whereas the liver tissue is a brownish-red. The presence of a solitary metastasis in the liver is unusual, numerous secondaries generally being present by the time the patient dies. In this case the primary was in the small intestine. **5.30 Lymphosarcoma: liver.** This shows both the capsular surface and a cut surface. There are numerous subcapsular nodules which on section are seen to be spherical. Histology showed that the deposits were centred on the portal tracts and consisted of small lymphocytes.

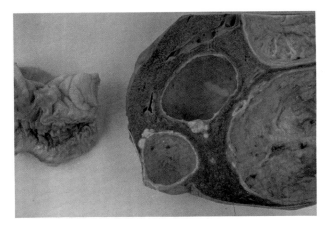

5.31 Pyaemic abscesses: liver

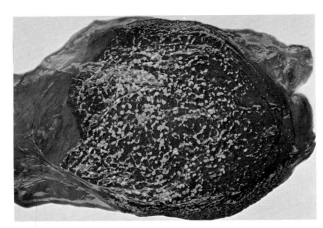

5.32 Chronic cholecystitis (strawberry gall-bladder)

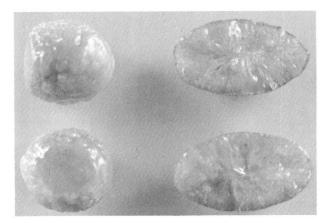

5.33 Cholesterol gall-stones

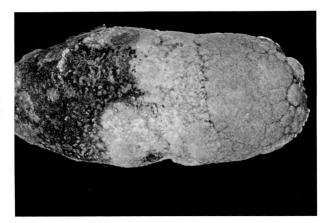

5.34 Cholesterol gall-stone

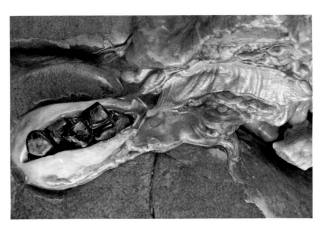

5.35 Chronic cholecystitis and cholelithiasis: gall-bladder

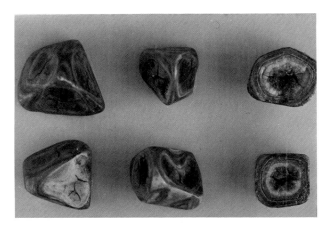

5.36 Mixed gall-stones

5.31 Pyaemic abscesses: liver. The liver contains many thick-walled abscess cavities, which are lined with a shaggy greenish-yellow purulent exudate. The abscesses developed as a result of spread of bacterial infection via the portal vein from a focus of diverticulitis in the sigmoid colon (left). Infected emboli may reach the liver from any suppurative process in the tissues drained by the portal vein. **5.32 Chronic cholecystitis (strawberry gall-bladder).** The gall-bladder is thick-walled and fibrous from chronic inflammatory change. However the mucosal folds are bright yellow, an appearance caused by the presence within the mucosa of large numbers of cholesterol-filled macrophages. **5.33 and 5.34 Cholesterol gall-stone.** **5.33** This shows three cholesterol stones. The two on the left are spherical and have bosselated surfaces. The stone on the right has been cut in two to show that it consists throughout of yellow material except for a small amount of darker material in the centre. Analysis showed the yellow material to be almost pure cholesterol. **5.34** This shows a large oval solitary cholesterol stone which was lodged in the neck of the gall-bladder in Hartman's pouch and obstructed the cystic duct, the gall-bladder being filled with clear white watery bile (hydrops of the gall-bladder). The crevices on the surface of the stone are visible (right) but for

the most part they have become obscured by deposition of white calcium carbonate and dark-brown calcium bilirubinate (left). **5.35 Chronic cholecystitis and cholelithiasis: gall-bladder.** This shows the inferior surface of the liver, gall-bladder and common bile duct. The bladder is contracted. Its wall is markedly thickened and fibrosed, and the serosal surface white and opaque. The lumen is full of facetted mixed gall-stones. The common bile duct is dilated, and the mucosal surface bright yellow from bile-staining. The lumen of the distal 1 cm (right) is narrowed. This is an old inflammatory stricture which followed an earlier episode of obstruction at the lower end of the duct by a gall-stone. **5.36 Mixed gall-stones.** These gall-stones were closely packed in a fibrosed gall-bladder, the facetted surfaces being in close apposition. The varied composition of the stones is evident in the two half-sections on the right: a brownish material is present in the centre surrounded by multiple laminae, some pale and others darker in colour. Chemically, mixed stones contain cholesterol, calcium carbonate and calcium bilirubinate in varying proportions. They constitute about 80% of biliary calculi. The association with chronic cholecystitis is very close.

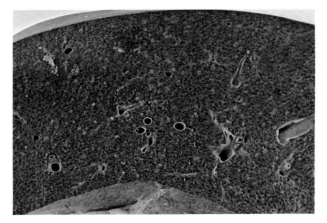

5.37 Extrahepatic bile duct obstruction: liver

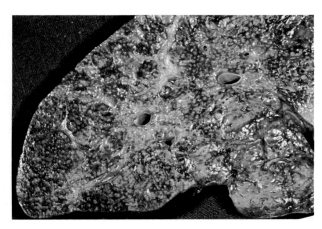

5.38 Extrahepatic bile duct obstruction: liver

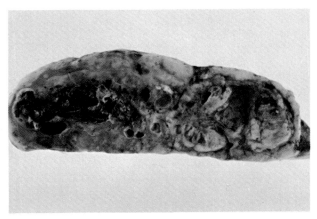

5.39 Suppurative cholangitis: liver

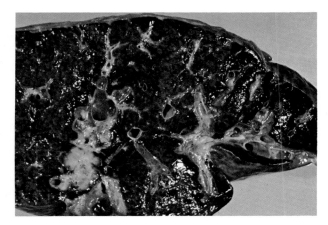

5.40 Carcinoma of common bile duct: liver

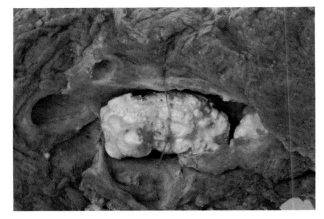

5.41 Carcinoma: gall-bladder

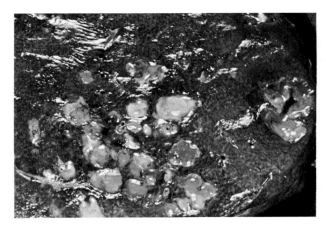

5.42 Calculus: pancreatic duct

5.37 and 5.38 Extrahepatic bile duct obstruction: liver. 5.37 The organ is coloured deep green from bile-staining. The hepatic tissue around the centrilobular veins is pale brown and the bile-staining is most intense in the portal areas. **5.38** This is biliary cirrhosis, a much more advanced lesion than that shown in 5.37. Although a cuff of unstained liver remains in the centrilobular zones, the hepatic tissue around the portal tracts is deep green. In addition there are fairly large pinkish-brown areas of hyperplastic liver, situated mainly beneath the capsule of the liver (at left top and bottom right). The patient was a child of seven years with mucoviscidosis (fibrocystic disease). **5.39 Suppurative cholangitis: liver.** Many yellow and white abscesses are present, centred on bile ducts. The largest abscess on the right has a necrotic partly cystic centre. The small intrahepatic bile ducts are greatly dilated and plugged with green bile, and the liver parenchyma has a distinct trabecular pattern, with pale grey connective tissue alternating with brown liver cells, a manifestation of increased periportal fibrosis following obstruction of the common bile duct by a carcinoma of the head of the pancreas. Ascending infection has led to the formation of the abscesses. **5.40 Carcinoma of common bile duct: liver.** Pale yellowish tumour is infiltrating the main bile ducts

within the liver. It has spread here from a primary carcinoma of the common bile duct (not illustrated) which caused complete obstruction of the duct. There is also tumour in the porta hepatis. Some of the bile ducts (centre) are dilated. Most of the hepatic tissue is a deep green colour from bile-staining but the cells around the central veins are much less affected. **5.41 Carcinoma: gall-bladder.** The gall-bladder is seen in longitudinal section. Almost no lumen remains, the specimen consisting largely of pale malignant tissue which is bile-stained and necrotic in places. Primary carcinoma of the gall-bladder is uncommon and it is often associated with chronic cholecystitis and cholelithiasis. It tends to invade the liver locally. **5.42 Calculus: pancreatic duct.** The main pancreatic duct has been opened. It is greatly dilated and contains an ovoid white calculus. Its wall is thickened and fibrous. The cut surface of the pancreas shows loss of the normal lobular appearance, with a marked increase in fat and fibrous tissue. Pancreatic calculi may be formed in association with chronic relapsing pancreatitis, in which there is progressive destruction of the pancreas as the result of repeated episodes of necrosis of the exocrine tissue.

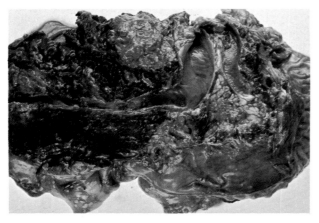

5.43 Acute haemorrhagic pancreatitis

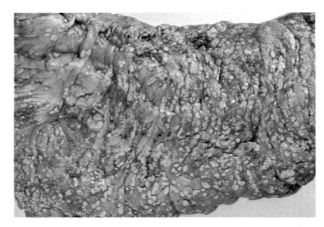

5.44 Acute haemorrhagic pancreatitis: omentum

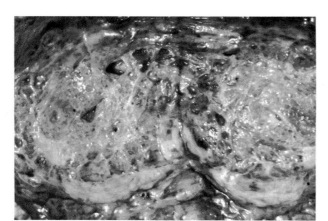

5.45 Cystadenoma: pancreas

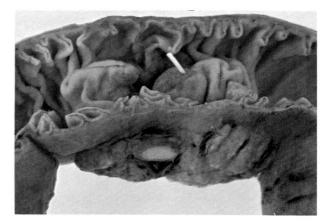

5.46 Carcinoma: pancreas

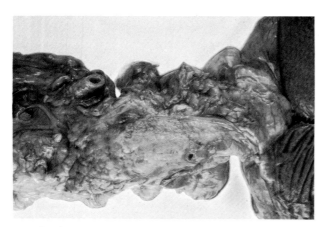

5.47 Carcinoma: pancreas

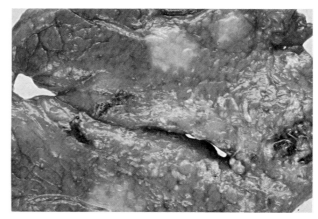

5.48 Histiocytic lymphoma: pancreas

5.43 and 5.44 Acute haemorrhagic pancreatitis. 5.43 This is the posterior aspect of the second part of the duodenum (right), the common bile duct, and the main pancreatic duct. The pancreas is swollen and oedematous and extensive haemorrhagic necrosis of the body and tail of the organ has occurred (left), with the formation of a dark brown haematoma. Small ovoid yellow-white foci of fat necrosis are visible in the peripancreatic fat (lower border). Acute haemorrhagic pancreatitis almost always affects adults between the ages of 40 and 60. The pathogenesis is not fully understood but duct obstruction, reflux of bile, ischaemia, and trauma are thought to be possible factors. **5.44** This shows part of the greater omentum ensheathing the transverse colon from the case shown in 5.43. It is studded with small yellow-white foci of fat necrosis. These foci appear rapidly in an attack of acute pancreatitis and are due to the release of pancreatic enzymes into the peritoneal cavity.
5.45 Cystadenoma: pancreas. The tumour is pinkish-white and has a gelatinous and partly fibrous surface. Multiple small cysts impart a sponge-like appearance to the cut surface. Cystadenomas are rare slow-growing benign tumours arising from duct epithelium and are generally rounded or coarsely lobulated, as in this example. They are more common in women and tend to be located in the tail of the pancreas. **5.46 and 5.47**

Carcinoma: pancreas. 5.46 This is the second part of the duodenum. A lobulated pinkish-white tumour is infiltrating the wall of the duodenum in the region of the ampulla of Vater (probe). Part of the tumour, grey-white in colour, is visible in the cut surface of the head of the pancreas at the lower border of the specimen. The majority of pancreatic carcinomas arise in the larger ducts and about 70% of them are located in the head of the organ. By obstructing the pancreatic and bile ducts they tend to cause obstructive jaundice. **5.47** This tumour is in the tail of the organ, close to the splenic hilum (right), where it appears as an ill-defined grey-white lesion. The cut end of a pancreatic duct can be seen within the mass. The lack of surface architecture in the tumour contrasts markedly with the well-defined lobular pattern of the adjacent normal parenchyma. Tumours of the body and tail of pancreas have a poorer prognosis than those of the head, since they frequently do not produce early symptoms and dissemination has often occurred by the time they present clinically.
5.48 Histiocytic lymphoma (reticulum cell sarcoma): pancreas. Three ill-defined plaque-like nodules of histiocytic lymphoma are present. Lymphomas generally disseminate by the bloodstream in their terminal stages and widespread deposits are found in many viscera. The patient is usually an elderly man.

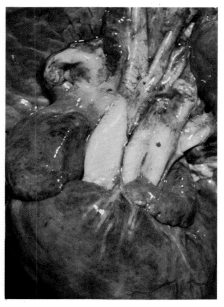

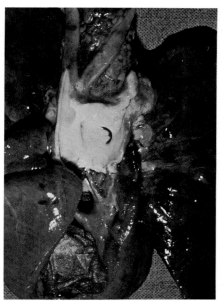

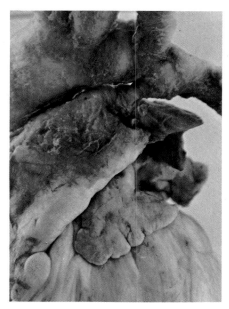

6.1 Transposition of great vessels:
    heart

6.2 Persistent truncus arteriosus

6.3 Persistent ductus arteriosus

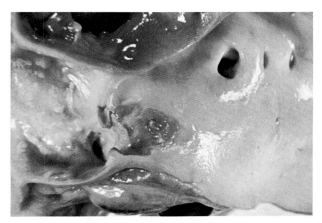

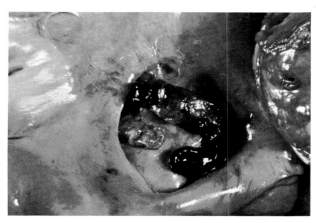

6.4 Coarctation: aorta

6.5 Paradoxical embolus: heart

6.1 Transposition of great vessels: heart. In this condition, the aorta arises from the right ventricle and the pulmonary trunk from the left ventricle. Other defects are often present, including atrial, ventricular and ductal shunts. In this example the right atrium is enlarged and dilated, and the aorta arises from a hypertrophied right ventricle and the pulmonary trunk from a hypertrophied left ventricle. **6.2 Persistent truncus arteriosus.** The heart has been opened to display the right ventricle. A common truncus arises from the junction of the left and right ventricles giving origin to the main systemic arteries and pulmonary arteries. A ventricular septal defect is also present (centre). **6.3 Persistent ductus arteriosus.** This shows the aortic arch (top) and pulmonary trunk. A short thick ductus arteriosus joins the aorta and left pulmonary artery. It was patent. In the patent ductus arteriosus complex, there is a left-to-right shunt at the level of the ductus, with increased blood flow in the pulmonary artery and increase in volume in the left side of the heart. Any ductus arteriosus which is patent after three months of age is abnormal. **6.4 Coarctation: aorta.** The usual site for a coarctation (a region of stenosis) is the isthmus; that is, the segment of aorta between the origin of the left subclavian artery and the ligamentum arteriosum. There are three types of coarctation: fetal, transitional, and adult (constrictive). This is an example of the adult type. The ascending aorta is on the left, and at the isthmus the aorta is considerably narrowed by a constrictive fold. Immediately beyond the coarctation there is a small red-brown mural thrombus (centre) on the descending aorta. The origin of the subclavian artery (upper right) is also visible. **6.5 Paradoxical embolus: heart.** A paradoxical embolus is one which arises in the venous circulation but enters the arterial side through an arteriovenous communication such as a patent foramen ovale

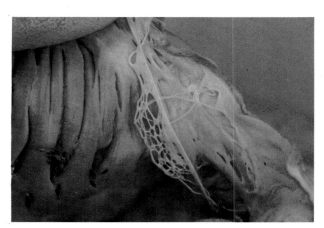

6.6 Chiari network: heart

or septal defect. This close-up view of the left atrium shows a patent fossa ovalis. Lying within the fossa and projecting into the left atrium is a coiled embolus which has come from a systemic vein. **6.6 Chiari network: heart.** A Chiari network is an irregular muscular reticulum within the auricle of the right atrium which represents the vestigial remnant of a valve formed during the embryological development of the heart. In this case it takes the form of a fine grey-white fenestrated network within the right atrium.

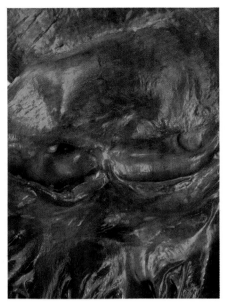

6.7 Bicuspid aortic valve: heart

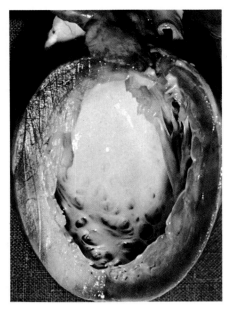

6.8 Endocardial fibroelastosis: heart

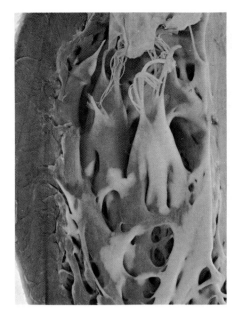

6.9 Idiopathic endocardial fibrosis: heart

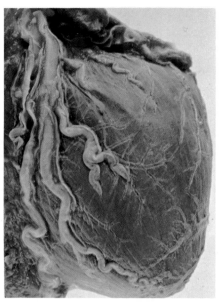

6.10 Brown atrophy: heart

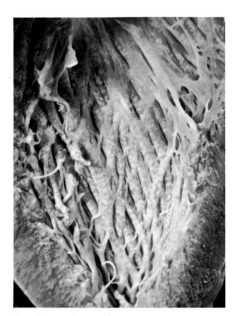

6.11 Fatty change: heart

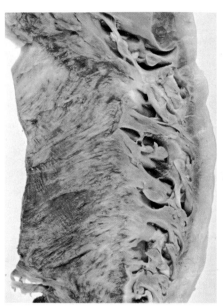

6.12 Fibrosis of myocardium

6.7 Bicuspid aortic valve: heart. The outflow tract of the left ventricle is opened to show a bicuspid aortic valve. This was a congenital lesion and an adult type of aortic coarctation was also present. The patient died from a dissecting aneurysm of the proximal aortic arch which was probably related to the hypertension caused by the constrictive effect of the coarctation. Congenital bicuspid aortic valve is a rare anomaly. **6.8 Endocardial fibroelastosis: heart.** This is the heart of a neonate. The endocardial surface of the left ventricle is covered with a layer of pearly grey-white tissue which histology showed to consist of collagen and elastic tissue. The wall of the ventricle is hypertrophied. This is the primary type of fibroelastosis, a disease of obscure origin which predominantly occurs in infants and children. The left ventricle is the chamber most frequently affected and in about 50% of cases there is valvular involvement. **6.9 Idiopathic endocardial fibrosis: heart.** At necropsy the heart was markedly dilated and hypertrophied. Irregular white patches are present on the endocardial surface of the left ventricle, including the trabeculae carneae and papillary muscles. Histologically the patches are areas of fibrosis confined to the endocardium, the myocardium being normal. The patient, a 67-year-old man, developed progressive cardiac failure with a markedly dilated heart for which no cause could be found clinically. **6.10 Brown atrophy: heart.** At necropsy the heart was small and atrophic. This shows the anterior surface of the left ventricle. There is a striking absence of epicardial fat and the colour is mahogany-brown. The colour is due to accumulation of a granular yellow-brown pigment (lipofuscin) within the muscle fibres. The branches of the left coronary artery are tortuous as a result of the shrinkage of the underlying myocardium. Brown atrophy is seen in the elderly, in patients with cancer and chronic wasting diseases, and in endocrine disorders such as Addison's disease and Simmond's disease. **6.11 Fatty change: heart.** The subendocardial muscle of the trabeculae carneae and papillary muscles of the left ventricle shows a patchy mottling, irregular yellow streaks and lines alternating with unaffected muscle to produce a 'tigroid', 'tabby-cat' or 'thrush-breast' pattern. This appearance is caused by patchy fatty change, in which lipid droplets collect within the myocardial fibres. Fatty change of this type is characteristic of anaemia and this patient had pernicious anaemia. There is a diffuse form which is usually found in severe infections and toxic states. **6.12 Fibrosis of myocardium.** This section through the wall of the left ventricle shows the presence of a considerable amount of greyish fibrous tissue. The fibrosis is diffuse and has resulted from chronic ischaemia of the myocardium, secondary to atherosclerotic narrowing of the coronary arteries. Diffuse fibrosis is often encountered in patients with a history of repeated anginal attacks or who have died suddenly from myocardial insufficiency without gross infarction. However in the present instance the patient, a 56-year-old man, did have a recent apical myocardial infarct, part of which is visible as a haemorrhagic area at the lower border.

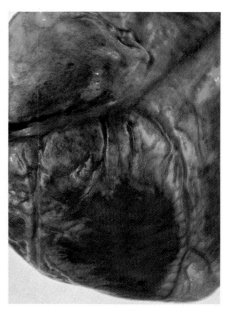

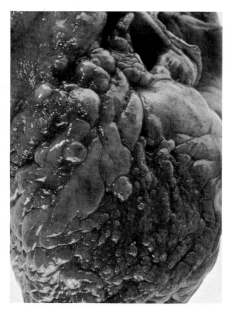

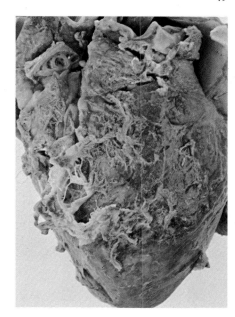

6.13 Petechial haemorrhages: heart   6.14 Sarcoidosis: heart   6.15 Uraemic pericarditis: heart

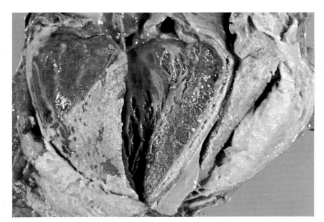

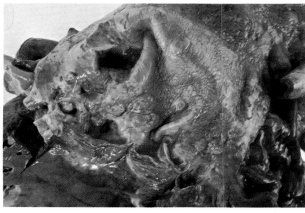

6.16 Acute suppurative pericarditis: heart   6.17 Syphilitic aortitis: heart and aorta

6.13 Petechial haemorrhages: heart. There are multiple small petechial haemorrhages in the epicardium, particularly noticeable in the fat. Petechiae and mucosal haemorrhages were present in other organs. The patient had aplastic anaemia, with reduced numbers of platelets in the blood. **6.14 Sarcoidosis: heart.** Small grey-white nodules cover much of the epicardium and epicardial fat. Histologically these were granulomas consisting of epithelioid cells and multinucleated giant cells. Myocardial involvement and subsequent fibrosis of the lesions may cause conduction defects, cardiac failure and sudden death. **6.15 Uraemic pericarditis: heart.** The epicardial surface is covered with grey-white strands of fibrin some of which appear contracted and white as a result of organisation. Uraemic pericarditis is a sterile form of pericarditis which is characteristically 'dry' and lacking a serous component. **6.16 Acute suppurative pericarditis: heart.** Purulent pericarditis is caused by pyogenic organisms such as staphylococci and streptococci. The parietal and visceral pericardium is covered with a yellowish-green purulent exudate. The exudate does not usually undergo complete resorption, and organisation may result in fibrosis and calcification and adhesive pericarditis. The organism in this case was the pneumococcus. **6.17 Syphilitic aortitis: heart and aorta.** The aorta is dilated and the wall looks wrinkled ('tree-bark') from the presence of longitudinal furrows and depressions interspersed with raised greyish-white fibrous plaques. The orifice of a saccular aneurysm is present in the ascending aorta. The aortic valve is incompetent, the valve ring is dilated, the cusps are thickened and rolled, and the commissures are widened. One coronary ostium is patent (left) but the other is stenosed. Aortitis, aortic valve disease and aneurysm formation are the major manifestations of

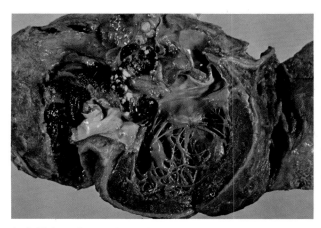

6.18 Tuberculous pericarditis: heart

cardiovascular syphilis. **6.18 Tuberculous pericarditis: heart.** The left ventricle and left atrium are displayed. The left ventricle is hypertrophied. The parietal and visceral pericardium is covered with a thick shaggy exudate of fibrin which is being organised and shows a tendency to form ridges (upper right). The adjacent mediastinal lymph nodes are caseous. The pericardial sac tends to become thick and leathery as a result of reparative fibrosis, and calcification occurs in the later stages. Chronic constrictive pericarditis may develop.

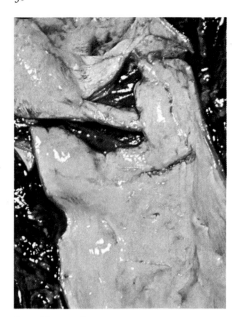

6.19 Traumatic rupture: aorta

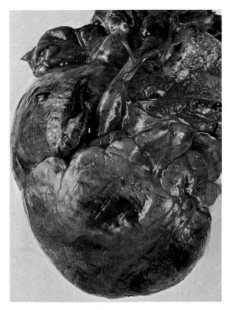

6.20 Idiopathic cardiomyopathy: heart

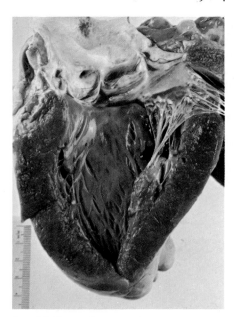

6.21 Malignant hypertension: heart

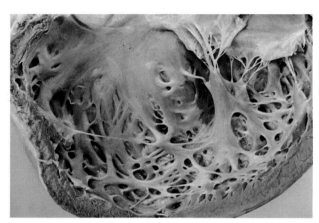

6.22 Fibroelastosis and mural thrombus: heart

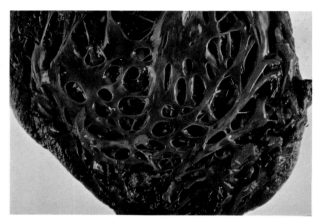

6.23 Viral myocarditis: heart

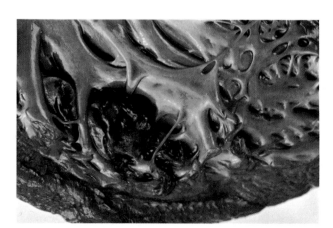

6.24 Mural thrombus: heart

6.19 Traumatic rupture: aorta. This shows the descending thoracic aorta. Several deep irregular transverse tears are present (top). This type of lesion is commonly found in cases of traumatic injury, especially motor and aviation accidents where sudden deceleration causes tearing of the aorta with subsequent rupture and haemothorax. **6.20 Idiopathic cardiomyopathy: heart.** Idiopathic cardiomyopathy occurs in children and young adults and they present with signs of intractable heart failure. The average weight of the heart is about 600 g. Mural thrombi are frequently present. This shows the anterior aspect of such a heart. It is very large and globular in shape. Although there is enlargement of all chambers, the right atrium and right ventricle appear to be most severely affected. **6.21 Malignant hypertension: heart.** The left ventricle is markedly hypertrophied, the wall measuring 2.2 cm in thickness, but its capacity is not increased (concentric hypertrophy). The trabeculae carneae are prominent. There is a close correlation between the severity of the hypertension and heart weight: the average weight is about 600 g but weights up to 1000 g are not uncommon. This patient died from an intracerebral haemorrhage. **6.22 Fibroelastosis and mural thrombus: heart.** The left ventricle is greatly dilated and greyish-white fibroelastic tissue covers the endocardial surface, including that of the papillary muscles of the mitral valve. A few small pale thrombi are visible in the crevices between the trabeculae below the left ventricular outflow tract (centre). It is probable that some cases of this type are adult examples of primary endocardial fibroelastosis of infancy (see 6.8). Mural thrombus formation is common in the adult but rare in the infantile and childhood cases. **6.23 Viral myocarditis: heart.** The ventricle is dilated, flabby-looking and minimally hypertrophied. The muscle is red-brown and haemorrhagic, the haemorrhagic mottling being well seen over the trabeculae carneae (upper centre). Small portions of mural thrombi are present. Inflammation in true viral myocarditis is restricted to the muscular layer of the heart. **6.24 Mural thrombus: heart.** This is the apex of the left ventricle. It is greatly hypertrophied and dilated and the trabeculae carneae are widened and hypertrophied. Red-brown mural thrombus is attached to the endocardium. There is no associated fibroelastosis. The cut surface of the myocardium is pale. The patient had idiopathic cardiomyopathy and the heart weighed 615 g.

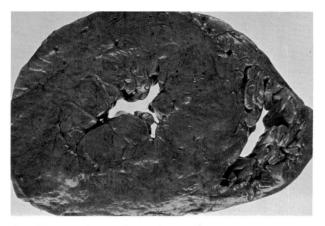

6.25 Hypertensive cardiomegaly

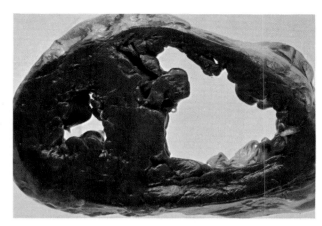

6.26 Biventricular hypertrophy: heart

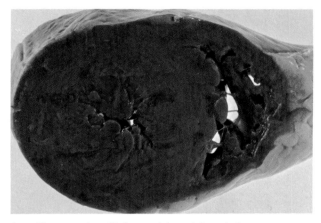

6.27 Hypertrophy of left ventricle and fungal abscess: heart

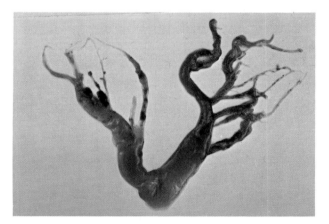

6.28 Post-mortem clot

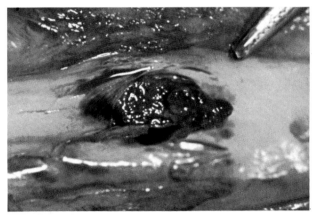

6.29 Thrombosis: femoral vein

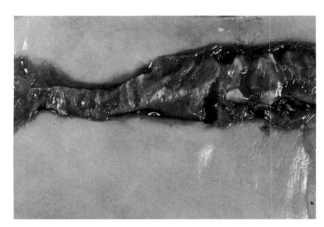

6.30 Thrombosis: inferior vena cava

6.25 Hypertensive cardiomegaly. Hypertrophy is characterised by an increase in mass of the myocardium, leading to increase in the weight of the heart and thickening of the walls of the affected chambers. Enlargement of the heart is an important sign of cardiac disease. In this case longstanding systemic hypertension has caused massive concentric hypertrophy of the muscle of the ventricle and septum (left). The right ventricle (right) shows secondary hypertrophy. The lumen of both ventricles appears smaller than normal. **6.26 Biventricular hypertrophy: heart.** This coronal section of the heart shows hypertrophy of the left and right ventricles. The right ventricle (right) is also dilated. The patient, a chronic bronchitic, died in congestive cardiac failure. No cause for the left ventricular hypertrophy was ascertained. **6.27 Hypertrophy of left ventricle and fungal abscess: heart.** This coronal section of the heart shows pronounced concentric hypertrophy of the left ventricle and to a lesser degree of the right ventricle. The small haemorrhagic area within the interventricular septum was found on microscopy to be a monilial abscess. **6.28 Post-mortem clot.** At necropsy it is important to distinguish between a thrombus and a post-mortem clot, and this shows some of the characteristics of the latter. It is a glistening semi-translucent, homogeneous pale yellow (chicken-fat) clot which formed a cast of the pulmonary trunk and its branches. Post-mortem clot may also appear deep red (red-currant jelly clot). Post-mortem clot does not adhere to the endothelial lining of the blood vessel and the lines of Zahn are absent. In contrast a thrombus tends to be dry, friable, mottled, greyish-white or red, and adherent to the endothelium. **6.29 Thrombosis: femoral vein.** This is a segment of the common femoral vein. An orifice of a tributary vein is visible (right). A pale brown thrombus is attached to a valve and fills the pocket behind the cusp. Formation of thrombus in veins often starts in this way, at points in the vessel where side-branches or valves produce turbulence and eddy currents which facilitate deposition of platelets on the endothelium and thus initiate thrombosis. **6.30 Thrombosis: inferior vena cava.** The inferior vena cava contains a long pale tapering thrombus which is attached firmly to the wall (mural or parietal thrombus) but does not occlude the lumen. Thrombi may be classified as red, white or mixed. The thrombus shown here is mixed, with alternating pale grey and pink areas, and the lines of Zahn can be seen (centre right) as distinct linear surface markings.

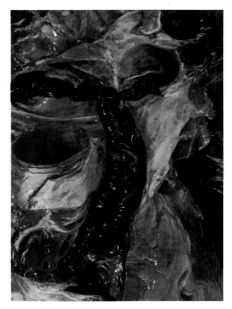

6.31 Pulmonary embolism

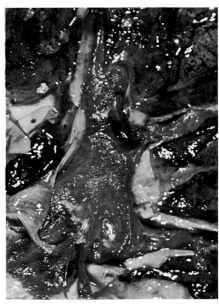

6.32 Thrombosis: pulmonary artery

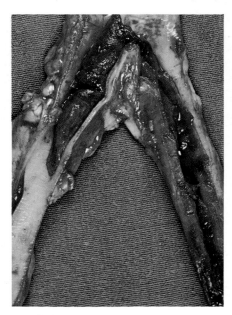

6.33 Saddle embolus: aorta

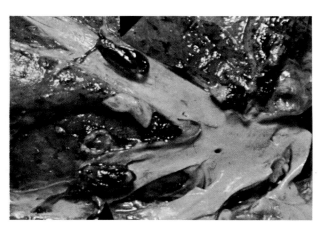

6.34 Recurrent pulmonary embolism

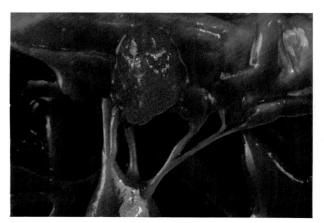

6.35 Lambl's excrescence: tricuspid valve

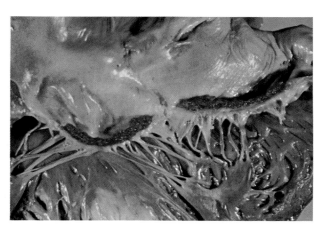

6.36 Terminal (abacterial) endocarditis: mitral valve

embolus of comparable size (6.31). Being of arterial origin the thrombus is drier, paler and more granular than a venous thrombus. This patient had a carcinoma of the common bile duct and an association between visceral carcinoma and an increased incidence of arterial and venous thrombi is well-recognised. **6.33 Saddle embolus: aorta.** A large brown embolus lies across the aortic bifurcation (saddle embolus) and thrombus extends into both common iliac arteries. The thrombus in the iliac artery (left) has completely occluded the vessel and red (propagating) thrombus has formed beyond the obstruction. The embolus probably originated in a thrombus on an atherosclerotic plaque in the abdominal aorta. The patient developed gangrene of both feet. **6.34 Recurrent pulmonary embolism.** The secondary branches of a pulmonary artery have been opened to reveal two small emboli wedged within the vessels. Both have tapering distal extensions. Minor recurrent embolic episodes are common in patients in hospital, and in massive fatal embolism it is usual to find several smaller emboli which preceded the final fatal episode but were not detected clinically. **6.35 Lambl's excrescence: tricuspid valve.** A globular red mass is attached to the free border of the valve cusp and projects onto the superior surface. This is a giant form of Lambl's excrescence. Small Lambl's excrescences are fairly common and are thought to result from repeated minor trauma during closure of the valve cusps. **6.36 Terminal (abacterial) endocarditis: mitral valve.** Conglomerate vegetations are present on the line of closure of both valve cusps. Vegetations of this type tend to occur on thickened or scarred valves such as those of healed rheumatic valvulitis, and the aortic cusp of the mitral valve (left) and adjacent chordae tendineae are thickened. It is not clear why the vegetations form but they frequently occur in patients with malignant disease and disseminated intravascular coagulation.

6.31 Pulmonary embolism. The right ventricle and pulmonary trunk are opened to display the bifurcation and first parts of the left and right pulmonary arteries. A large coiled-up embolus lies within the right ventricular outflow tract, filling the pulmonary trunk and straddling the bifurcation, with extension into both pulmonary arteries (saddle embolus). The embolus contains pale grey and dark red thrombus areas and its shape and size differ from the configuration of the pulmonary trunk. Massive pulmonary embolism as depicted here produces sudden death. **6.32 Thrombosis: pulmonary artery.** Thrombosis of the pulmonary artery is a rare event. Thrombus fills the main pulmonary artery and its branches and forms a cast of the lumen, in contrast to an

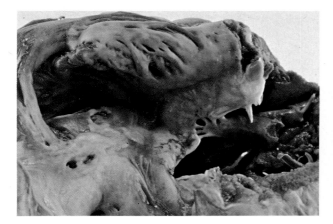

6.37 Carcinoid heart disease: tricuspid valve

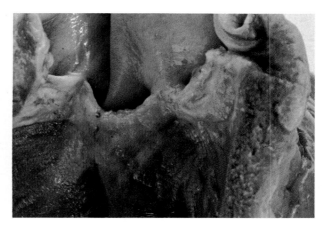

6.38 Carcinoid heart disease

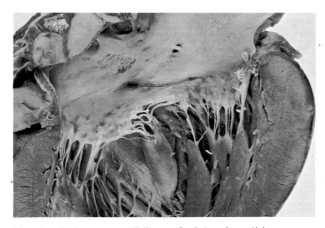

6.39 Atypical verrucous (Libman-Sacks) endocarditis: mitral valve

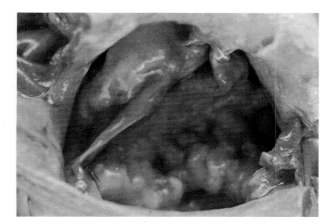

6.40 Calcific stenosis: aortic valve

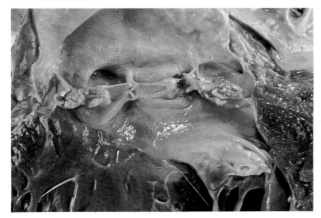

6.41 Chronic rheumatic endocarditis: aortic valve

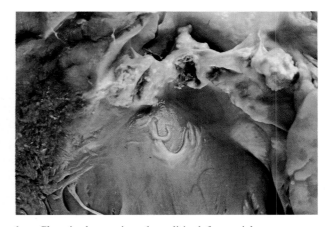

6.42 Chronic rheumatic endocarditis: left ventricle

6.37 and 6.38 Carcinoid heart disease. In most cases of carcinoid disease, the distinctive lesions are limited to the right side of the heart. **6.37** This shows stenosis of the tricuspid valve. The cusps are irregularly contracted and thickened and the chordae (right of centre) are shortened. The greyish-white fibrous tissue extends over the superior surface of the valve to involve the right atrial wall which is thickened and yellowish-grey. The fibrous tissue which forms on the endocardium in this condition is devoid of elastic tissue. **6.38** The right ventricle, pulmonary valve and first part of the pulmonary trunk are shown. The ventricle is hypertrophied, and there is distortion and stenosis of the pulmonary valve due to irregular fibrous contracture of the cusps. The margins of the cusps are rolled and the commissures fused. **6.39 Atypical verrucous (Libman-Sacks) endocarditis: mitral valve.** The superior surface of the mitral valve is covered with flat tawny-grey vegetations typically small though somewhat larger than those found in acute rheumatic endocarditis. They are not confined to the line of closure of the valves and the acute inflammatory process has spread over the surface of the valve to involve its base (right). The chordae are normal. Libman-Sacks endocarditis is a manifestation of systemic lupus erythematosus, being found in about 50% of cases. The patient was a 22-year-old woman. **6.40 Calcific stenosis: aortic valve.** This shows the superior surface of the aortic valve, viewed from the first part of the ascending aorta. The

three cusps are thickened and nodular due to fibrosis and calcification. The commissures are fused and the free margins of the valve roughened. The orifice is reduced to a slit-like orifice. Nodular calcific aortic stenosis occurs predominantly in middle-aged men. Some cases are considered to be 'rheumatic' but the condition in the majority of cases is probably 'degenerative', especially when it is an isolated lesion. **6.41 to 6.44 Chronic rheumatic endocarditis. 6.41** This shows the aortic valve. Healing following acute rheumatic valvulitis has resulted in fibrosis with varying degrees of distortion of the valve leaflets. The commissures are fused and the anterior and right posterior cusps (left) show irregular fibrous thickenings at the valve nodule and lunulae. The left posterior cusp (centre) is less affected. The anterior cusp of the mitral valve is thickened and the chordae contracted and stouter (right). The left ventricle is hypertrophied and dilated, and the endocardial surface of the outflow tract is thickened and greyish-white. **6.42** The aortic valve cusps are greatly thickened, calcified and ulcerated, producing a stenotic and incompetent valve. The degree of commissural fusion is extreme. Two crescentic bands of fibrous tissue are situated beneath the valve, on the endocardium of the dilated and hypertrophied left ventricle. These are the endocardial pockets of Zahn and their openings are directed towards the aortic orifice. They are formed by regurgitant jets of blood impinging onto the left ventricular wall as a result of the valve's incompetence.

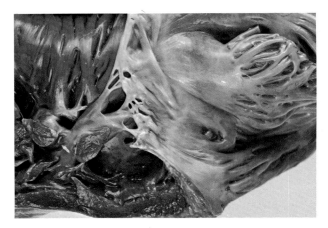

6.43 Chronic rheumatic endocarditis: tricuspid valve

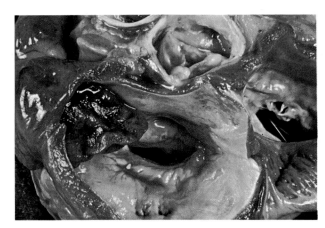

6.44 Chronic rheumatic endocarditis: left and right atria

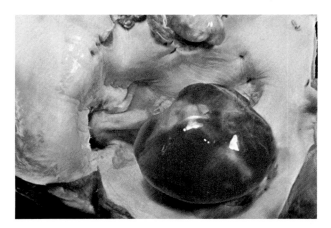

6.45 Ball thrombus: left atrium

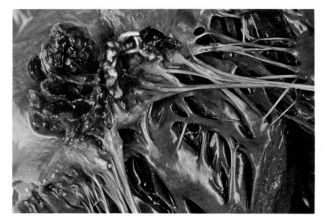

6.46 Subacute bacterial endocarditis: mitral valve

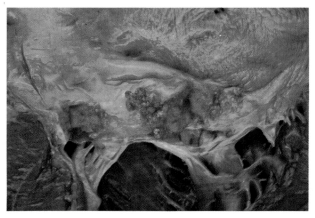

6.47 Subacute bacterial endocarditis: mitral valve

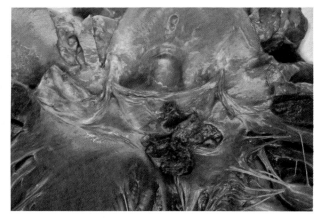

6.48 Acute bacterial endocarditis: aortic valve

6.43 and 6.44 Chronic rheumatic endocarditis. 6.43 This shows the tricuspid valve. There is stenosing fibrosis and fenestration (centre), and the chordae are thickened and shortened, with approximation of the margin of the valve cusp and papillary muscle. The right atrium is dilated and thick-walled. Its endocardial surface is greyish-white and the pectinate muscles hypertrophied (top right). The right ventricle is hypertrophied and the trabeculae (top left) are prominent. Tricuspid stenosis is almost always rheumatic in origin and the patient also had mitral stenosis. **6.44** This is a view from above of both atria, the mitral valve (lower left), tricuspid valve (right), and aortic valve (top centre). The left atrium is aneurysmally dilated and the wall is thickened and pearly-grey in colour. Polypoid thrombus (centre left) protrudes from the left atrial appendage. The mitral valve cusps show severe nodular thickening, with a narrow central opening. The tricuspid valve is also stenotic, but the aortic valve shows the most advanced changes. The patient had atrial fibrillation, in which thrombus frequently forms in the left atrium. **6.45 Ball thrombus: left atrium.** The dilated left atrium is viewed from above. The wall is thickened and greyish-white. The underlying mitral valve orifice is stenosed. A globular red thrombus ('ball' thrombus) lies free within the atrial lumen. This type of thrombus arises from a pedunculated mural thrombus which becomes detached from the wall of the atrium. A ball thrombus is sometimes found in association with mitral stenosis. It tends to obstruct the mitral valve

orifice intermittently. **6.46 and 6.47 Subacute bacterial endocarditis. 6.46** This shows a large, globular, friable red-brown mass of vegetations on the superior surface of the mitral valve. The chordae are thicker and show minimal fusion. *Streptococcus viridans* was grown on blood culture. Subacute bacterial endocarditis is caused by low-virulence microorganisms and it is characterised by a milder course and longer duration (endocarditis lenta) than the acute form. In the majority of cases the causative organism is *Streptococcus viridans*. Common predisposing factors are transient episodes of bacteraemia and underlying heart disease. **6.47** Recurrent bouts of rheumatic endocarditis have caused severe mitral stenosis. The valve cusps are wrinkled and greatly thickened, with fusion and contraction of the chordae. The fibrosis extends into the papillary muscles. Infective endocarditis has developed in the damaged valve cusps and the surface of the cusps is covered with bulky red-brown vegetations. The left atrial wall is wrinkled, with diffuse grey-white fibrosis. **6.48 Acute bacterial endocarditis: aortic valve.** The valve is bicuspid, a congenital defect. A large globular vegetation is present. The vegetations in acute bacterial endocarditis are smooth and often ulcerated, and in this example there is necrosis of the cusp with suppuration and perforation. The vegetations are friable and liable to release embolic fragments. The causative organism is generally virulent and invasive, e.g. *Staphylococcus aureus,* and capable of producing the disease in a heart without a pre-existing valvular lesion.

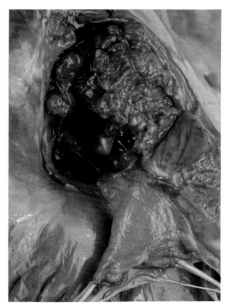

6.49 Fungal endocarditis

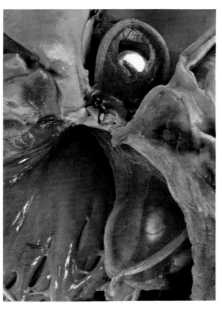

6.50 Starr-Edwards prostheses: aortic and mitral valves

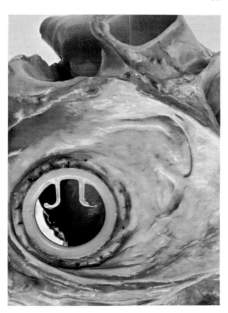

6.51 Abrams-Lucas prosthesis: mitral valve

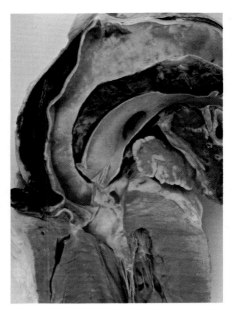

6.52 Dissecting aneurysm: aorta

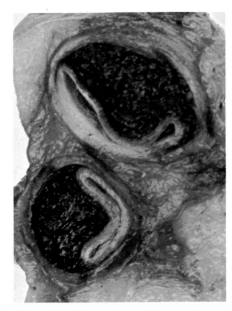

6.53 Dissecting aneurysm: iliac arteries

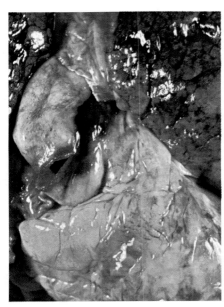

6.54 Dissecting aneurysm: heart and aorta

6.49 Fungal endocarditis. This shows the ventricular aspect of the aortic valve from a 62-year-old woman who had recently had an aortic valve displacement. A mass of pale brown vegetations (1 × 0.5 cm) with superimposed red thrombus virtually occludes the valve orifice. The aortic cusp of the mitral valve (bottom) is thick and fibrotic, evidence of chronic rheumatic endocarditis. *Aspergillus fumigatus* was cultured from the vegetations. Fungal endocarditis, previously rare, has recently increased as a result of widespread use of antibiotics, steroids and the advent of cardiac surgery. **6.50 Starr-Edwards prostheses: aortic and mitral valves.** Starr-Edwards prostheses have been inserted to replace mitral (bottom) and aortic (top) valves severely damaged by chronic rheumatic endocarditis. The valve cages are covered with a delicate pink fibrinous membrane. This membrane is seen frequently *post mortem* in these cases. Its significance and pathogenesis are obscure, and it is probably an agonal event. **6.51 Abrams-Lucas prosthesis: mitral valve.** An Abrams-Lucas prosthesis has been used to replace a stenosed and incompetent mitral valve. The hooks of the suspensory mechanism of the valve flap disengaged from the valve ring 6½ years after insertion through mechanical wear-and-tear, resulting in sudden death. **6.52 to 6.54 Dissecting aneurysm.** Dissecting aneurysm is produced by

haemorrhage into the media of a vessel and in about 75% of cases the lesion starts in the ascending aorta a few cm above the aortic valve. Degeneration of the media, often mucoid in nature, predisposes to the condition. Men are affected twice as often as women and most cases occur in patients between 40 and 60 years of age. **6.52** The wall of the ascending aorta and arch of the aorta has been split and contains a mass of dark blood clot. There is pronounced concentric hypertrophy of the left ventricle, evidence of the systemic hypertension which had been present for many years and which was an important predisposing factor. **6.53** This is a transverse section of the internal and external iliac arteries. It shows more or less complete obliteration of the lumen of each vessel by the blood within the media, the blood having tracked down the aorta from the aortic arch. **6.54** The external aspect of the heart, great vessels and parts of the lungs is shown. A transverse tear is present in the ascending aorta (left of centre). This tear, the margins of which are blood-stained, was the point at which a dissecting aneurysm of aorta ruptured into the pericardial sac to cause death by cardiac tamponade. In about 50% of cases of dissecting aneurysm the terminal event is haemorrhage of this type.

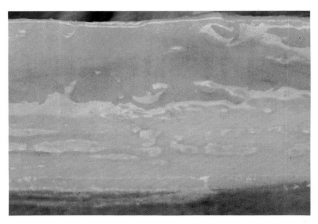

6.55 Fatty streaks: carotid artery

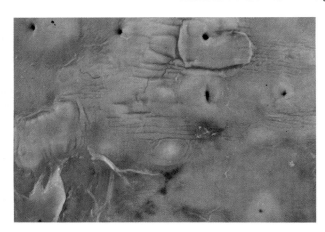

6.56 Atherosclerosis: aorta

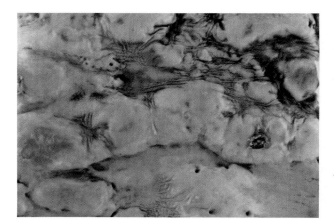

6.57 Atherosclerosis: aorta

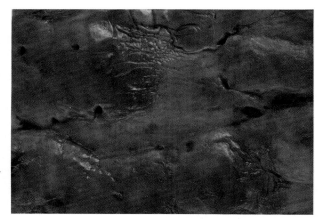

6.58 Atherosclerosis: aorta

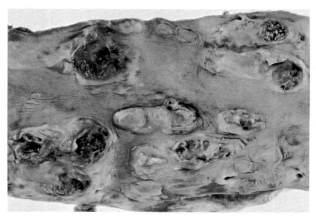

6.59 Atherosclerosis: aorta

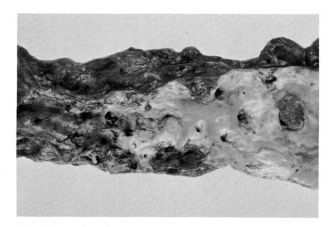

6.60 Atherosclerosis: aorta

6.55 to 6.61 Atherosclerosis. 6.55 These are fatty streaks—linear lesions in the intima. They run longitudinally, and histologically they consist of lipid, intracellular and extracellular. Fatty streaks, which are not infrequently found in young subjects and even in infants, have a haphazard distribution but show a predilection for sites which in later life tend to be affected by atherosclerosis. Few are believed to progress to form elevated permanent plaques. **6.56** This shows fibrous plaques in the aorta. Flat greyish-white fibrous plaques are present in relation to the openings of intercostal arteries. The adjacent intima is wrinkled. Histologically the plaques consist of collagen and elastic tissue and a central core of amorphous material. Plaques begin to appear in the aorta after the third decade and are probably permanent. Some may be derived from lipid streaks. **6.57** These are complicated plaques in the aorta. As the atherosclerotic process advances, it is probable that the fibrous plaques develop into large complicated plaques which tend to be orientated along the vessel. There is abundant fat within complicated plaques, as confirmed by the yellow colour of the lesions shown here. The

plaques tend to ulcerate, as seen in one area (right). **6.58** The aorta has been immersed in Sudan stain to demonstrate the lipid content of the plaques. The bright red staining of the lipid-rich raised fibrous and complicated plaques contrasts with the unstained intervening intima. **6.59** This illustrates a later stage of the development of the atherosclerotic process in the aorta. Most of the plaques show central ulceration, and the yellow fatty debris of complicated lesions is seen in the plaque at the top right. The brown colour of the ulcerated plaques on the left is due to old episodes of intimal haemorrhage and thrombosis. The mural thrombi that form on the roughened surface of ulcerated plaques are an important source of emboli. **6.60** In the aorta, atherosclerosis tends to be most severe on the posterior wall of the distal abdominal aorta. This shows the abdominal aorta down to the iliac bifurcation (left). The infrarenal segment of aorta (centre to left margin) is dilated and the intima appears grey-white because of massive dystrophic calcification. The orifice of the coeliac artery is occluded by a pale red-coloured thrombus (right) which had formed on an atherosclerotic lesion at that point.

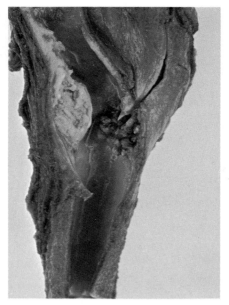

6.61 Atherosclerosis: carotid arteries

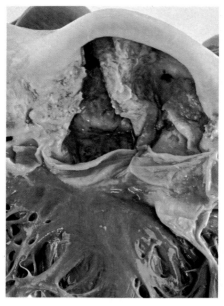

6.62 Aneurysm: sinuses of Valsalva

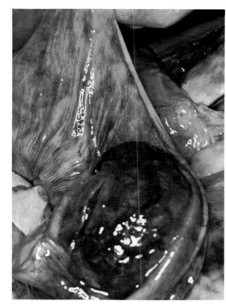

6.63 'False' aneurysm

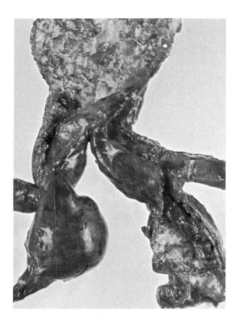

6.64 Aneurysm: iliac arteries

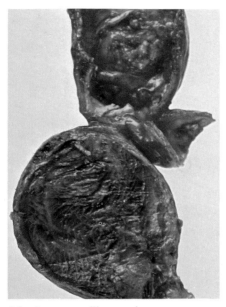

6.65 Aneurysm: iliac arteries

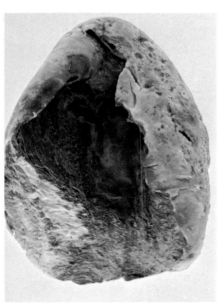

6.66 Thrombus from aneurysm

6.61 Atherosclerosis. Atherosclerosis is commonly found in the region of the carotid sinus. This shows part of the right common carotid artery (bottom centre), the carotid sinus (centre) and the internal carotid artery (top left). A yellow-white calcified plaque at the origin of the internal carotid artery is causing marked stenosis of the lumen. Opposite the plaque, at the origin of the external carotid artery, there is a small irregular brown mass of mural thrombus. **6.62 to 6.66 Aneurysm.** An aneurysm is an abnormal circumscribed dilatation of an artery due to structural weakening. **6.62** This shows aneurysmal dilatation of the aortic sinuses of Valsalva. The intimal surface of the aortic arch is greyish-white and roughened. The aortic cusps are normal, but the aortic valve ring is dilated and the patient had aortic incompetence. About 80% of aortic arch aneurysms are syphilitic and most are saccular. However the progressive dilatation of the arch found in syphilitic aortitis very rarely causes aneurysms of the sinuses of Valsalva and in this case the pathogenesis was considered to be atherosclerotic. **6.63** This is a 'false' aneurysm, which is essentially an encapsulated perivascular haematoma that retains its communication with the arterial lumen. A loop of terminal ileum has been opened to reveal a haemorrhagic mass bulging into the lumen. A fatal haemorrhage from the aneurysm into the

ileum occurred through the small slit-like hole visible on the surface of the mass. An atherosclerotic aneurysm of the abdominal aorta had been resected some days previously, but post-operative bleeding had resulted in a false aneurysm around the vascular prosthesis. **6.64 and 6.65** In the following instance the lesion developed as a consequence of weakening of the arterial wall by atherosclerosis. **6.64** The aorta (top) shows extensive ulcerative atherosclerosis. Both common iliac arteries are dilated and the left internal iliac artery (right) contains a mural thrombus attached to underlying atherosclerotic plaques. The right common iliac (left) is dilated and the first part of the internal iliac artery is expanded into a saccular aneurysm with a smooth outline. **6.65** The saccular aneurysm involves the left common and external iliac arteries. The aneurysm sac is filled with antemortem thrombus, the cut surface of which is reddish-brown and shows the grey-white striations of Zahn. Atherosclerotic aneurysms most commonly occur in the lower abdominal aorta and these may extend into the iliac arteries. **6.66** This shows a large mass (measuring 20 × 12 × 12 cm) of thrombus removed from an atherosclerotic aneurysm of aorta. The laminated structure of the thrombus is clearly evident (lower left). A large central channel through which the blood continued to flow can also be seen.

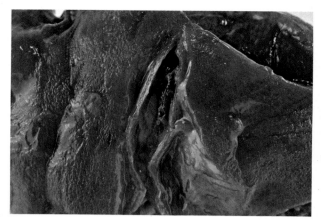

6.67 Coronary artery: thrombosis

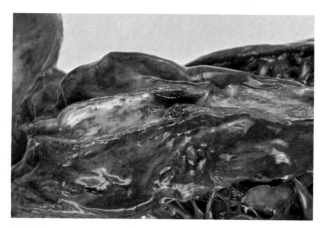

6.68 Coronary artery: atherosclerosis

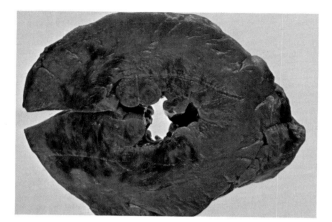

6.69 Infarct of myocardium

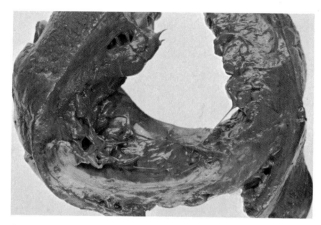

6.70 Infarct of myocardium

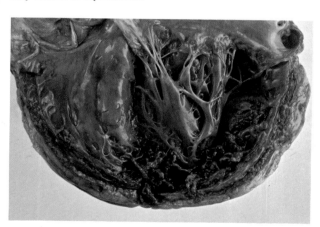

6.71 Infarct of myocardium

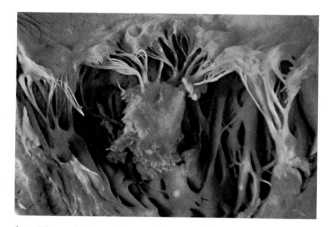

6.72 Myomalacia cordis: papillary muscle

6.67-6.72 Coronary occlusion and myocardial infarction. In some cases of myocardial infarction, a coronary artery or one of its major branches is occluded by thrombus, generally in association with atherosclerosis, although occasionally haemorrhage into an atherosclerotic plaque appears to be the cause. **6.67** The epicardial surface of the left ventricle is covered with a granular fibrinous exudate. The left anterior descending coronary artery contains a recent thrombus (above left of centre) and the vessel distal to the thrombus (below the thrombus) is narrowed by atherosclerosis. The patient had a recent extensive infarct of the anterior part of the interventricular septum. **6.68** The right coronary artery (top) is widely patent but a calcified atherosclerotic plaque has produced a stenosed segment (top centre). Stenosis has been greatly increased by haemorrhage into the plaque, which accordingly is red in colour. Haemorrhage into a plaque is an important cause of coronary occlusion, even in the absence of thrombus formation on the plaque. **6.69** This is a coronal section through the left ventricle and interventricular septum (right) close to the apex. A massive recent infarct is present in the posterolateral wall of the left ventricle. The infarcted muscle appears haemorrhagic. Myocardial infarcts generally develop this blotchy red appearance 2 or 3 days after the onset. **6.70** This coronal section shows a yellow-white infarct of the anterior part of the interventricular septum (bottom). It takes 6 to 8 days for a myocardial

infarct to develop the colour evident here. Between the 8th and 10th days a reddish-purple zone appears at the periphery of the necrotic muscle, and such a zone is just visible (lower left) around this lesion. The patient a woman of 44, sustained a clinical infarct 8 days before her death. **6.71** The heart has been opened to display the left ventricle. There is an extensive recent full-thickness antero-septal infarct of the myocardium which involves the endocardial surface. Greyish-brown mural thrombus has formed over the infarcted area. This type of mural thrombus is an important source of systemic emboli. **6.72-6.74 Myomalacia cordis.** An infarct of myocardium sometimes undergoes marked softening and ruptures to produce haemopericardium, cardiac tamponade and sudden death. This complication occurs most frequently 10 to 14 days after the onset of the lesion, and rupture is more likely in hypertensive subjects than in normotensive or shocked patients. The majority of cases involve the anterior wall of the left ventricle. It is estimated to be the cause of death in 8 to 20% of cases of myocardial infarction. **6.72** This shows the superior papillary muscle of the left ventricle and mitral valve. Part of the muscle has undergone infarction and the necrotic part has ruptured. Rupture of the papillary muscle is a rare complication of infarction affecting the left ventricle. It leads to mitral insufficiency from failure of anchorage of the valve during ventricular systole and is usually rapidly fatal.

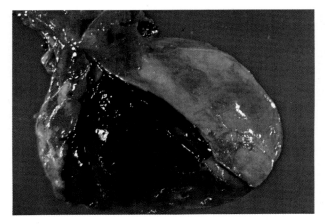

6.73 Myomalacia cordis

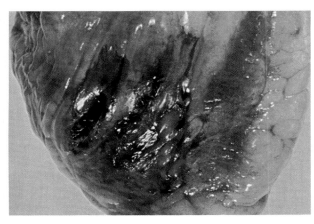

6.74 Myomalacia cordis

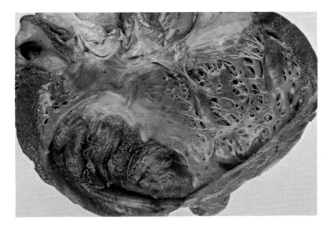

6.75 Aneurysm of the left ventricle

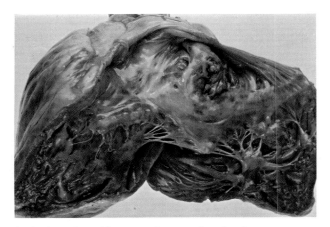

6.76 Disseminated intravascular coagulopathy: heart

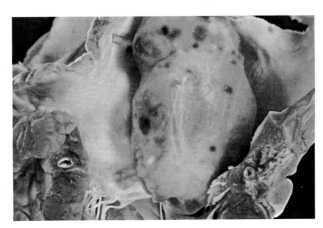

6.77 Myxoma: atrium

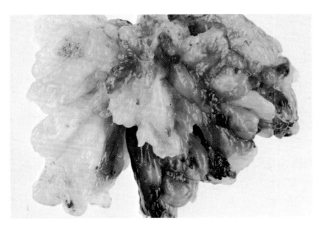

6.78 Myxoma: atrium

6.73 and 6.74 Myomalacia cordis. 6.73 The pericardial sac is partly reflected to reveal a large haematoma distending the sac (haemopericardium), the patient having died from cardiac tamponade. The blood came from a ruptured infarct of the anterior wall of the left ventricle. **6.74** This is the heart shown in 6.73. The source of haemorrhage is two slit-like tears in the heart wall over the infarct. The epicardial fat adjacent to the tears appears red and bruised. **6.75 Aneurysm of the left ventricle.** There is a large thin-walled aneurysm at the apex of the left ventricle (below left). It contains laminated mural thrombus. The underlying lesion is a massive infarct of the septum which has become fibrosed. The fibrous tissue, which gives the septal wall above the aneurysm a greyish-white colour, has yielded to produce the aneurysmal sac. Aneurysms of the heart are most commonly located at the apex of the left ventricle. **6.76 Disseminated intravascular coagulopathy: heart.** The heart has been opened to display the interventricular septum (left) and the right atrium and right ventricle (right). Multiple small haemorrhagic areas are visible in the subendocardium of the ventricle

and atrium. They are well seen over the inferior papillary muscle of the tricuspid valve (centre). Histology showed these to be small infarcts, caused by microthrombi within the intramyocardial arterioles and capillaries. The patient had thrombotic thrombocytopenic purpura. **6.77 and 6.78 Myxoma: atrium.** The nature of this lesion is controversial. Some regard it as organised mural thrombus but others believe that it is a true neoplasm. It is the commonest primary intracardiac 'tumour', and about 75% occur in the left atrium near the fossa ovalis. **6.77** The atrium contains a large smooth ovoid gelatinous pale-yellow tumour, 10 cm long and 5 cm in diameter. The myxoma, the surface of which shows focal areas of haemorrhage, projects into the mitral valve orifice. The atrium is dilated and its wall shows endocardial fibrosis. A tumour of this size may intermittently obstruct the mitral valve orifice. **6.78** This is a pedunculated lobular villous myxoma. The surface is glistening and cream-coloured with pale brownish areas of haemorrhage. The tumour was located in the left atrium of a 16-year-old girl.

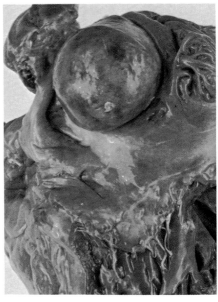

6.79 Secondary carcinoid tumour: heart

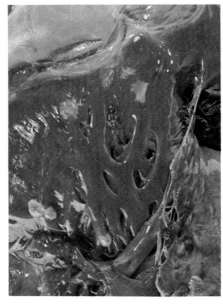

6.80 Secondary carcinoma: heart

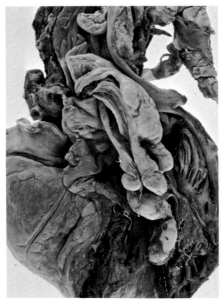

6.81 Secondary sarcoma: heart

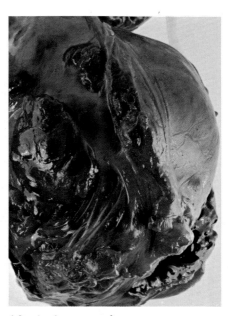

6.82 Angiosarcoma: heart

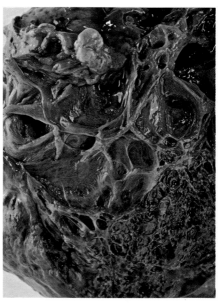

6.83 Haemangioma: retroperitoneum

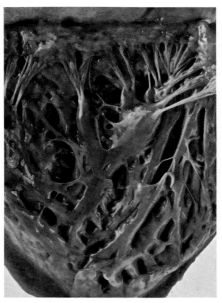

6.84 Leukaemic infiltration: heart

6.79 Secondary carcinoid tumour: heart. A large smooth round pink-brown tumour projects into the right atrium. The primary tumour was in a main bronchus and it had infiltrated the wall of the atrium directly from the lung. Malignant tumours in the heart are usually metastatic, primary cardiac neoplasms being very rare. **6.80 Secondary carcinoma: heart.** This is the right ventricle. Four small pinkish-white secondary deposits are present at the infundibulum (below centre). The primary was a carcinoma of breast. Carcinoma of lung may give rise to similar metastases, although pericardial involvement is more usual than myocardial. **6.81 Secondary sarcoma: heart.** The superior vena cava, right atrium and right ventricle contain smooth elongated polypoid creamy-brown tumour masses. Invasion of the cava and right heart is typical of the way that peripheral sarcomas spread by the venous system and histologically this was a leiomyosarcoma. Two years earlier a primary paratesticular leiomyosarcoma had been removed. **6.82 Angio-**sarcoma: heart. At necropsy this appeared to be a primary neoplasm of heart. Nodular haemorrhagic tumour fills the pericardial sac over the right ventricle and atrium. Polypoid masses of tumour have invaded the heart and project into the atrium and ventricle. Histologically the tumour was an angiosarcoma. **6.83 Haemangioma: retroperitoneum.** Haemangiomas are congenital in origin and comprise the largest group of childhood tumours. Three main types are recognised; capillary, cavernous, and mixed. This specimen, a large haemorrhagic mass, was located in the retroperitoneum of a 26-year-old woman. The cut surface has a sponge-like appearance from the presence of large numbers of cavernous spaces. Some of these are dark green from old haemorrhage. **6.84 Leukaemic infiltration: heart.** The endocardial surface of the left ventricle is covered with a thick plaque-like mass of creamy-white tumour. This is an extreme example of leukaemic infiltration in a patient with acute granulocytic leukaemia.

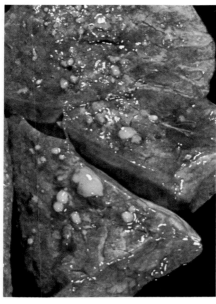

7.1 Suppurative bronchitis: lung

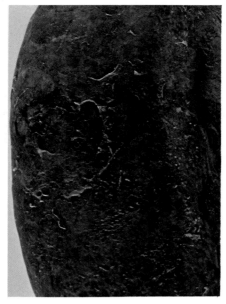

7.2 Pneumococcal pneumonia

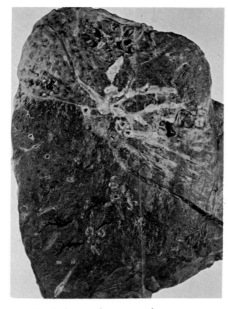

7.3 Staphylococcal pneumonia

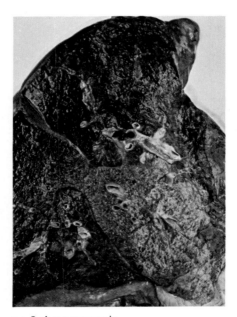

7.4 Lobar pneumonia

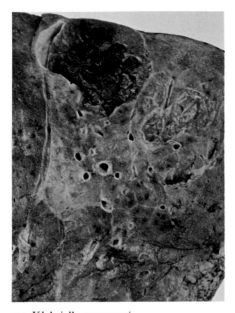

7.5 Klebsiella pneumonia

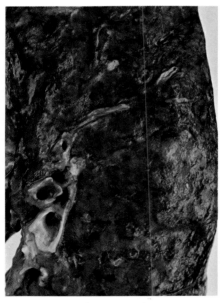

7.6 Acute bronchopneumonia

7.1 Suppurative bronchitis: lung. Beads of greenish mucopus are exuding from the cut ends of the large and small bronchi and there is bronchopneumonic consolidation of the lower lobe (bottom). The patient suffered from mucoviscidosis (fibrocystic disease), a congenital defect in which the bronchi fill with viscid mucus. Eventually secondary infection supervenes, often by low-virulence staphylococci, giving rise to suppurative bronchitis and bronchopneumonia. Bronchiectasis usually also develops. **7.2 Pneumococcal pneumonia.** This is the lower lobe. It is uniformly consolidated and smooth in outline. The surface is red-brown and yellowish-white strands of fibrinous exudate give it a dry granular appearance. Untreated pneumococcal lobar pneumonia passes through four phases: an initial phase of congestion; early consolidation (red hepatisation); late consolidation (grey hepatisation); and if the patient recovers, resolution. Classical lobar pneumonia is now rare. It occurs in patients with pulmonary congestion from chest injuries or after exposure to cold, and chronic alcoholism also predisposes. **7.3 Staphylococcal pneumonia.** This is the right lung. The middle and lower lobes are red-brown and the cut surface is dry and granular from extensive bronchopneumonic consolidation. Multiloculated abscess cavities have formed in the apex and basal segments of the upper lobe. About 5% of bacterial pneumonias are staphylococcal. They tend to follow viral

pneumonia or occur in debilitated patients infected with antibiotic-resistant organisms. In some cases, multiple small foci of consolidation may form a honeycomb of abscess cavities. **7.4 Lobar pneumonia.** The right middle lobe (centre right) is grey and airless and completely consolidated. Its appearance contrasts with that of the dark red congested lower lobe and part of the upper lobe. Histology showed large amounts of fibrin within the alveoli, with many disintegrating neutrophil polymorphs. In untreated lobar pneumonia this late stage of consolidation (grey hepatisation) occurs between 4 and 8 days. **7.5 Klebsiella pneumonia.** This shows the apex of the upper lobe. There is extensive confluent greyish-white consolidation, and a large irregular abscess cavity (top) containing blood clot is situated beneath the pleura. Two other abscesses are present. Klebsiella pneumonia accounts for 1 to 2% of all cases of lobar pneumonia. The acute form commonly affects men over 50 years of age who are generally diabetic and have severe oral and dental sepsis. Initially lobular, the process soon becomes lobar in distribution and large abscesses tend to form, as in this case. The cut surface may have a sticky mucoid appearance. **7.6 Acute bronchopneumonia.** The patient had a carcinoma of the stomach and developed a terminal acute bronchopneumonia. This is a section of the left lower lobe showing a well-defined lobular pattern of consolidation.

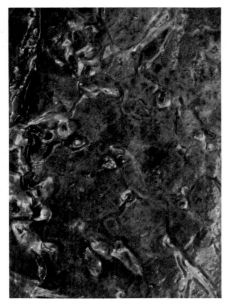

7.7 Ventilator lung and bronchopneumonia

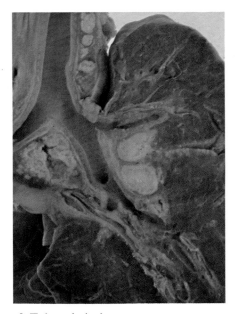

7.8 Tuberculosis: lung

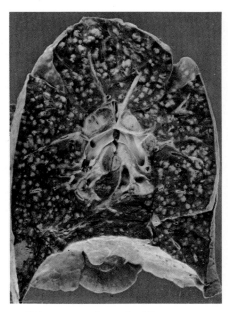

7.9 Primary complex and miliary
tuberculosis: lung

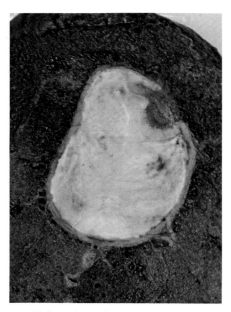

7.10 Tuberculoma: lung

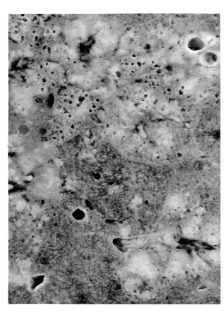

7.11 Tuberculous bronchopneumonia

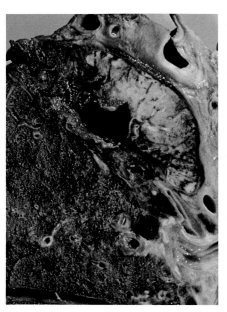

7.12 Fibrocaseous tuberculosis: lung

7.7 Ventilator lung and bronchopneumonia. The cut ends of the bronchi (bottom centre) are plugged by mucopus. A lobular pattern of consolidation is apparent, the pinkish-white areas of consolidated lung being delineated by prominent septa. There are also areas of haemorrhage. The patient sustained severe crush injuries to his chest two weeks prior to his death and for that time he was artificially ventilated on a respirator because of intractable pulmonary oedema which terminated in secondary bronchopneumonia. **7.8 Tuberculosis: lung.** These are the lungs of a child with primary tuberculosis. Two caseous masses constituting the primary (Ghon) focus are present in the basal segment of the left upper lobe (right of centre). There is also enlargement and caseous necrosis of a number of hilar and tracheobronchial lymph nodes. The lung lesion and the caseous nodes make up the primary complex. The primary focus occurs with equal frequency in either lung and tends to be subpleural, in the mid-portion of a lobe rather than apical. Rarely multiple foci may be found. **7.9 Primary complex and miliary tuberculosis: lung.** This also is the lung of a young child. There is a primary (Ghon) focus measuring about 1 cm in diameter beneath the pleura at the base of the lower lobe (bottom left). The hilar nodes are caseous (centre), and in addition the cut surface of the lung is studded with greyish-white miliary tubercles each about 1 mm in diameter. There were similar tubercles in many other organs. The miliary spread had occurred

following rupture of a caseous hilar node into a pulmonary vein. **7.10 Tuberculoma: lung.** This is the apex of the upper lobe. It contains a solitary caseous mass enclosed within a thick grey-white fibrous capsule. The cut surface has a faintly lamellated appearance. The surrounding lung is normal. Tuberculoma occurs in adults with reinfection tuberculosis. It is often solitary and usually situated in an upper lobe. The size varies from 0.5 to 4 cm in diameter and the capsule may be calcified. The lesion is usually inactive but it may become reactivated. **7.11 Tuberculous bronchopneumonia.** This close-up view shows semi-confluent irregular nodules of caseation, each centred on a thick-walled bronchus. Acinar tuberculosis results from spread of infection by the respiratory bronchioles, following aspiration of tuberculous material from elsewhere in the lung. The lesions may progress to lobular bronchopneumonia (top). Pulmonary tuberculosis is a recognised hazard of prolonged steroid therapy and this patient had been receiving this form of treatment for scleroderma. **7.12 Fibrocaseous tuberculosis: lung.** The apex of the upper lobe (top) contains a large greyish-white caseous focus which has cavitated. A thin fibrous capsule is present around the focus and the pleura and mediastinum (right and top) show dense white fibrous thickening. Chronic fibrocaseous tuberculosis develops in progressive reinfection (reactivation) tuberculosis and usually involves an upper lobe. Ulceration into a bronchus leads to cavity formation.

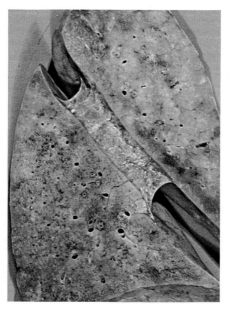

7.13 *Pneumocystis carinii* pneumonia

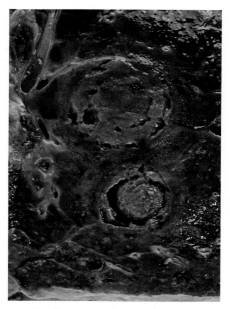

7.14 Confluent bronchopneumonia and fungal infection

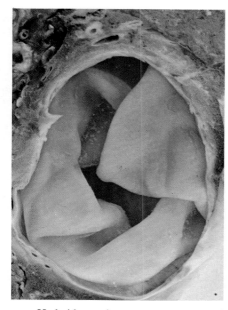

7.15 Hydatid cyst: lung

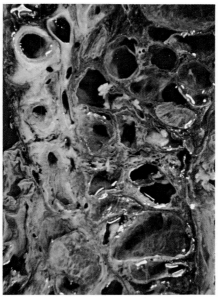

7.16 Bronchiectasis

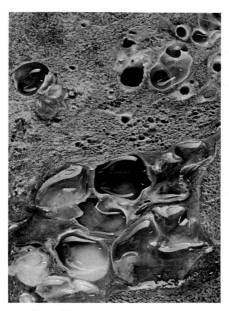

7.17 Bronchiectasis

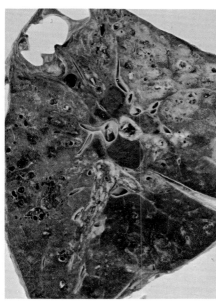

7.18 Bronchiectasis

7.13 Pneumocystis carinii pneumonia. The upper and lower lobes are completely consolidated and a uniform grey colour. Fine adhesions are present between the lobes. At necropsy the tissues felt firm, rubbery and rather 'dry', and histologically the alveoli were filled with a pale eosinophilic foamy substance enclosing the protozoon *Pneumocystis carinii*. This is a rare type of pneumonia which may be found in infants during the early months of life, or in adults often in association with leukaemia, lymphoma or cytomegalovirus inclusion disease. **7.14 Confluent bronchopneumonia and fungal infection.** The pleural surface (bottom) is covered with an opaque grey organising fibrinous exudate and the lung shows confluent bronchopneumonic consolidation. Its cut surface is a dark rusty-brown colour. Two round chronic abscess cavities (centre) contain grey-brown fungal 'balls'. The patient had acute granulocytic leukaemia treated with cytotoxic drugs. He developed an acute pyogenic bronchopneumonia and then terminal mycotic infection of the bronchopneumonic abscess cavities supervened. **7.15 Hydatid cyst: lung.** The cyst has a thick white fibrous capsule and is surrounded by compressed lung. It contains a folded partially-separated opaque membrane which represents the laminated germinal layer. This

layer contains numerous papillae, not seen here, which become pedunculated vesicles (brood capsules) containing scolices. Primary hydatid cysts may also be found in the liver. Hydatid cysts represent the phase in the intermediate host of the larval (cysticercal) stage of *Echinococcus granulosus* (dog tapeworm). **7.16-7.18 Bronchiectasis. 7.16** This is the lower lobe. The bronchi are thick-walled and dilated into fusiform and cylindrical cavities. There is severe peribronchial fibrosis and the intervening lung is almost completely collapsed. Chronic (atelectatic) bronchiectasis follows obstruction of a major lobar bronchus. The bronchiectatic changes involve whole lobes and lung abscesses may develop. **7.17** This is the saccular type of bronchiectasis. Large smooth-walled saccular bronchi are full of gelatinous inspissated mucus. The adjacent lung does not show collapse or peribronchial fibrosis. Saccular bronchiectasis often follows an attack of bronchopneumonia in early childhood. The left lower lobe is most frequently involved. **7.18** The left lower lobe (lower right) is consolidated and red-brown in colour. Many small bronchi are ectatic (centre left) and semi-confluent yellowish-green abscesses are present in the apex of the upper lobe (top). These abscesses have cavitated.

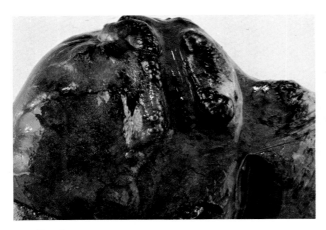

7.19 Emphysema

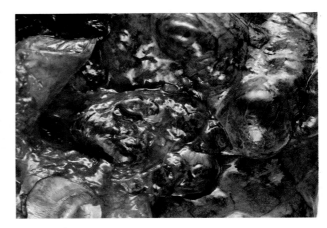

7.20 Emphysema

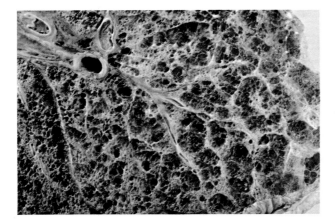

7.21 Emphysema

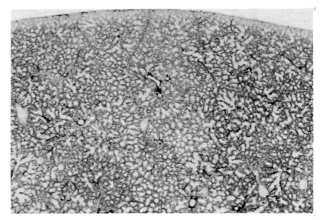

7.22 Panacinar emphysema

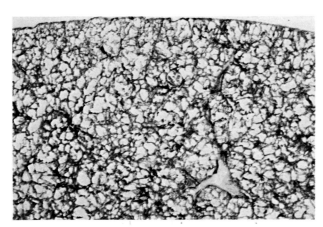

7.23 Panacinar emphysema

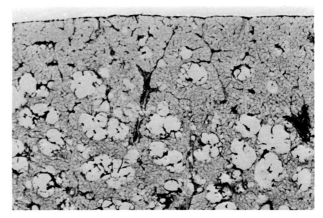

7.24 Centrilobular emphysema

7.19-7.26 Emphysema. 7.19 This is the pleural surface of the apex of the lung. It is a mottled red-black colour, from the presence of carbonaceous pigment (anthracosis). There are several very large cystic emphysematous bullae, with the intervening lung appearing contracted. Giant bullae are generally a manifestation of advanced panacinar emphysema arising from progressive dilatation and destruction of alveolar walls, whereby large subpleural air sacs bounded by lobular septa are formed. They may rupture and cause spontaneous pneumothorax. Occasionally they are seen in young adults without a history of lung disease or emphysema. Isolated bullae ('blebs') of this type are thought to result from rupture of alveoli into the subpleural interstitial tissues. **7.20** The lung is red-black and anthracotic. Many large bullous cysts are present, with thin semi-translucent walls. The subpleural cysts are causing gross distortion of the pleural surface of the lung, and fibrous septa due to pleural adhesions increase the distortion. The patient had severe chronic bronchitis and panacinar emphysema. **7.21** This is the cut surface of a lung which has been infused with formalin via the bronchi. It shows severe panacinar emphysema, with marked

dilatation of the whole acinus. The emphysematous spaces thus formed are of variable size, and retraction of the damaged and distended acini causes the bronchi and septa to appear prominent. Panacinar emphysema tends to involve the whole lung and affects men more than women. **7.22-7.26** are thin (about 400 μm) sections of lung prepared by the Gough and Wentworth technique, which is a particularly useful method for studying emphysema and the 'dust' diseases. **7.22** This is an example of mild panacinar emphysema. The notable feature is the uniform distension of the whole of the acinus. **7.23** This is a more advanced stage of panacinar emphysema. Each lobule is greatly enlarged and the distended acini are several mm in diameter. All acini are affected. It is not certain whether panacinar emphysema is a late stage of centrilobular emphysema or is a distinct entity. **7.24** This is centrilobular emphysema. The peripherally situated alveoli within each lobule are normal but those in the centre are enlarged, measuring up to 1 cm in diameter. The distribution of the affected lobules may be segmental, lobar or generalised. The lesions are more common in the upper lobes.

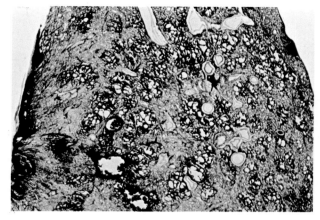

7.25 Simple coalminers' pneumoconiosis and focal emphysema

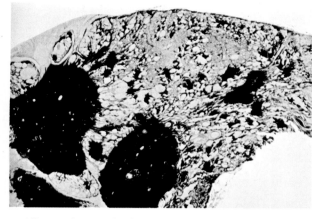

7.26 Progressive massive fibrosis: lung

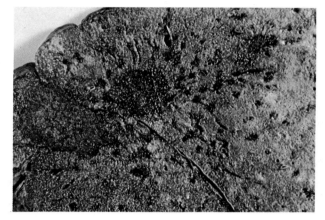

7.27 Silicosis: lung

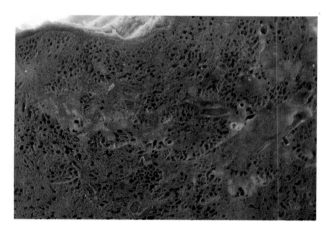

7.28 Haematite lung

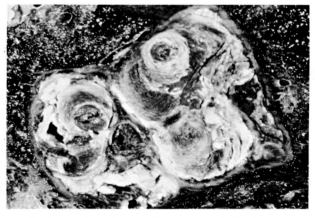

7.29 Caplan's lesion (rheumatoid pneumoconiosis): lung

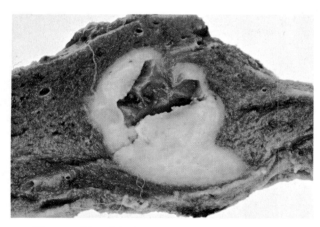

7.30 Rheumatoid nodule: lung

7.25 Simple coalminers' pneumoconiosis and focal emphysema. The emphysema is centrilobular ('focal emphysema') and closely associated with heavy deposition of coal dust. In this type of pneumoconiosis, the particles of coal dust are phagocytosed and deposited in the interalveolar septa, subpleural septa and around bronchioles and arteries producing a network (coal-dust reticulation). The association of the focal centrilobular emphysema with dust reticulation may be coincidental. There are also focal rheumatoid lesions beneath the pleura on the left. **7.26 Progressive massive fibrosis: lung.** The lung shows severe centrilobular emphysema and in addition there are several large solid black areas of progressive massive fibrosis. The latter lesion is thought to develop following the onset of tuberculosis. The relationship to silica dust is obscure. The centre of the large fibrotic masses may break down and cavitate. Concomitant emphysema may lead to cor pulmonale and death. **7.27 Silicosis: lung.** There are two large sharply-demarcated silicotic nodules at the apex of the upper lobe (left and centre) which contain much anthracotic pigment and are a deep black colour. Silica provokes marked fibrous tissue formation and in a silicotic nodule the collagen fibres are often arranged in concentric bands, with a clearly demarcated border and much carbon pigment in the periphery of the nodule. **7.28 Haematite lung.** The cut surface of the lung is uniformly

brick-red and diffuse centrilobular emphysema is present. Rounded solid fibrous red-brown nodules are visible (upper right). The red colour is due to the deposition of iron oxide. Silica dust produces the fibrous nodules and the result is a type of modified silicosis. These changes are seen in the lungs of haematite miners, welders, boiler scalers and other iron workers. **7.29 Caplan's lesion (rheumatoid pneumoconiosis): lung.** In Caplan's lesion the rheumatoid process produces a marked cellular and necrotising reaction at the periphery of silicotic nodules. In this example, the grey-white lesion is large and complex, and composed of nodules which are lamellated and show concentric whitish areas of calcification. Calcification is common in rheumatoid pneumoconiosis. The Caplan lesion is found in miners with silicosis who develop rheumatoid arthritis and the pulmonary lesion may antedate those in other systems. **7.30 Rheumatoid nodule: lung.** The nodule is whitish with a necrotic brown area. It is rounded and well-demarcated from the pulmonary tissue. Histologically the necrotic part was surrounded by a 'palisade' of macrophages, scanty giant cells, lymphocytes and plasma cells. Fibroblasts and fibrous tissue were also present peripherally. The patient was a 30-year-old woman who had had rheumatoid arthritis for 10 years. Rheumatoid nodules in the lung rarely exceed 2 cm in diameter and this one was 1.5 cm.

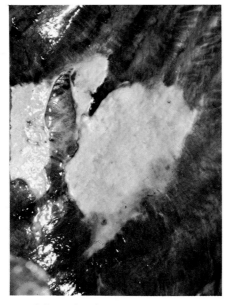

7.31 Asbestosis: pleura

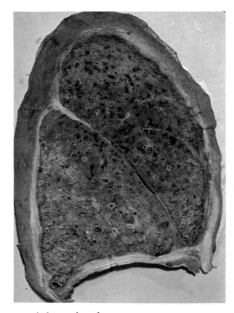

7.32 Asbestosis: pleura

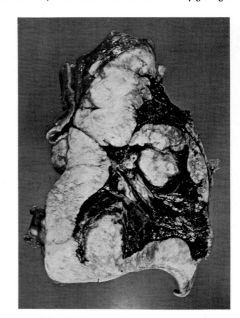

7.33 Mesothelioma: pleura

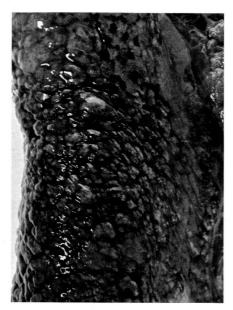

7.34 Idiopathic pulmonary fibrosis
(honeycomb lung)

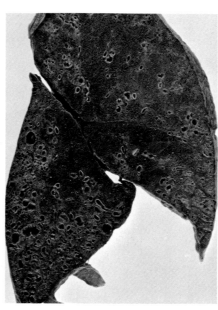

7.35 Idiopathic pulmonary fibrosis
(honeycomb lung)

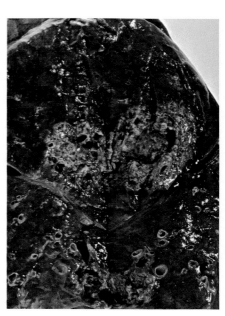

7.36 Wegener's granulomatosis: lung

7.31 and 7.32 Asbestosis: pleura. 7.31 This shows the parietal pleura over the posterior thoracic wall. Several yellowish plaques are present. These plaques are common findings in people exposed to asbestos and they are firm and often of cartilaginous consistence. Histologically they are composed of dense laminated acellular collagen. This man had worked in a shipyard for many years. **7.32** A markedly thickened visceral pleura encases the whole lung and the fibrosis extends into the interlobar fissure. There is also diffuse greyish-white fibrosis and bronchiectasis affecting the basal segments of the lower lobe (lower left). The lung is smaller than normal. The asbestotic process more often involves the lower lobes than the upper. **7.33 Mesothelioma: pleura.** A thick layer of pinkish-white tumour ensheaths most of the lung, and compresses and infiltrates the upper and lower lobes. The basal portion of the lung is, however, particularly severely affected. Mesothelioma of the pleura is a malignant tumour which often shows a mixed histological structure, with fibrosarcoma-like areas and 'epithelial' patterns consisting of tubules or papillary structures. A history of industrial exposure to asbestosis is obtained in over 80% of the cases. **7.34 and 7.35 Idiopathic pulmonary fibrosis (honeycomb lung). 7.34** This shows the pleural surface of the lower lobe. It is markedly 'nodular', the raised areas measuring up to 1 cm in diameter. These areas are formed by the presence within the lung of many fibrous-walled cystic structures. There is some resemblance to 'hobnail' liver. The changes are greatest in the lower and outer zones. **7.35** There is red-brown fibrosis and consolidation in the upper and middle lobes and the upper part of the lower lobe. Multiple large and small cysts are also present, being especially numerous in the basal segment of the lower lobe (below left). In the development of honeycomb lung, a chronic inflammatory process affecting mainly the interstitial tissues of the lung leads in time to fibrous obliteration of many terminal bronchioles and 'compensatory' dilatation of the unaffected alveoli and respiratory bronchioles. **7.36 Wegener's granulomatosis: lung.** Wegener's granulomatosis consists of the triad of lesions: necrotising granulomas in the nose, paranasal sinuses and lung; a vasculitis affecting small arteries and veins; and glomerulitis. This shows a pulmonary lesion. A large ill-defined yellowish-grey lesion is situated in the base of the upper lobe, and a similar smaller focus is present in the lower lobe. The centres of both lesions are necrotic and cavitation has occurred. The lung appears congested.

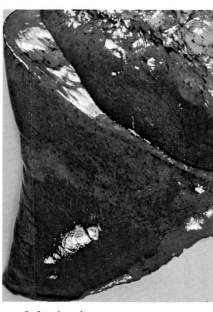

7.37 Infarction: lung

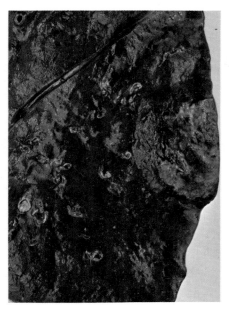

7.38 Infarction: lung

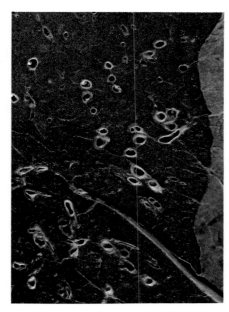

7.39 Recurrent pulmonary embolism and pulmonary hypertension: lung

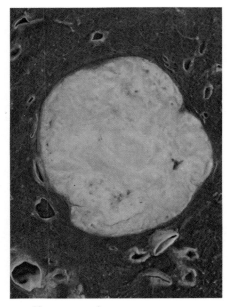

7.40 Hamartoma: lung

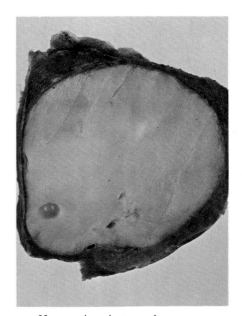

7.41 Haemangiopericytoma: lung

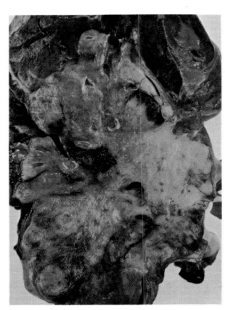

7.42 Carcinoid tumour: bronchus

7.37 and 7.38 Infarction: lung. Infarction of lung rarely occurs in previously healthy persons. As a rule those affected have had cardio-respiratory disease for some time and are usually over 40 years of age. Recent infarcts are dark-red in colour and haemorrhagic, becoming paler as the red cells within them lyse and organisation proceeds. Most infarcts result from impaction of an embolus in a branch of the pulmonary arteries. **7.37** There is a large triangular dark-red infarct at the base of the left lower lobe (lower left) and another in the upper lobe. Pulmonary infarcts are often multiple and about 75% are located in the lower lobes. **7.38** The pale pink infarct is wedge-shaped and located in the lower lobe beneath the pleura. It is surrounded by a dark-red congested border. The infarct is swollen and the pleural surface is raised over it. **7.39 Recurrent pulmonary embolism and pulmonary hypertension: lung.** This lung was fixed by infusion of formalin into the air passages. It is dark brown and the pulmonary arteries are thick-walled and unduly prominent. Many contain pale emboli, which have shrunk and retracted from the vessel wall. Recurrent showers of small pulmonary emboli may cause obstruction of the pulmonary arterial tree and eventually chronic pulmonary hypertension. Local formation of thrombus may be superimposed on the embolic process. Most cases occur in young or middle-aged women and pregnancy is often a factor. It is often difficult to distinguish between obliterative pulmonary hyper-

tension resulting from thromboembolic obstruction and primary (idiopathic) pulmonary hypertension. **7.40 Hamartoma: lung.** The lesion is a solitary well-circumscribed creamy-white mass. Its cut surface has a lobulated pattern and looks somewhat cartilage-like, with foci of calcification. The hamartoma contains the normal tissues of the bronchial wall but cartilage, myxoid connective tissue and gland-like clefts lined by cuboidal epithelium are usually present. It is a solitary lesion as a rule, situated subpleurally, and usually a chance finding during routine chest radiography. **7.41 Haemangiopericytoma: lung.** The neoplasm is a smooth rounded yellowish mass, with tiny areas of cystic degeneration (lower left). Multiple similar lesions were present elsewhere in the lungs on X-radiography. The primary tumour was in the uterus. Primary sarcoma of lung is very rare. **7.42 Carcinoid tumour: bronchus.** The tumour is a large irregular pinkish-white mass. It is invading the hilum, adjacent lung and hilar lymph nodes extensively. Carcinoid tumours account for about 90% of all so-called adenomas of bronchus. They usually arise from major bronchi and behave as slow-growing carcinomas, often showing marked local invasion, as here, but only occasionally forming distant metastases. Neurosecretory granules similar to those found in oat cell carcinoma have been demonstrated within the tumour cells.

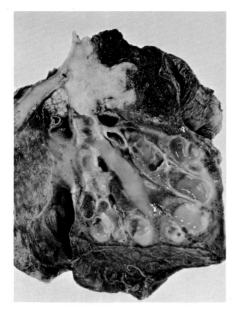

7.43 Squamous carcinoma: bronchus

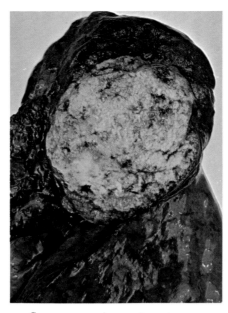

7.44 Squamous carcinoma: bronchus

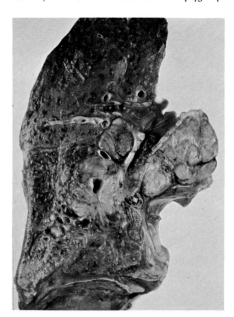

7.45 Oat cell carcinoma: bronchus

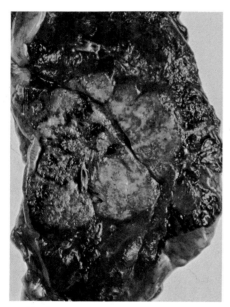

7.46 Peripheral carcinoma: bronchus

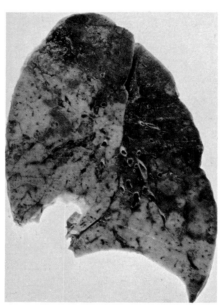

7.47 Alveolar cell carcinoma: bronchus

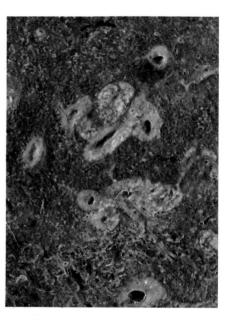

7.48 Carcinomatous lymphangitis

7.43-7.47 Carcinoma: bronchus. About 75% of carcinomas involve a main bronchus close to the carina. Obstruction of the lumen is caused either by intraluminal growth or by a stenosing tumour encircling the wall and may lead to abscess or gangrene in the lung distal to the lesion. **7.43** This is a squamous carcinoma. It is an irregular pale growth which obstructs the lower lobe bronchus producing collapse of the lung distal to the growth and (atelectatic) bronchiectasis. The dilated bronchi are full of greenish mucopus. **7.44** A large yellowish-white and almost totally necrotic squamous carcinoma fills most of the upper lobe. The yellow granular cheesy appearance is typical of squamous carcinoma. 40-60% of all bronchial cancers are of this type. They are prone to undergo central cavitation and mimic lung abscess. **7.45** This is an oat cell carcinoma. Oat cell carcinoma constitutes about 10% of all bronchial primary tumours. It is a highly malignant growth, typically situated in a major bronchus and showing a marked tendency to early spread. In this case the pinkish-white neoplasm has arisen in the right lower lobe bronchus. 'Warty' tumour growth protrudes through the bronchial mucosa, and extension into the lung has occurred, with tumour encircling the pulmonary artery. Massive involvement of the hilar lymph nodes is present. The lower lobe shows extensive consolidation with yellowish-white nodules of endogenous lipoid pneumonia. **7.46** This is a

peripheral carcinoma. The pleural surface of the lung is thickened over a circumscribed, subpleural, lobulated growth, the cut surface of which is yellowish-white and necrotic. Roughly one-third of bronchial carcinomas occur in the periphery of the lung. They often appear to be well-demarcated spherical masses, firm on the outside and friable centrally, but they invade the lung and lymphatic invasion is commonly present at the time of diagnosis. **7.47** This is an 'alveolar cell' carcinoma. Greyish-white tumour involves two-thirds of the left upper lobe and one-third of the lower lobe. The colour of the growth and the lobar distribution suggest pneumonic consolidation. Secondary tumours can produce the same appearance and this should always be borne in mind before the diagnosis of primary alveolar cell carcinoma is made (see 7.51) **7.48-7.50 Carcinomatous lymphangitis.** Diffuse infiltration of the pulmonary lymphatics by carcinoma is often referred to as carcinomatous lymphangitis or lymphangitis carcinomatosa. Many different types of primary tumour can give rise to this form of spread within the lungs. **7.48** This shows the cut surface of the lung in close-up. The walls of the small bronchi are extensively invaded and thickened by white tumour tissue, producing a pipestem appearance. A similar pattern of spread by peribronchial lymphatics may be seen in metastatic growths, especially from breast and stomach.

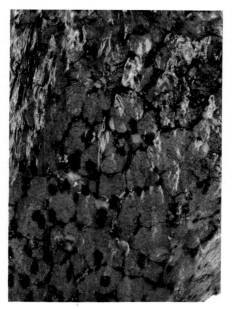

7.49 Carcinomatous lymphangitis

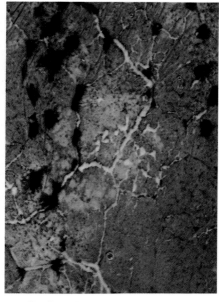

7.50 Carcinomatous lymphangitis

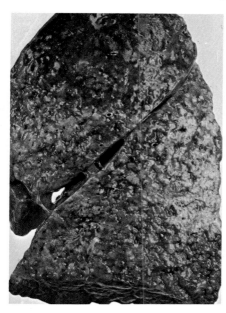

7.51 Diffuse secondary carcinoma: lung

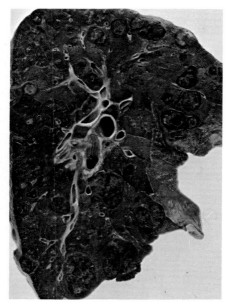

7.52 Secondary choriocarcinoma: lung

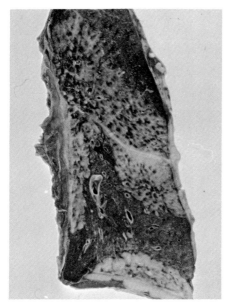

7.53 Histiocytic lymphoma: lung

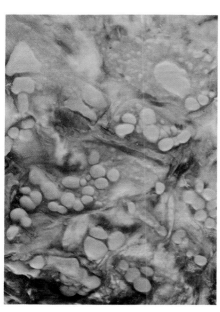

7.54 Histiocytic lymphoma: lung

7.49 and 7.50 Carcinomatous lymphangitis. 7.49 This is the visceral pleura. Multiple small discrete yellow-white deposits of tumour are present in the subpleural lymphatics. The primary tumour was a carcinoma of breast. The black pigment is inhaled carbonaceous dust (anthracosis). **7.50** This is a more advanced lesion than that shown in 7.49. The lympatic vessels over the pleura are extensively permeated by secondary tumour which causes them to stand out in relief from the surface. **7.51 Diffuse secondary carcinoma: lung.** The entire lung is consolidated by gelatinous raised greyish-green nodules of secondary carcinoma. Stomach, pancreas and ovary are the usual sites of the primary growth and the primary in this case was a mucus-secreting carcinoma of pancreas. It is often difficult to distinguish this pattern of secondary dissemination from primary alveolar cell carcinoma and the diffuse consolidation and mucoid appearance may also be mistaken for a Klebsiella pneumonia. **7.52 Secondary choriocarcinoma: lung.** The lung contains multiple round (cannon-ball) haemorrhagic and necrotic secondary deposits of choriocarcinoma. The primary was in a teratoma

of testis. Most metastatic tumours in the lung arise from blood-borne spread, and the pulmonary metastases are found in about 30% of patients dying from malignant disease. Primary tumours which metastasise readily to the lungs are carcinomas of kidney, stomach, breast, colon and thyroid and sarcomas of bone. **7.53 and 7.54 Histiocytic lymphoma (reticulum cell sarcoma).** About 7% of malignant lymphomas originate in the lungs, though these tumours account for less than 0.5% of all malignant tumours. Lymphomas are commoner in the upper lobes and grow as nodular masses or growths that involve the whole lobe. Pleural extension is common. Histiocytic lymphoma is commoner in women, with an average age of around 40. **7.53** The upper and lower lobes are diffusely infiltrated by greyish-green tumour. The pleura is thickened and diffusely infiltrated, especially over the diaphragmatic surface (bottom). **7.54** The patient died from disseminated histiocytic lymphoma. This is the pleural surface of the diaphragm. It is studded with smooth raised yellowish-white plaques of tumour.

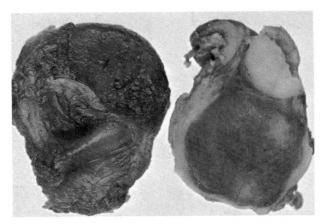

8.1 Regeneration of pituitary

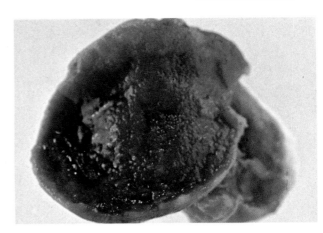

8.2 Pressure atrophy: pituitary

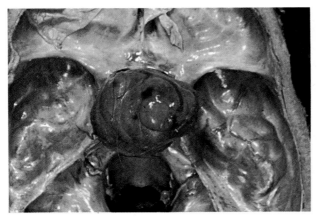

8.3 Adenoma: pituitary

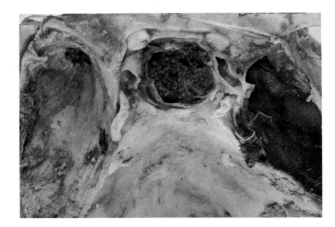

8.4 Chromophobe carcinoma: pituitary

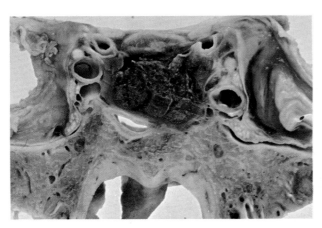

8.5 Chromophobe carcinoma: pituitary

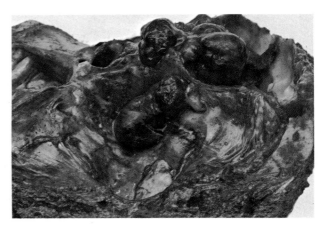

8.6 Chromophobe carcinoma: pituitary

8.1 Regeneration of pituitary. The patient had undergone a transphenoidal hypophysectomy 6 years previously for Cushing's syndrome, and histology showed a normal pituitary containing a small basophil adenoma. Over the next 6 years the pituitary regenerated to the size shown here (1 cm diameter). It has been bisected. The external aspect is on the left, along with a thickened pituitary stalk. The cut surface on the right shows a thick greyish-white capsule. The pars anterior is light brown in colour and the pars nervosa white (upper right). **8.2 Pressure atrophy: pituitary.** The patient had signs of mild acromegaly. The gland has been cut in mid-sagittal section. The posterior lobe is a pinkish-white colour. The anterior lobe is brown and congested; it is flattened as a result of pressure by a suprasellar craniopharyngioma. Pressure atrophy and necrosis of the pituitary may be a complication of intracranial tumours, especially when they are located around the pituitary fossa. Lesions which may do so include tumours and cysts of parapituitary epithelial rests. **8.3 Adenoma: pituitary.** A large pink fleshy mass with a lobulated surface is bulging out of the pituitary fossa. An adenoma may cause enlargement of the sella and then, as here, bulge upwards through the diaphragma sellae as a suprasellar extension into the cranial cavity, hypothalamus or midbrain. Adenomas are classified according to their cell type. The commonest is the chromophobe adenoma,

which accounts for about 65% of all adenomas. It tends to attain a large size and is found in adults between the ages of 30 and 50. **8.4-8.6 Chromophobe carcinoma: pituitary.** An adenoma of the pituitary occasionally shows considerable local invasion and a few, nearly always of the chromophobe type, are classified as carcinomas. They show extensive local bone invasion and may spread diffusely over the base of the skull but haematogenous dissemination is extremely rare. **8.4** This is an example of such a neoplasm in a man of 62. The sella is filled with haemorrhagic tumour and extrasellar extension of the growth over the right clivus and greater wing of sphenoid involves the floor of the right middle cranial fossa (right). **8.5** This is the lesion shown in 8.4 and it is a coronal section through the sphenoid bones of the middle cranial fossa. The sella is expanded by dark haemorrhagic tumour which is eroding the underlying basi-sphenoid. The cavernous sinuses, containing the internal carotid arteries, third, fifth and sixth cranial nerves are seen in cross-section. **8.6** The middle cranial fossa is seen from above. A polypoid haemorrhagic tumour extends over the basisphenoid (centre) and right posterior clinoid process and greater wing of sphenoid (right). Histologically the tumour was a chromophobe carcinoma which showed marked nuclear pleomorphism and frequent mitoses. The patient was a 34-year-old woman.

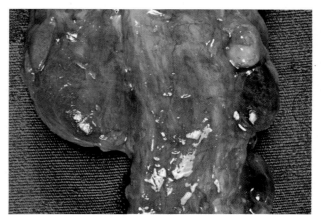

8.7 Adenoma: parathyroid

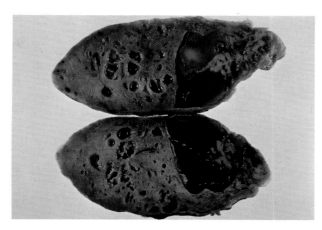

8.8 Adenoma: parathyroid

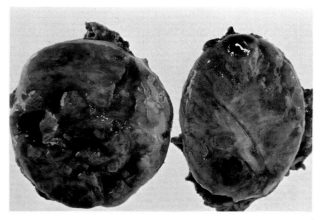

8.9 Phaeochromocytoma: adrenal

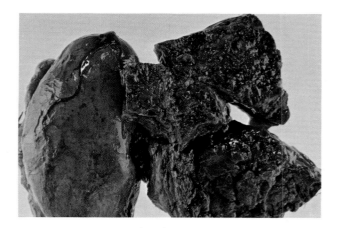

8.10 Ganglioneuroma: adrenal

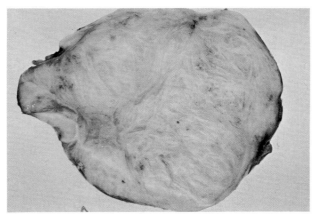

8.11 Ganglioneuroma: adrenal

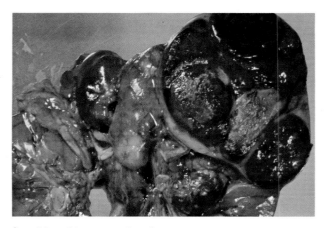

8.12 Neuroblastoma: adrenal

8.7 and 8.8 Adenoma: parathyroid. Primary hyperparathyroidism is caused by an adenoma in about 80% of cases, and two or more adenomas are found in 3 to 6% of patients with primary hyperparathyroidism. The adenomas are usually small and only rarely exceed a few g in weight. They are typically spherical to oval, soft tan to reddish-brown, smoothly-encapsulated tumours. The cut surface may be focally cystic and haemorrhagic, with fibrosis and calcification in places. **8.7** Most of these features are visible in this case. The posterior aspect of the larynx and trachea is shown. One lobe of the thyroid is at the upper left. The other lobe has been removed, to reveal two oval dark-brown parathyroid adenomas (lower right) with a paler lymph node just above them. Both adenomas are encapsulated. **8.8** This adenoma, which has been bisected, is an ovoid smooth tan-coloured tumour in which there are multiple foci of cystic degeneration. One large cystic cavity (right) is filled with recent blood clot. **8.9 Phaeochromocytoma: adrenal.** The tumour which measured 6 cm in its greatest diameter has been bisected. It is spherical, with a smooth capsule. The cut surface is yellow-brown, with areas of recent haemorrhage and cystic change. A phaeochromocytoma is a tumour of the adrenal medulla and typically secretes adrenalin and noradrenalin. It may also occur at other extra-adrenal sites. About 5% of the sporadic tumours are bilateral, as are 50% of familial phaeochromocytomas. Slices of the tumour immersed in potassium dichromate characteristically turn a dark mahogany-brown colour (chromaffin reaction). **8.10 and 8.11 Ganglioneuroma: adrenal.** A ganglioneuroma

is a benign neoplasm of mature nerve cells and their related fibres. It occurs usually in young adults, is commoner in women and is frequently discovered on routine examination. It may be found at any site where sympathetic ganglion cells occur. 40% are located within the adrenal and 20% in the ganglia of the upper abdominal sympathetic chain. The following two examples were in the adrenal. **8.10** This specimen is somewhat atypical. It is a very large haemorrhagic mass, somewhat larger than the adjacent kidney (left). The patient, a 40-year-old woman, presented with paroxysmal hypertension and a pre-operative diagnosis of phaeochromocytoma was made. She became normotensive three days pre-operatively and histological examination of the tumour showed it to be a ganglioneuroma that had undergone spontaneous massive haemorrhagic necrosis. **8.11** The appearance of this tumour is more typical of ganglioneuromas. It is roughly spherical with a capsule and a smooth, mildly bosselated surface. The cut surface is greyish-white, with a characteristic whorled fibrous appearance. **8.12 Neuroblastoma: adrenal.** A large coarsely lobular haemorrhagic tumour has destroyed the adrenal, infiltrated the upper pole of the kidney, and metastasised to the para-aortic lymph nodes. Neuroblastoma is the commonest adrenal tumour in infants, 30% occurring under the age of 1 year and 80% below 5 years. Typically it is a greyish-red vascular tumour, with necrosis and haemorrhage prominent. It is highly malignant, with a marked propensity for metastasising to the liver and bone.

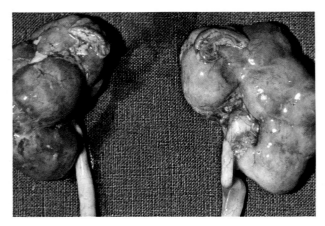

8.13 Congenital hypoplasia: adrenals

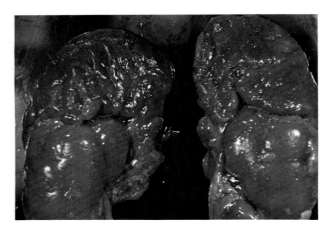

8.14 Congenital hyperplasia: adrenals

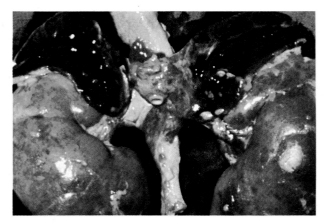

8.15 Haemorrhage: adrenals

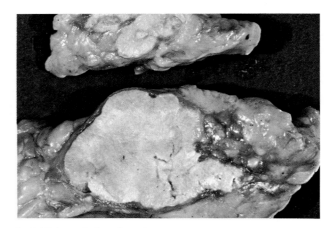

8.16 Tuberculosis: adrenal

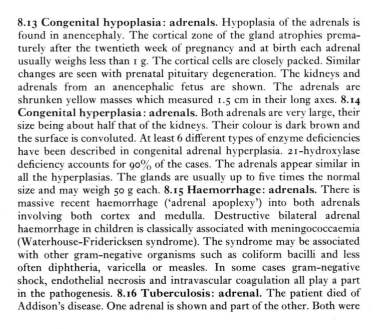

8.17 Iatrogenic cortical atrophy: adrenals

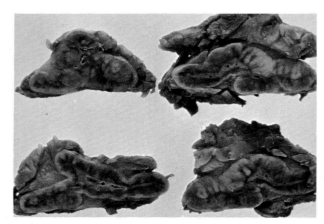

8.18 Diffuse cortical hyperplasia: adrenals

8.13 Congenital hypoplasia: adrenals. Hypoplasia of the adrenals is found in anencephaly. The cortical zone of the gland atrophies prematurely after the twentieth week of pregnancy and at birth each adrenal usually weighs less than 1 g. The cortical cells are closely packed. Similar changes are seen with prenatal pituitary degeneration. The kidneys and adrenals from an anencephalic fetus are shown. The adrenals are shrunken yellow masses which measured 1.5 cm in their long axes. **8.14 Congenital hyperplasia: adrenals.** Both adrenals are very large, their size being about half that of the kidneys. Their colour is dark brown and the surface is convoluted. At least 6 different types of enzyme deficiencies have been described in congenital adrenal hyperplasia. 21-hydroxylase deficiency accounts for 90% of the cases. The adrenals appear similar in all the hyperplasias. The glands are usually up to five times the normal size and may weigh 50 g each. **8.15 Haemorrhage: adrenals.** There is massive recent haemorrhage ('adrenal apoplexy') into both adrenals involving both cortex and medulla. Destructive bilateral adrenal haemorrhage in children is classically associated with meningococcaemia (Waterhouse-Fridericksen syndrome). The syndrome may be associated with other gram-negative organisms such as coliform bacilli and less often diphtheria, varicella or measles. In some cases gram-negative shock, endothelial necrosis and intravascular coagulation all play a part in the pathogenesis. **8.16 Tuberculosis: adrenal.** The patient died of Addison's disease. One adrenal is shown and part of the other. Both were enlarged, but on section they are found to consist of yellowish-white caseous material. In the adrenal, the cellular response, granuloma formation and fibrosis are deficient compared with other tissues, and parenchymal destruction and necrosis are correspondingly greater. In the past 70% of Addison's disease was caused by tuberculosis, but idiopathic adrenocortical atrophy now predominates. **8.17 Iatrogenic cortical atrophy: adrenals.** Both glands are markedly atrophic, the combined weight being 3.7 g and the absence of peri-adrenal fat noteworthy. Histologically the cortex appeared collapsed with considerable reduction in thickness of the zona fasciculata, associated with areas of cytolysis. The zona glomerulosa and zona reticularis were relatively unaffected. The cause of the atrophy was long-term corticosteroid therapy for rheumatoid arthritis. **8.18 and 8.19 Cortical hyperplasia: adrenals.** Adrenocortical hyperplasia may be diffuse or nodular. It is present in about 70% of patients with Cushing's syndrome, and nonspecific hyperplasia is commonly found in acromegaly, thyrotoxicosis, hypertension and diabetes mellitus. In most adult patients with bilateral hyperplasia, the hyperplasia is diffuse. **8.18** This is an example of diffuse hyperplasia. Two sections of each adrenal are shown. Both glands are much enlarged (combined weight 30 g) and they show diffuse cortical hyperplasia. The cortex has a broad irregular brown inner layer and a well-demarcated yellow lipid-rich outer zone. The nodular foci in the cortex measure up to 1 cm in diameter.

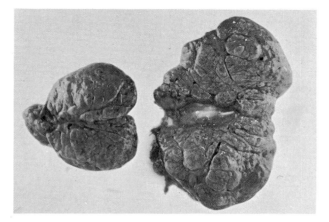

8.19 Adenomatous cortical hyperplasia: adrenals

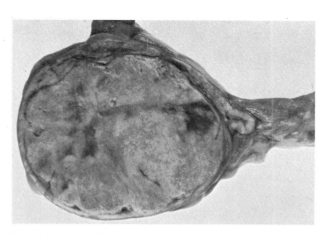

8.20 Adenoma: adrenal cortex

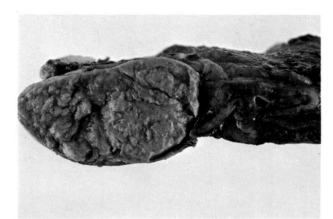

8.21 Adenoma: adrenal cortex

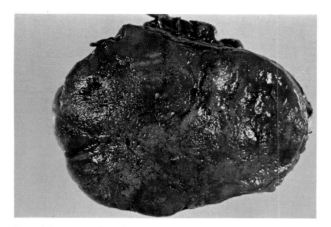

8.22 Adenoma: adrenal cortex

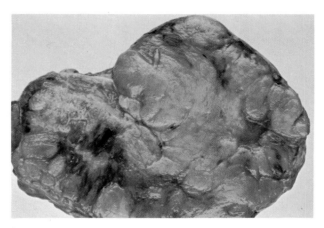

8.23 Carcinoma: adrenal cortex

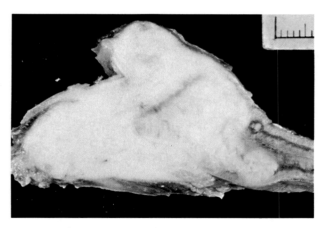

8.24 Secondary carcinoma: adrenal

8.19 Cortical hyperplasia: adrenals. This is an example of adenomatous hyperplasia. Both adrenals are enlarged. One measures 11 cm in its longest axis and the other 6 cm. Their combined weight was 90 g. Each has been bisected, to show a bright yellow nodular tissue, with disappearance of recognisable cortical structure. The term adenomatous, or nodular hyperplasia is confined to nodules up to about 2.5 cm in diameter which compress and displace the overlying cortex. Adenomatous hyperplasia occurs in 15% of cases of bilateral hyperplasia in Cushing's syndrome. The majority of cases are in women. **8.20-8.22 Adenoma: adrenal cortex. 8.20** This was a non-functioning 'adenoma', which was an incidental finding at necropsy in a patient with chronic bronchitis and cor pulmonale. It is a large oval faintly-lobulated bright yellow mass 2.5 cm in diameter with areas of haemorrhage on its cut surface. A thin layer of cortex is stretched over it. The true incidence of non-functioning 'adenomas' is unknown but the lesion is related to nodular hyperplasia. Sometimes a lesion may become sufficiently large as to present as an abdominal swelling. **8.21** This gland is from a patient with primary aldosteronism (Conn's syndrome). A golden-yellow, encapsulated adenoma (2 x 1.5 x 1 cm) is attached to an otherwise normal adrenal (right). Solitary adenomas are found in 90% of patients with Conn's syndrome. 60% weigh less than 6 g and about 80% measure less than 3 cm in diameter. The histological pattern varies but the commonest cell type resembles the clear cells of the zona fasciculata. In some

adenomas, cells of the zona glomerulosa type are predominant, forming solid trabeculae or alveoli. **8.22** This tumour was found in an 8-year-old boy with virilism. It is a large oval brown mass which weighed 250 g. In children most adrenal tumours are functional, and about 75% of the functioning tumours are benign adenomas, the remaining 25% being carcinomas. They are commoner in girls and develop in the first four years of life. Clinical signs usually appear between 4 and 8 years. In boys, virilisation occurs in about 6% of the cases. The brown colour is often due to the presence of lipochrome pigment. **8.23 Carcinoma: adrenal cortex.** Carcinomas of the adrenal cortex are usually large tumours, weighing up to 2000 g, and haemorrhage, necrosis and calcification are common features. This one, a large irregular lobulated pale yellow mass, weighed 390 g and the cut surface shows areas of haemorrhage and necrosis. About 90% of adrenal carcinomas are functional. 50% are associated with Cushing's, 20% with virilisation and 12% with feminisation. This specimen was removed from a 66-year-old woman and there was evidence of oestrogen secretion by the tumour. **8.24 Secondary carcinoma: adrenal.** A large part of the gland has been replaced by whitish tumour. The appearances suggest that the secondary deposit first appeared in the medulla. Metastatic carcinoma is often bilateral. The true incidence is not known, some series reporting an overall incidence of around 10%. Carcinomas of lung and breast give rise to adrenal metastases in 40% and 25% of cases respectively at necropsy.

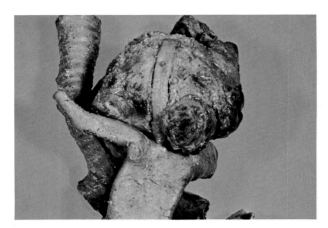

8.25 Aortic body tumour

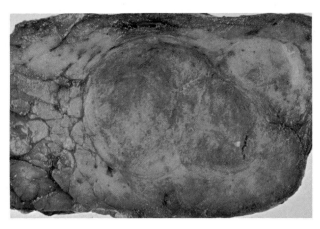

8.26 Islet cell tumour: pancreas

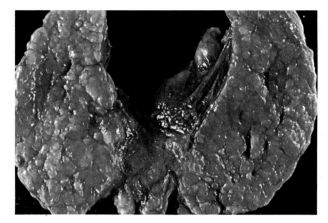

8.27 Primary thyrotoxicosis: thyroid

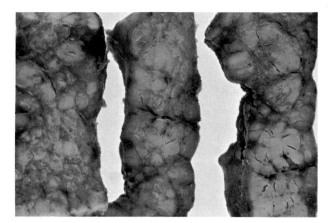

8.28 Hashimoto's thyroiditis

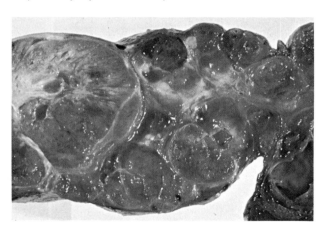

8.29 Multinodular goitre: thyroid

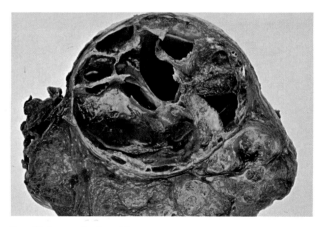

8.30 'Adenoma': thyroid

8.25 Aortic body tumour. A large lobulated greyish tumour is situated above the aortic arch, displacing and compressing the trachea and innominate artery. The left common carotid artery (centre) is closely applied to the front of the mass. An aortic body tumour (non-chromaffin paraganglioma; chemodectoma) is a tumour of chemoreceptor tissue. It occurs slightly more often in women and about 5% are bilateral. Histologically the neoplasm is lobulated, with nests of polyhedral cells arranged in an alveolar or organoid pattern. Characteristically it has a righly vascular stroma. **8.26 Islet cell tumour: pancreas.** The lobular structure of the exocrine pancreatic tissue (left) contrasts with an ovoid pale tawny yellow islet cell tumour located in the tail of the pancreas. The tumour is well-circumscribed and bilobed, measuring approximately 0.5 x 0.5 x 2 x 2 cm. Histologically it was composed of beta cells (insulinoma). Beta cell tumours are commonest in the body and tail of the pancreas. They are usually encapsulated but may range from less than 1 cm up to 10 cm in diameter. **8.27 Primary thyrotoxicosis: thyroid.** The gland in primary thyrotoxicosis usually weighs between 30 and 60 g. This one is shown in section. It is symmetrically enlarged, pinkish-red from increased vascularity, and 'fleshy', with no colloid visible. The histological picture is one of intense hyperplasia with papilliform epithelial ingrowths into many follicles. **8.28 Hashimoto's thyroiditis.** In this condition, the thyroid may weigh up to 200 g and the gland shown here was enlarged, firm and rubbery. Three slices of the gland are shown. The cut surface is opaque and yellowish-white and a lobulated structure is evident. Histologically there was destruction of the gland's architecture with a lymphocytic infiltrate, including follicles with germinal centres, and Askanazy-cell change of the thyroid epithelium. There is evidence to suggest that the condition results from an auto-immune process. **8.29 Multinodular goitre: thyroid.** The gland is very large and composed of nodules which vary greatly in size. There is a high concentration of colloid within the nodules which gives the cut surface a brownish gelatinous appearance. Darker areas of haemorrhage are present, and there are paler areas of fibrosis (centre). Cystic degeneration has also occurred in places. The patient was mildly thyrotoxic. Nodular goitre complicated by secondary hyperplasia mainly affects older patients and in whom the signs of hyperthyroidism are often atypical. **8.30 'Adenoma': thyroid.** The thyroid is enlarged and nodular, and the cut surface has the gelatinous pale tan-brown colour of a colloid goitre. A large (5 cm diameter) encapsulated 'adenoma' is present in one lobe. This adenoma shows old and recent haemorrhage, and marked cystic degeneration. Though often clinically referred to as adenomas, these nodules in over 90% of cases are found on histological examination to be areas of colloid adenomatous hyperplasia within a diffusely nodular gland.

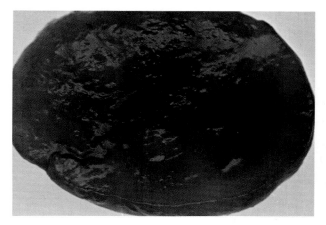

8.31 Follicular adenoma: thyroid

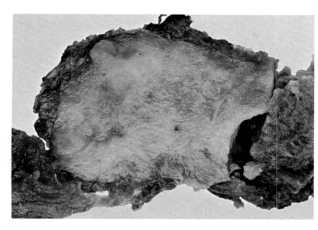

8.32 Medullary carcinoma: thyroid

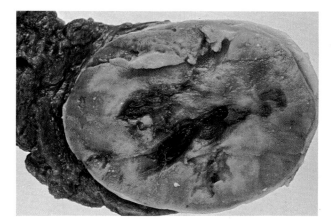

8.33 Follicular carcinoma: thyroid

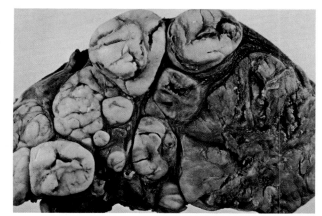

8.34 Follicular carcinoma: thyroid

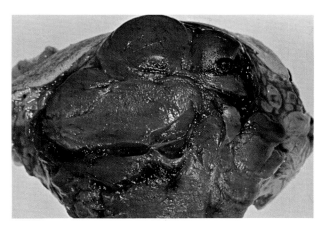

8.35 Askanazy-cell carcinoma: thyroid

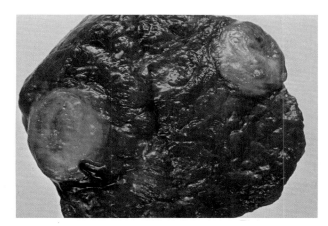

8.36 Histiocytic lymphoma: thyroid

8.31 Follicular adenoma: thyroid. This was a smooth encapsulated solitary oval tumour measuring 3 cm in diameter. The cut surface is a light tan-brown colour and the consistence appears soft and gelatinous. The surface bulges as a result of compression by the fibrous capsule. Follicular adenomas may be fetal, colloid, simple, embryonal or Askanazy-cell in type. This is a fetal adenoma which is the commonest type. Such an adenoma consists of very small 'fetal' follicles and an oedematous fibrovascular stroma. **8.32 Medullary carcinoma: thyroid.** The thyroid contains a small oval yellowish-white tumour which lacks a fibrous capsule. The cut surface is smooth and uniform. Medullary carcinomas arise from the calcitonin-secreting parafollicular cells and vary in size from 1.5 cm to large tumours. Microscopically they consist of spindle cells arranged in a hyalinised stroma in which amyloid is frequently present. **8.33 and 8.34 Follicular carcinoma: thyroid. 8.33** This thyroid is from a 36-year-old man. It contains an ovoid solid yellowish-white tumour with a smooth regular outline but lacking a fibrous capsule. The cut surface shows central necrosis and haemorrhage. Microscopically the tumour consisted of solid cellular areas interspersed with a microfollicular pattern typical of a well-differentiated follicular adenocarcinoma. **8.34** The thyroid gland is infiltrated and distorted by multiple creamy-white nodules of tumour, the largest of which (bottom right) shows central necrosis and haemorrhage. The nodules are not encapsulated. Follicular carcinoma tends to invade blood vessels but lymph node metastases also occur. Rarely a follicular carcinoma causes secondary hyperthyroidism. **8.35 Askanazy-cell carcinoma: thyroid.** The tumour is lobulated and a pinkish colour, with areas of haemorrhage. Extensive local permeation has occurred, with infiltration of the adjacent fat beneath the skin of the neck (top left and top right). About 20% of follicular carcinomas are of the Askanazy-cell type and their pattern of bahaviour varies a good deal. Some show blood vessel invasion, with metastasis to bones and lungs. **8.36 Histiocytic lymphoma (reticulum cell sarcoma): thyroid.** Lymphomas, especially Burkitt's (African) tumour, quite commonly involve the thyroid in the presence of disseminated disease. This patient died from disseminated histiocytic lymphoma. The thyroid contains two yellowish-white deposits. Metastases are also found fairly frequently in the thyroid at necropsy in cases dying with widely disseminated carcinoma or melanoma.

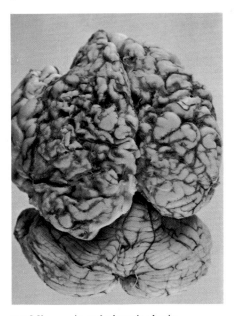

9.1 Microgyria and ulegyria: brain

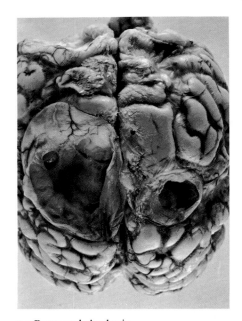

9.2 Porencephaly: brain

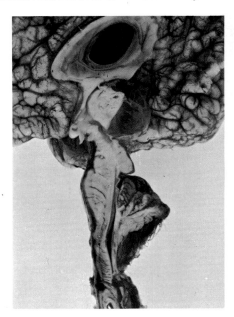

9.3 Arnold-Chiari malformation: brain and spinal cord

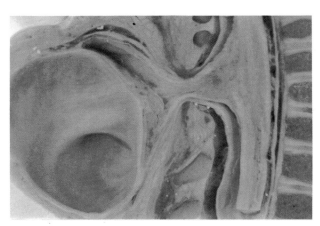

9.4 Meningocele: spinal cord and vertebral column

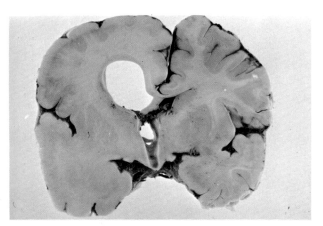

9.5 Ulegyria: brain

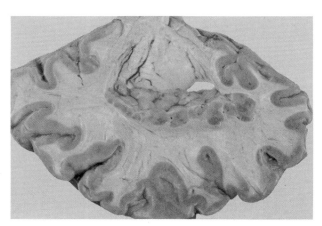

9.6 Ectopic grey matter: brain

9.1 Microgyria and ulegyria: brain. The term microgyria is used to describe abnormally small convolutions irrespective of whether they are a consequence of prenatal malformation or of a destructive process occurring at birth or in infancy. Ulegyria refers to general preservation of the convolutional pattern but with individual gyri showing shrinkage and sclerosis. Both types of lesion are commonly found in subjects with cerebral palsy following birth injury and this brain is from a child who suffered from such a lesion. Both cerebral hemispheres are small. Some gyri are normal but most are shrunken. The cerebellum is normal. **9.2 Porencephaly: brain.** The term porencephaly describes a congenital defect extending from the surface of the cerebral hemisphere into the subjacent ventricle. It includes cystic cavities which have resulted from pre- or post-natal vascular lesions associated with birth injury. This

brain is from a 20-year-old man who suffered ischaemic damage to his brain at birth and had a life-long history of epilepsy. Two large cystic cavities are seen on the superior surface of both occipito-parietal lobes. The roof of each cyst consists of a thin fibrous membrane. The cysts communicated with the lateral ventricles. **9.3 Arnold-Chiari malformation: brain and spinal chord.** Arnold-Chiari malformation is a congenital malformation of the lower brain-stem and lower part of the cerebellum which is constantly present in cases of meningomyelocele. A median sagittal section of the brain shows the right cerebral hemisphere and brain-stem. There is elongation of the medulla and pons, with downward herniation of the cerebellum into the upper cervical spinal canal. The finger-like processes of cerebellar tissue are bound down to the back and sides of the medulla and spinal cord by arachnoidal adhesions (bottom centre). **9.4 Meningocele: spinal cord and vertebral column.** This is a close-up view of a spina bifida. A narrow-necked sac has herniated through a defect in the vertebral arch to form a large thick-walled subcutaneous sac (left). The sac (meningocele) is derived from the meninges but does not contain the spinal cord. In a meningomyelocele the spinal cord also passes into the sac. **9.5 Ulegyria: brain.** The patient was a 2-year-old girl with spastic tetraplegia caused by severe antepartum anoxia. This coronal section of the brain shows loss of the gyral pattern of the right parieto-temporal lobes and greyish-white sclerosis of the left hemisphere due to extensive gliosis of central white matter and cortex (compare with the normal on the right side). The left lateral ventricle and third ventricle are dilated. Sclerosis and/or cavitation of the centrum semiovale is the most characteristic central lesion of birth trauma. **9.6 Ectopic grey matter: brain.** This is a rare congenital anomaly. A coronal section of the brain at the level of the occipital horn of the lateral ventricle shows ectopic grey matter situated around the ventricle. The ectopic islands of cortex project into the ventricular cavity and cause the ventricular surface to appear lobulated. Ectopic foci of grey matter may act as epileptogenic foci and this patient was an epileptic.

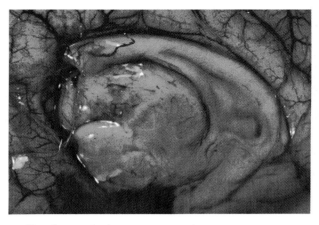

9.7 Kernicterus: brain

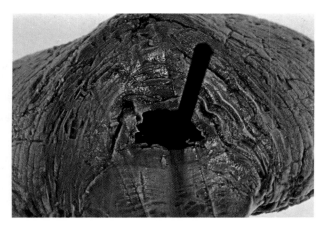

9.8 Syringobulbia: pons and cerebellum

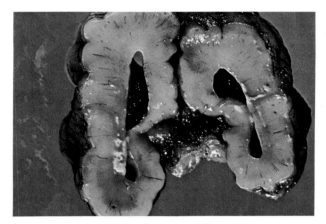

9.9 Cytomegalovirus disease and periventricular calcification: brain

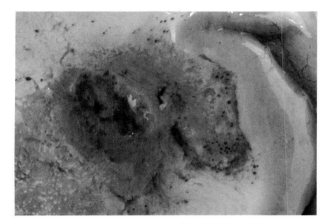

9.10 Acute abscess: brain

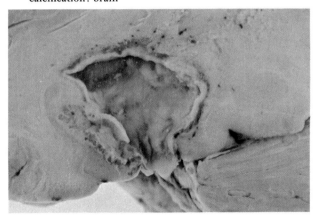

9.11 Chronic abscess: brain

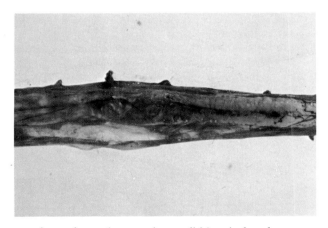

9.12 Acute abscess (suppurative myelitis): spinal cord

9.7 Kernicterus: brain. Kernicterus (nuclear jaundice) is the staining of the basal ganglia by bile pigments, and in the newborn a high concentration of bile pigment is most frequently due to severe haemolytic disease resulting from rhesus incompatibility. Some children may subsequently show signs of damage to neurons in the affected ganglia. This shows the medial aspect of a parasagittal section of the brain of a neonate. The corpus callosum, thalamus and subthalamic basal ganglia are stained pale yellow colour by bile pigment. **9.8 Syringobulbia: pons and cerebellum.** Syringomyelia is characterised by the presence of a cavity (syrinx) within the spinal cord, and when the cavity is within the medulla and pons the condition is termed syringobulbia. The cavity is usually filled with xanthochromic fluid. In this case the cavity, which contains a probe, is large and located in the pons. There are multiple causes of this type of lesion. One form is thought to be due to a failure of closure of the spinal cord. Other causes include old haemorrhage or infection. **9.9 Cytomegalovirus disease and periventricular calcification: brain.** Intrauterine infection by cytomegalovirus may arrest cerebral development at about the fourth month of fetal life, causing microcephaly, hydrocephaly and periventricular calcification. The calcified lesions have to be distinguished from congenital toxoplasmosis. In this coronal section of the brain from an immature fetus, white foci of calcification are present around the occipital horns of both lateral ventricles. The ventricles are dilated due to associated hydrocephalus. **9.10 Acute abscess: brain.** A large pinkish-red abscess is situated beneath the cerebral cortex of the parietal lobe. It involves the subcortical white matter and adjacent thalamus (lower left). The centre is necrotic and cavitating. The surrounding brain is swollen and oedematous and there are focal haemorrhages. There is no evidence of encapsulation. Brain abscesses may originate from infected arterial emboli (usually in the distribution of the middle cerebral artery) or by direct extension from infections of bone or sinuses. **9.11 Chronic abscess: brain.** An irregular ragged abscess cavity has formed in the inferior part of the temporal lobe. The inner wall of the cavity is covered with greyish-green purulent exudate, and the abscess is enclosed in a capsule which consisted, on histological examination, of granulation tissue, fibrous tissue and reactive glial tissue. In chronic abscesses, necrosis of the wall is common, with formation of satellite lesions (lower left centre). Most temporal lobe abscesses result from extension of a chronic mastoiditis but this one followed a purulent leptomeningitis. **9.12 Acute abscess (suppurative myelitis): spinal cord.** This is part of the thoracic cord. A localised fusiform swelling is present which has been opened to show the contents of green pus. The cord segments adjacent to the abscess are discoloured from chronic meningitis. *Listeria monocytogenes* was cultured from the blood. Cord abscesses are very rare and, like cerebral abscesses, may result from arterial emboli or extension from adjacent infection, either meningitic or osteomyelitic. Direct implantation of infection following trauma or lumbar puncture may also be responsible.

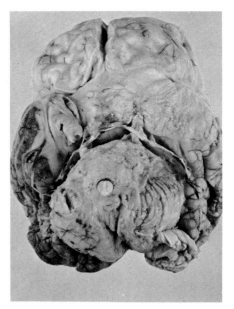

9.13 Acute purulent meningitis: brain

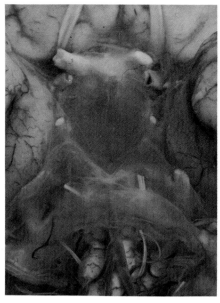

9.14 Leptomeningeal fibrosis: brain

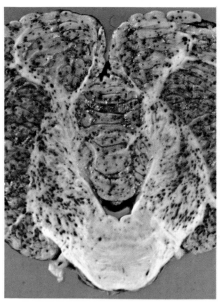

9.15 Cerebral malaria: brain

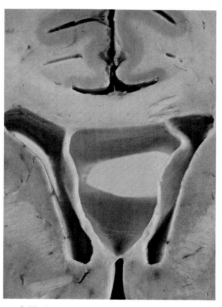

9.16 Hydrocephalus: brain

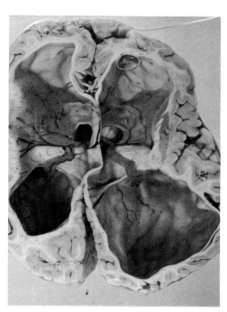

9.17 Hydrocephalus: brain

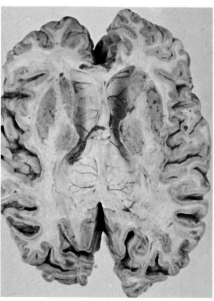

9.18 Ventricular dilatation and cortical atrophy: brain

9.13 Acute purulent meningitis: brain. This shows the undersurface of the brain of a 5-month-old boy. The surface is covered by a shaggy greyish-green purulent exudate. A recent ventriculo-atrial shunt had been inserted for obstructive internal hydrocephalus secondary to a craniopharyngioma. The organism responsible for the diffuse meningitis was *Streptoccocus pneumoniae*. In children the most common causative organisms of leptomeningitis are *Haemophilus influenzae* and *Escherichia coli*. **9.14 Leptomeningeal fibrosis: brain.** There is marked fibrotic thickening of the leptomeninges over the base of the cerebrum and brain-stem. Leptomeningeal fibrosis is frequently attributed to previous episodes of leptomeningitis in which the exudate has been organised into a fibrous scar, with post-inflammatory hydrocephalus resulting. This patient had a past history of acute meningitis. **9.15 Cerebral malaria: brain.** Cerebral malaria occurs when *Plasmodium falciparum* parasitizes large numbers of red cells, and the capillaries in the brain become blocked by agglutinated masses of parasite-containing erythrocytes. Small necrotic and haemorrhagic foci result, within the cortex of the cerebrum and cerebellum, and foci of this type are present in larger numbers in the cerebellar hemispheres and peduncles. A few are also present in the pons. **9.16 and 9.17 Hydrocephalus: brain.** The term hydrocephalus indicates dilatation of, and an increased amount of cerebrospinal fluid within, the ventricles. When the fluid increase is restricted to the ventricles, the condition is that of internal hydrocephalus. Obstruction to fluid flow is a common cause of internal hydrocephalus and the cause may be developmental or inflammatory. Ventricular dilatation is limited to that part of the brain proximal to the obstruction. **9.16** This brain shows a minimal degree of symmetrical dilatation of the lateral ventricles but the septum lucidum is split to enclose a thin-walled cavity (centre) which is sometimes referred to as the 'fifth' ventricle. The cavity of the septum lucidum does not communicate with the ventricles of the brain. The symmetrical internal hydrocephalus in this patient was caused by leptomeningeal carcinomatosis and obliteration of the foramina in the roof of the fourth ventricle. **9.17** The brain here shows gross internal hydrocephalus with marked symmetrical dilatation of the lateral ventricles and interventricular foramina, with subsequent atrophy of the periventricular white matter. **9.18 Ventricular dilatation and cortical atrophy: brain.** This is a horizontal section of the brain (weight 1090 g) of an 81-year-old woman who died from a haemorrhage from a chronic gastric ulcer. She also had ischaemic heart disease and cerebral atherosclerosis. There is marked generalised atrophy of the cortex of the senile type, with pronounced compensatory dilatation of the lateral ventricles. The gyri are greatly widened and the sulci shrunken and irregular. A few small cystic softenings are visible in the lentiform nucleus (upper right).

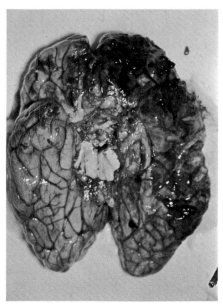

9.19 Contusions: brain

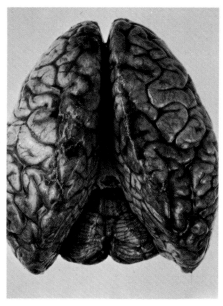

9.20 Traumatic subarachnoid
haemorrhage: brain

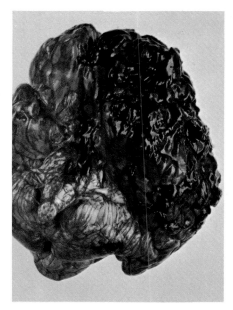

9.21 Subdural haemorrhage (subdural
haematoma): brain

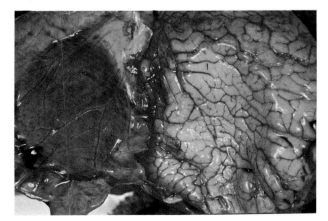

9.22 Subdural haemorrhage (subdural haematoma): brain

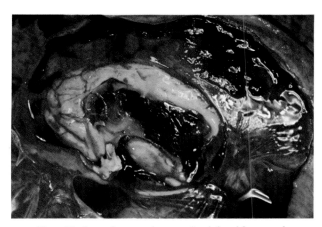

9.23 Choroid plexus haemorrhage and subdural haemorrhage:
brain

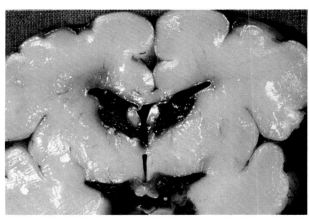

9.24 Intraventricular haemorrhage: brain

9.19 Contusions: brain. Contusions and lacerations are most commonly found at the tips and orbital portions of the frontal lobes and tips and lateral portions of the temporal lobes. Contusions of the brain are caused by blunt trauma. This patient sustained severe trauma to the left occipital region of the head which has caused extensive fronto-temporal (contre-coup) contusions and lacerations of the brain (top centre and bottom right). Contre-coup lesions occur at some distance from the impact area and are usually more extensive than the coup lesions which are at the point of impact. **9.20 Traumatic subarachnoid haemorrhage: brain.** The brain is swollen and oedematous and the superior surface of both cerebral hemispheres shows yellowish discolouration following breakdown of the extravasated blood. Multiple focal subarachnoid haemorrhages are present, particularly in the parasagittal region. The patient sustained a closed head injury 2 weeks before death. **9.21 and 9.22 Subdural haemorrhage (subdural haematoma): brain. 9.21** A massive subdural haemorrhage over the left frontal and temporo-parietal region extends over the inferior surface of the hemisphere. The cause was an extensive fracture of the skull. Most subdural haemorrhages follow blunt injury to the skull without fracture; and in the elderly especially, they may occur without a history of direct injury to the head. The usual source of bleeding is a torn vein and most lesions begin in the parasagittal region because the majority of veins that cross the subdural space do so in the vicinity of the superior sagittal sinus. **9.22** This is a chronic lesion, and organisation and encapsulation of the extravasated blood by vascular granulation tissue derived from the dura has occurred, with formation of a smooth-looking dark brown mass (left). The parietal lobe (right) which lay beneath the mass is deeply depressed as a result of pressure atrophy. When large, a chronic subdural haematoma may produce brain displacement herniations and fatal secondary brain-stem haemorrhages. **9.23 Choroid plexus haemorrhage and subdural haemorrhage: brain.** This is a sagittal section of the brain of a neonate showing the falx cerebri in situ. An extensive subdural haemorrhage is present over the convexity of the falx. Further haemorrhage is present within the choroid plexus of the lateral ventricle with extension into the third ventricle. Tentorial lacerations associated with subdural and choroidal haemorrhages commonly occur in complicated labours. **9.24 Intraventricular haemorrhage: brain.** Intraventricular haemorrhage is a frequent complication of extreme degrees of prematurity. This is a coronal section of the brain of an immature fetus. The lateral ventricles are filled with blood clot, and haemorrhage is also present over the base of the brain (lower centre) having spread there via the foramina in the roof of the fourth ventricle.

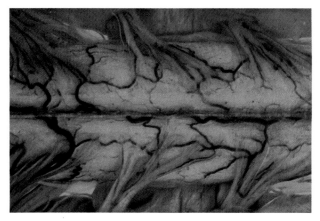

9.25 Motor neuron disease: spinal cord

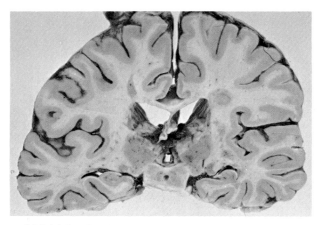

9.26 Multiple sclerosis: brain

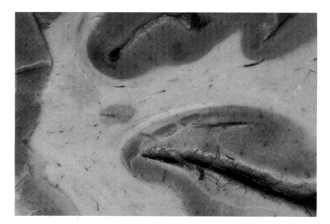

9.27 Multiple sclerosis: brain

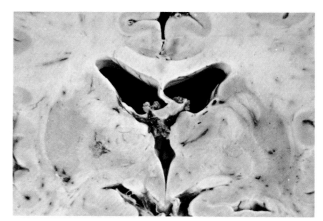

9.28 Carbon monoxide poisoning: brain

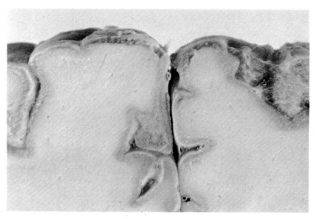

9.29 Anoxic encephalopathy: brain

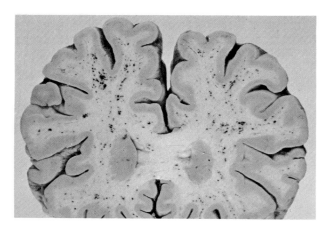

9.30 Fat embolism: brain

9.25 Motor neuron disease: spinal cord. This shows the anterior (ventral) surface of spinal cord. The anterior spinal nerve roots are atrophic and thin. Motor neuron disease primarily affects the pyramidal or motor system and the clinical syndrome depends on the motor level predominantly affected. In the form known as progressive (spinal) muscular atrophy it is the anterior horn cells which are primarily affected. The gross appearance of the spinal cord is generally not particularly helpful in making the diagnosis and a decrease in size of the ventral roots of the lumbar and cervical segments of the cord is only occasionally seen. **9.26 and 9.27 Multiple sclerosis: brain.** In this disease, foci of demyelination (plaques) are found scattered irregularly, and usually asymmetrically, throughout the grey and white matter. **9.26** In this coronal section of the brain, well-defined greyish-brown chronic plaques of demyelination are present at the upper angles of both lateral ventricles within the white matter of the centrum semiovale. One plaque (right) consists of an older central clearly-demarcated darker zone surrounded by a more recent poorly-defined and paler zone of partial demyelination ('shadow plaque'). **9.27** This is a close-up view of the subcortical white matter of a frontal lobe. A recently-formed oval pinkish-grey plaque is present beneath the cortical ribbon, with apparent sparing of the subcortical arcuate fibres. This is a characteristic site. Although multiple sclerosis plaques are more easily visualised in the white matter they can be found in the cortex and in this case three small plaques can be detected in the grey matter at the top. **9.28 Carbon**

monoxide poisoning: brain. Carbon monoxide 'poisoning' produces anoxic damage in the brain. In the early stages (1–3 days after the episode), the globus pallidus shows oedema and petechial haemorrhages. This may progress to cystic necrosis and softening, and in the later stages bilateral lesions of the globus pallidus and substantia nigra are commonly found. The cerebral cortex shows laminar necrosis with neuronal loss. In this example the damage is largely unilateral, consisting of a cystic area of softening in the left globus pallidus. **9.29 Anoxic encephalopathy: brain.** There is almost total necrosis of the grey matter over both paracentral cortices. The cortical ribbon is shrunken and yellowish-brown. There were symmetrical softenings in both basal ganglia. The patient, a 43-year-old man, suffered from tetanus and was treated by muscular paralysis and artificial respiration. An episode of cardiac arrest was followed by deep unconsciousness for some weeks prior to death. The brain was atrophic, weighing 1150 g, as a result of anoxic damage. **9.30 Fat embolism: brain.** This is a coronal section of the frontal region. Small haemorrhagic foci are scattered throughout the subcortical white matter and centrum semiovale. Microscopically each focus consists of a capillary containing fat globules surrounded by a zone of infarction and haemorrhage—focal microinfarcts. Cerebral fat embolism usually follows fractures of long bones. This patient had recently undergone operative nailing of a fractured femur, a procedure not rarely complicated by fat embolism.

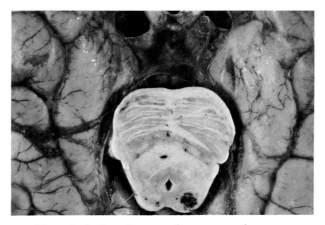

9.31 Thrombotic thrombocytopenic purpura and
microinfarcts: brain

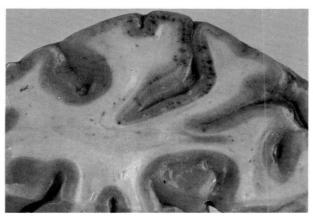

9.32 Thrombotic thrombocytopenic purpura and
microinfarcts: brain

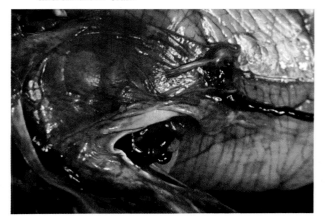

9.33 Sinus thrombosis: brain

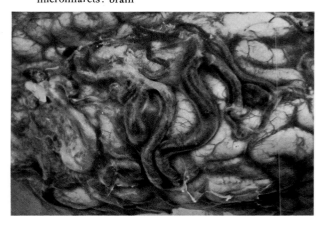

9.34 Venous angioma: brain

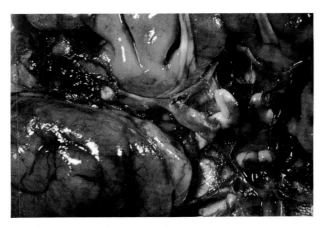

9.35 Arteriovenous hamartoma: brain

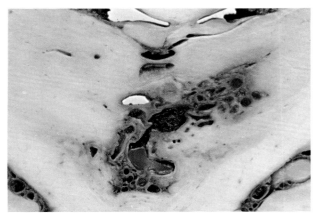

9.36 'Berry' aneurysm: middle cerebral artery

9.31 and 9.32 Thrombotic thrombocytopenic purpura and microinfarcts: brain. Thrombotic thrombocytopenic purpura is a rare condition characterised by fever, purpura, haemolytic anaemia, thrombocytopenia and bizarre cerebral symptoms. Thrombi composed of platelets and fibrin form in the small blood vessels of the brain and produce microinfarcts which are mainly confined to the grey matter. **9.31** This patient presented with epileptic fits and progressive loss of consciousness, resulting in death 12 hours after admission to hospital. Histological examination confirmed disseminated intravascular coagulation. In this transverse section of the midbrain and upper pons at the level of the inferior corpora quadrigemina, a collection of haemorrhagic microinfarcts is present in the right inferior corpus quadrigeminus. **9.32** The occipital cortex from the same patient shows crops of pin-point lesions confined to the cerebral cortex. Histologically the cortical capillaries were plugged by fibrin thrombi and surrounded by 'ball-and-ring' haemorrhages and a narrow zone of infarction. **9.33 Sinus thrombosis: brain.** This shows the posterior fossa of the skull of a neonate. The straight sinus (right) overlying the cerebellum and the left sigmoid sinus (lower centre) are both thrombosed, as is the left transverse sinus (lower left). Thrombosis of dural venous sinuses may occur alone or be associated with thrombosis of accompanying veins. Primary thrombosis may complicate dehydration, head injury or birth trauma. Secondary thrombosis results from local or remote pyogenic infections.

9.34 and 9.35 Vascular hamartoma: brain. Vascular malformations are found in about 5% of brains. The commonest are capillary telangiectases. The remainder are either arteriovenous or venous in type. The arteriovenous type is commoner in men and usually occurs in the territory of the middle cerebral artery. The pure venous type is rare. **9.34** This is an example of the venous type of angioma. It forms a complex tangle of dilated and thrombosed veins within the leptomeninges over the superior-lateral convexity of the left parietal lobe. **9.35** A large complex intracerebral arteriovenous hamartoma is present within the thalamus and basal ganglia. The greyish-white vessels are thick-walled and many are thrombosed. The adjacent brain (upper right) contains much brown haemosiderin as a result of previous haemorrhages. The hamartoma communicated with dilated vessels in the Sylvian fissure (lower right) which had bled and caused the patient to present on a number of occasions with evidence of subarachnoid haemorrhage. **9.36 'Berry' aneurysm: middle cerebral artery.** A saccular aneurysm (0.5 cm diameter) is situated on the trifurcation of the right middle cerebral artery within the Sylvian fissure. It has a greyish-white wall. The aneurysm has leaked, causing subarachnoid haemorrhage. Berry aneurysms are usually sited at points of branching. About 60% are located on the anterior portion of the circle of Willis, and are the commonest type of aneurysm of the circle of Willis, being found in about 5% of adults. They are commoner in females and in about 30% of cases are multiple.

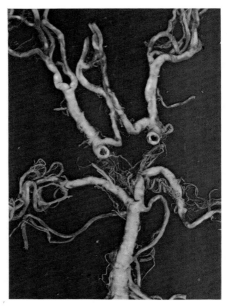

9.37 Atherosclerosis: cerebral arteries

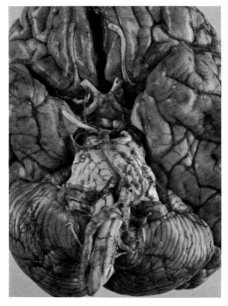

9.38 Atherosclerosis: basilar artery

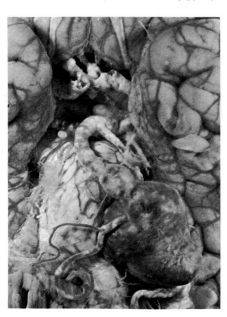

9.39 Aneurysm: basilar artery

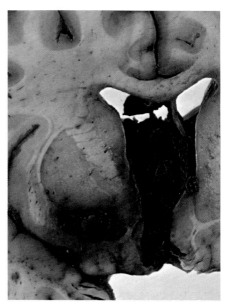

9.40 Subarachnoid haemorrhage: brain

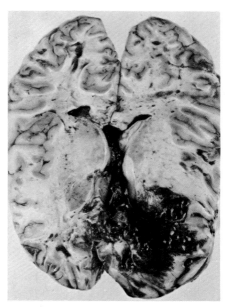

9.41 Intracerebral haemorrhage: brain

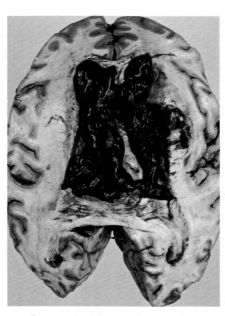

9.42 Intracerebral haemorrhage: brain

9.37 and 9.38 Atherosclerosis: cerebral arteries. 9.37 The basilar artery (bottom) and the vessels of the circle of Willis are thick-walled and yellow. The lesions are nodular but confluent in many parts. The cut ends of the internal carotid arteries (centre) show some narrowing of the lumen. The intracranial and extracranial arteries are often affected by atherosclerosis but in general the lesions develop at a later age than atherosclerosis of the coronary arteries. **9.38** The basilar artery (lower centre) is dilated and tortuous with yellowish-white nodular atherosclerotic lesions along its length. The terminal portion of the left vertebral artery is also severely atherosclerotic. Vertebro-basilar atherosclerosis is an important cause of cerebral ischaemia in the elderly and clinically may cause 'drop-attacks' due to transient episodes of brain-stem ischaemia. **9.39 Aneurysm: basilar artery.** Severe atherosclerosis may cause aneurysmal dilatation, fusiform or saccular, of the basilar artery. Thrombosis and calcification often occur but rupture is rare. This shows a large bluish-black part-fusiform and part-saccular aneurysm of the first part of the artery. The vessel rostral to the aneurysm is dilated and tortuous and scattered yellow atherosclerotic plaques are present. **9.40 Subarachnoid haemorrhage: brain.** About 80% of cases of subarachnoid haemorrhage follow rupture of a 'berry' aneurysm. This is a coronal section of the brain. Bleeding has occurred into the left Sylvian fissure

with massive extension into the third and lateral ventricles. There is also a recent haematoma in the left basal ganglia. Extension of the haemorrhage into the adjacent ventricles and brain is a frequent occurrence in subarachnoid haemorrhage. The two common sites for intracerebral haemorrhage are frontal and temporal, from aneurysms in the region of the anterior communicating artery or the middle cerebral artery in the Sylvian fissure (see 9.36). **9.41 to 9.44 Intracerebral haemorrhage: brain.** Massive intracerebral haemorrhage is a common cause of death in patients with uncontrolled systemic hypertension. About 70% of the haemorrhages are located in the cerebral hemispheres. The brain surrounding the haemorrhage is usually swollen and oedematous. **9.41** A large recent haemorrhage is present in the occipital pole of the right cerebral hemisphere. There is also blood clot within the lateral ventricles and scattered petechial haemorrhages in the opposite occipital pole. **9.42** In this example, the haemorrhage has ruptured into the ventricles, and both lateral ventricles are filled with soft gelatinous clot resembling red-current jelly. There is also a ragged haemorrhage in the region of the right lentiform nucleus (top centre). Intraventricular extension is a common event in hypertensive-type intracerebral haemorrhage. Minor initial intraventricular bleeding may be followed by tracking of the blood through the foramina of the fourth ventricle into the subarachnoid space.

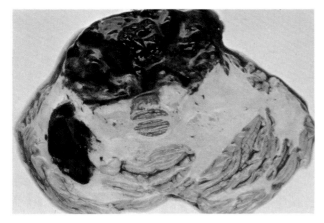

9.43 Intracerebral haemorrhage: brain

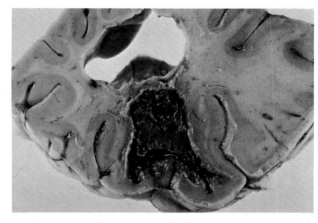

9.44 Intracerebral haemorrhage: brain

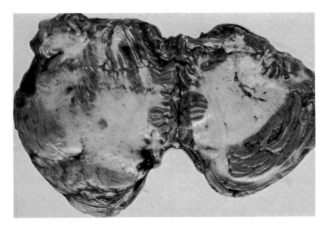

9.45 Infarction: brain

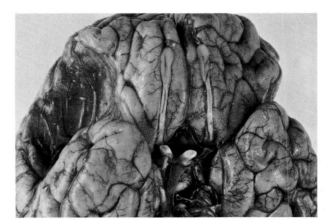

9.46 Infarction: brain

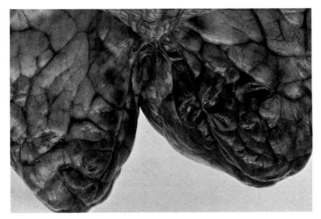

9.47 Infarction: brain

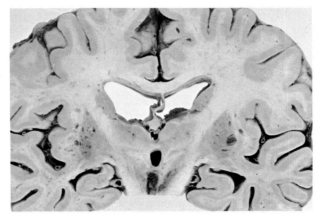

9.48 Infarction: brain

9.43 and 9.44 Intracerebral haemorrhage: brain. 9.43 About 20% of hypertensive haemorrhages are located in the deep white matter of the cerebellar hemispheres and 10% in the pons and midbrain. A massive recent haemorrhage has largely destroyed the pons, and another is present in the central white matter of the right cerebellar hemisphere. Massive haemorrhage (greater than 1.5 cm) into the cerebellum or pons and midbrain is almost always rapidly fatal. **9.44** This coronal section of the occipital lobe of one cerebral hemisphere shows a partly-organised old haemorrhage. The pale grey-brown haematoma has retracted from the surrounding brain. Astrocytic proliferation has occurred with formation of a glial reaction around the haemorrhage; and the thick capsule and the adjacent brain are stained golden-brown by breakdown products of haemoglobin. **9.45-9.48 Infarction: brain.** If a cerebral artery is suddenly occluded by thrombosis or by an embolus, an infarct is produced. **9.45** This is a recent infarct of cerebellum. One hemisphere (left) is infarcted. It is swollen compared with the normal hemisphere on the right. It is also paler than normal and the distinction between grey and white matter is indistinct. Two areas of haemorrhagic infarction are present in the cortex. **9.46** In large infarcts the quantity of necrotic tissue produced is considerable. The process of removing the dead material

proceeds from the periphery, and the end-stage is often a large 'cavity' which may be collapsed or filled with clear fluid. In this case a large depressed cavity is present over the inferior aspect of the right fronto-temporal region (left). The cavity is covered by a thin, brown-coloured membrane. This infarct was caused by an embolus in the middle cerebral artery. The patient had chronic rheumatic heart disease and the source of the embolus was thrombus in the left atrium. **9.47** This shows recent haemorrhagic infarction of the infero-medial aspects of both occipital lobes, especially affecting the calcarine area. Ischaemic lesions in the occipital lobes are commonly associated with supratentorial space-occupying lesions. The lesions are brought about by obstruction of the posterior cerebral arteries following tentorial herniation, and they are often confined to the distribution of the calcarine branches of the posterior cerebral artery. **9.48** In widespread atherosclerosis and hypertension, small irregular cystic softenings are often present in the brain, especially in the caudate nucleus and putamen. They are often called apoplectic cysts. In this example, multiple small brownish cystic lesions are present in the pallida, external capsules and claustra in both sides of the brain. The brain itself is atrophic, with dilated ventricles and widened sulci (note especially the temporal lobes).

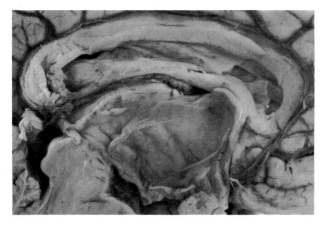

9.49 Suprasellar epidermoid cyst (craniopharyngioma): brain

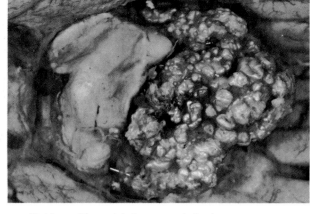

9.50 Epidermoid cyst (cholesteatoma): brain

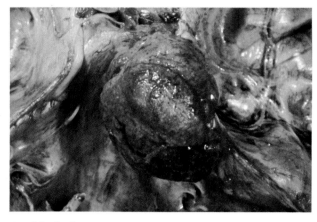

9.51 Meningioma

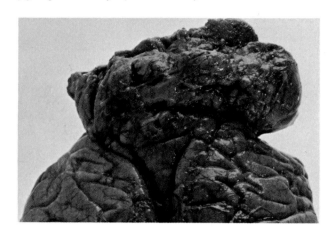

9.52 Meningioma

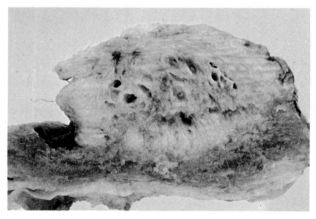

9.53 Meningioma

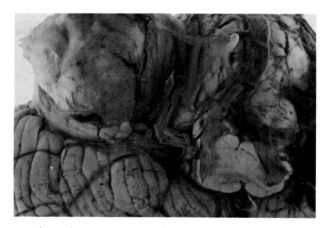

9.54 Acoustic nerve tumour (schwannoma): brain

9.49 Suprasellar epidermoid cyst (craniopharyngioma): brain. This lesion arises from small nests of squamous epithelium commonly found around the pituitary stalk. A thin-walled cyst projects upwards into the cavity of the third ventricle and forwards to compress the optic chiasma. It is customary to separate cystic or partly cystic tumours of the type shown here which are anatomically related to the pituitary gland from epidermoid cysts (see 9.50), although structurally they are closely affiliated. **9.50 Epidermoid cyst (cholesteatoma): brain.** A nodular mass is displacing the pons. It has the striking mother-of-pearl sheen ('pearly tumour') typical of this type of lesion. The appearance is caused by the presence of abundant cholesterol, in addition to keratinous material. Epidermoid cysts are usually sited in the cerebello-pontine angle but can occur in other sites. They vary in size but are invariably circumscribed, with a smooth nodular capsule. Dermoid cysts are rarer than epidermoids and tend to be found in the mid-line. Both types of cysts are thought to arise from ectodermal inclusions formed during closure of the neural groove. **9.51-9.53 Meningioma.** Meningiomas account for about 15% of all intracranial primary tumours. They are usually detected in middle age and are more common in women. Within the cranial cavity about 50% are situated near the sagittal sinus and tend to be located in the anterior half of the cranial cavity. **9.51** A large smooth lobulated pinkish-red tumour is situated at the clivus immediately posterior to the dorsum sellae. The cut surface of the lesion had a characteristic tough whorled pattern. **9.52** This is an example of the syncytial type of meningioma. A large oval lobulated partly necrotic tumour is situated over both frontal lobes. It has arisen from the parasagittal region between the hemispheres. **9.53** Some meningiomas erode bone and cause hyperostosis. The flattened 'meningioma-en-plaque' is especially prone to behave like this but involvement of the cranium is not confined to this type. Hyperostosis and/or bone erosion may be seen with the more classical forms of growth. This shows a section of an oval yellowish-white meningioma containing cystic cavities. Its base is eroding the underlying cranium to a depth of 2.5 cm. This form of meningioma is benign though it may invade dural sinuses and bone by direct spread. A few develop malignant characteristics. **9.54 and 9.55 Acoustic nerve tumour (schwannoma): brain.** Schwannomas are usually solitary. They arise on the cranial and spinal nerves as well as on peripheral nerves. The auditory nerve is most commonly involved. It is a lesion of middle life. Typically the tumour is encapsulated, firm and grey-white and attached to the cranial nerve which is stretched over it. The larger tumours often have an irregular lobulated surface with yellow, softened and sometimes haemorrhagic areas internally. **9.54** This shows, in close-up, a large yellowish-white lobulated spherical schwannoma which has arisen from the right auditory nerve and is lying within the cerebello-pontine angle.

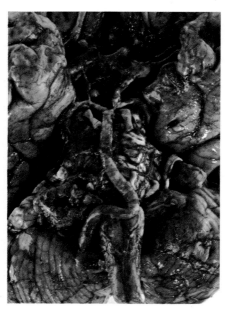

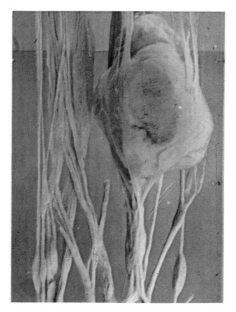

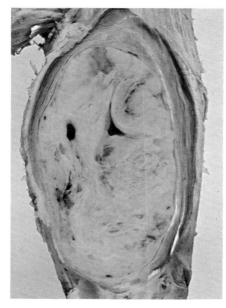

9.55 Acoustic nerve tumour (schwannoma): brain

9.56 Neurofibroma: cauda equina.

9.57 Neurofibrosarcoma

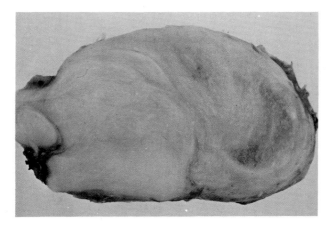

9.58 Ganglioneuroma: mediastinum

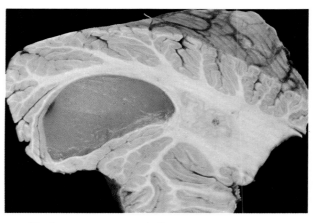

9.59 Cystic astrocytoma: cerebellum

9.55 Acoustic nerve tumour (schwannoma): brain. A small flat umbilicated pinkish tumour arising from the right auditory nerve is located within the cerebello-pontine angle. **9.56 Neurofibroma: cauda equina.** Neurofibromas are derived from the schwann cell but differ from schwannomas in texture, shape and the presence of a loose connective tissue stroma. The lesions are usually multiple (von Recklinghausen's neurofibromatosis) and the involved nerves display an irregular cylindrical or fusiform enlargement (plexiform neurofibroma). In this case a large ovoid lobulated neurofibroma has arisen from the nerve sheaths of the cauda. Several thickened nerves blend with the capsule of the tumour. Many of the other nerves show small fusiform swellings (lower right). **9.57 Neurofibrosarcoma.** The tumour is a large part-white and part-yellow mass, with areas of haemorrhage and cystic necrosis. It has a pseudocapsule of compressed muscle and was situated close to the knee-joint. Large neurofibromas of the peripheral nerves occasionally become malignant. The incidence of malignant change is not known but when the change does occur it is always in association with von Recklinghausen's disease. **9.58 Ganglioneuroma: mediastinum.** Ganglioneuroma is a benign tumour commonly found in the posterior mediastinum. It is derived from ganglion cells of the peripheral nervous system with a supporting schwann cell and connective tissue cell component. It is usually a large firm, well-circumscribed spherical or elliptical lobulated tumour. Growth is typically slow. The cut surface of this one has a uniform fibrous texture with a greyish-white and slightly yellowish tint and a semi-translucent ill-defined whorled pattern. A crescent-shaped area of cystic degeneration is present (right). **9.59-9.64 Astrocytoma: brain. 9.59** This is a cystic astrocytoma of the cerebellum. It occupies the lateral lobe of the cerebellar hemisphere and takes the form of a crescentic cystic cavity filled with gelatinous pale green fluid. The fluid had a high content of protein. Astrocytoma of the cerebellum is predominantly a tumour of children and young adults. It is slow-growing

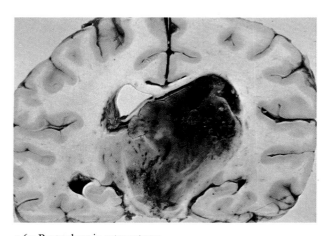

9.60 Protoplasmic astrocytoma

and frequently cystic. Involvement of the cerebral hemispheres is more common in the adult. In large cystic tumours, the cyst is fringed by soft gelatinous tumour. Histologically it is usually a pilocytic astrocytoma showing extensive spongy change. **9.60** This is a protoplasmic astro-cytoma. In this coronal section of brain it forms a large pale grey gelatinous mass with much old and recent brownish haemorrhage. Arising from the region of the third ventricle, it has extended into the thalamus and basal ganglia and upwards into the subependymal region of the right lateral ventricle. This variety of astrocytoma in its pure form is rarer than the other types and is usually located in the cerebrum. Degenerative changes are common.

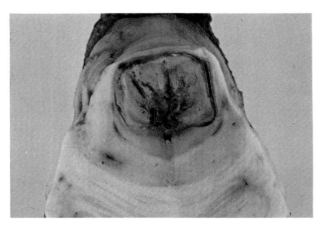

9.61 Protoplasmic astrocytoma

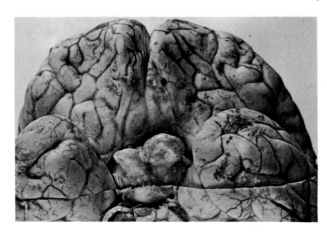

9.62 Pilocytic astrocytoma

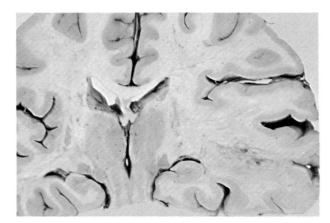

9.63 Fibrillary astrocytoma

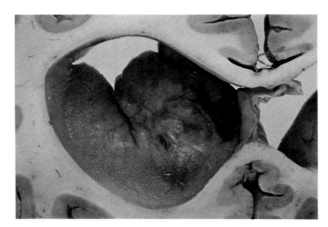

9.64 Giant-cell astrocytoma

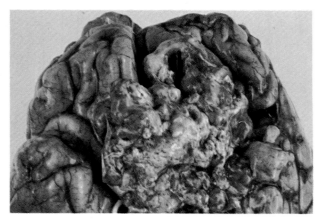

9.65 Spongioblastoma polare

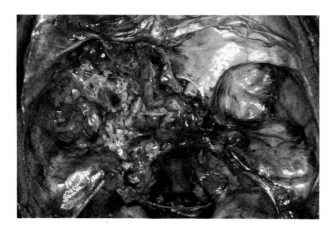

9.66 Spongioblastoma polare

9.61-9.64 Astrocytoma: brain. 9.61 Protoplasmic astrocytomas often invade the leptomeninges and may spread caudally to involve the ependyma of the fourth ventricle and into the spinal canal. This is a view of the pons from the case shown in 9.60. The greyish gelatinous tumour has grown into the fourth ventricle and is expanding the ventral portion. The patient was a 46-year-old woman. **9.62** This is a pilocytic astrocytoma. This type of astrocytoma is usually located in the region of the hypothalamus, third ventricle, optic chiasma or cerebellum. The nodular greyish-white neoplasm is situated in the optic chiasma. Histologically two types of pilocytic astrocytoma are recognised: one consisting of closely-packed interwoven bundles of broad bipolar fibrillated cells, the 'adult' type; and the other, termed 'juvenile' because it is essentially a growth of young subjects, consisting of cells which are morphologically simple. **9.63** This is a fibrillary astrocytoma. It is a common form of astrocytoma which particularly involves the cerebral hemispheres in adults, has a firm tough rubbery consistence, and the colour of which is such that it is often difficult to distinguish the lesion from adjacent white matter. The tumour cells contain large numbers of fine and coarse neuroglial fibrils. This lesion is a diffuse white mass which is expanding the right temporal lobe. The adjacent temporal cortex is pale and its demarcation from the subjacent white matter is blurred (compare the left temporal lobe). Central areas of cystic degeneration are present. **9.64**

This is a subependymal giant-cell astrocytoma, a tumour typically and frequently associated with tuberose sclerosis. It forms a mass in the wall of the lateral ventricles. A lesion of this size is prone to cause obstruction. Histologically the neoplasm contained many large fusiform or pyramidal cells among which there were giant bizarre forms. Most authorities regard this type of lesion, which differs from other astrocytomas in being benign, as being an astrocytoma or spongioblastoma, and its frequent association with tuberose sclerosis suggests an origin from the giant astrocytes found in this syndrome. The patient here was a boy of 10 years. **9.65 and 9.66 Spongioblastoma polare.** Confusion exists over this rare type of glioma, some regarding it as a pilocytic astrocytoma. So-called true polar spongioblastoma is a rare malignant growth occurring in children and young adults and often arising in the third ventricle, optic tracts or midbrain. It frequently spreads widely in the meninges to produce thick sheets of soft growth over the base of the brain and spinal cord. **9.65** This example forms a large irregular yellow mass which is extensively infiltrating the optic chiasma, hypothalamus and third ventricle and inferior surface of the left frontal lobe. **9.66** This shows the base of the skull from the previous case. Necrotic yellow tumour is invading the left sphenoid bone and floor of the middle cranial fossa, with extension into the left orbital cavity.

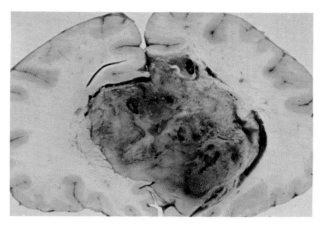

9.67 Glioblastoma multiforme

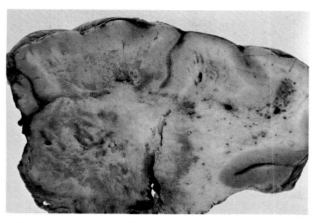

9.68 Mixed sarcoma and glioma

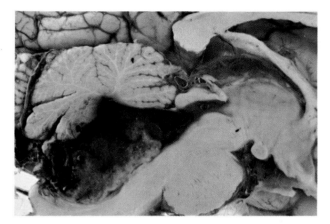

9.69 Ependymona: brain

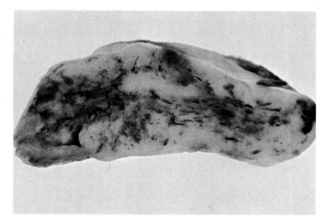

9.70 Ependymona: spinal cord

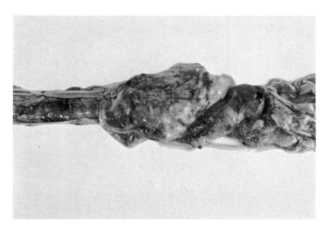

9.71 Metastatic ependymoma: spinal cord

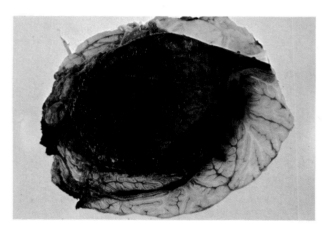

9.72 Medulloblastoma

9.67 Glioblastoma multiforme. This highly malignant tumour constitutes 50–60% of all gliomas. It is more common in older adult subjects. Arising typically in the cerebral hemispheres, it often extends into and across the corpus callosum into the opposite hemisphere (the so-called butterfly glioma). These features are seen in this coronal section of the brain. A massive tumour is infiltrating the corpus callosum and both cerebral hemispheres. The surface of the tumour has a variegated yellow-white (necrotic) and reddish-brown (haemorrhagic) appearance. **9.68 Mixed sarcoma and glioma.** This is a coronal section of the frontal lobe. A yellowish-white tumour, with areas of brownish discolouration, focal haemorrhages and cystic change, has replaced most of the left lobe and has burst through the parietal cortex (lower left) to the meningeal surface. Histologically the tumour was a glioblastoma with a sarcomatous component. A mixed sarcomatous and glioblastomatous pattern is a rare but well-recognised form of lesion to which the term gliosarcoma is sometimes applied. **9.69–9.71 Ependymoma.** Ependymomas account for 5% of all intracranial gliomas and 60% of them arise in the posterior fossa. Tumours of the 4th ventricle, which are predominantly tumours of childhood and adolescence, are usually solid and may arise from the ependymal cells, the choroid plexus or subependymal cells. **9.69** This is a sagittal section of cerebellum, brain-stem and posterior cerebral hemisphere. The fourth ventricle is occluded by a necrotic haemorrhagic red-brown tumour arising from the medulla, and obstructed internal hydrocephalus is present as shown by the dilated lateral ventricle (top right). The tumour is a subependymoma (subendymal glioma) a type of ependymoma in which fibrillary subependymal astrocytes are prominent. **9.70** Ependymomas predominate amongst the gliomas of the spinal cord and filum, and intramedullary ependymoma of the spinal cord is often well-circumscribed. The neoplasm arises from the cells lining the central canal or remnants of it, or from the cells of the ventriculus terminale of the filum terminale. This shows a small portion of the filum (bottom left) and an oval creamy yellow tumour, the cut surface of which shows recent haemorrhage, is present. Microscopically the tumour was a myxo-papillary ependymoma. **9.71** Irregular yellowish-white nodules of tumour are present in the cauda equina and lower lumbosacral cord, and there are small discrete deposits on the surface of the cord (left). This is not a primary growth arising in the cord, however, but metastases from a malignant ependymoma of the fourth ventricle. Though ependymomas are notably benign, malignant change occurs in about 5%. Evidence of subarachnoid spread with spinal seedlings is seen in some tumours of the fourth ventricle, especially if the cisterna magna is infiltrated or following surgical intervention. **9.72 Medulloblastoma.** Medulloblastoma is a malignant tumour of the cerebellum. It occurs predominantly in children aged 5 to 8 years and is commoner in boys. It is usually a soft friable mass with a tendency to haemorrhage and necrosis. This example is a large rounded fairly well-demarcated necrotic haemorrhagic red-brown lesion which is expanding the cerebellar hemisphere. There is often spread to the fourth ventricle and metastasis may take place via the ventricles and subarachnoid space, particularly in the region of the cauda equina.

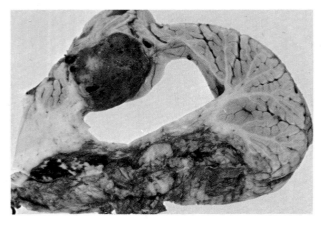

9.73 Haemangioblastoma: cerebellum

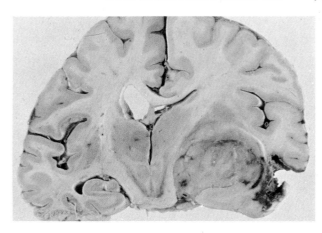

9.74 Microgliomatosis: brain

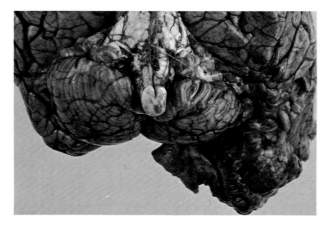

9.75 Secondary carcinoma: brain

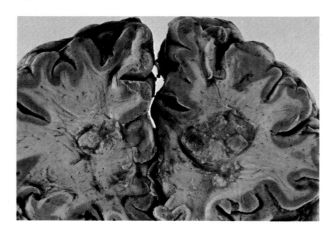

9.76 Secondary carcinoma: brain

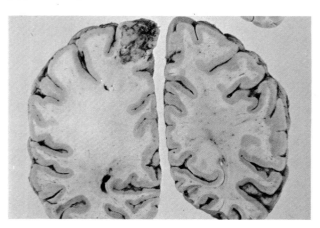

9.77 Secondary carcinoma: brain

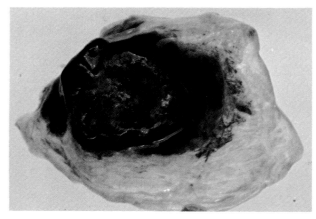

9.78 Secondary carcinoma: brain

9.73 Haemangioblastoma: cerebellum. Haemangioblastomas are usually benign and are typically located in the cerebellum. In this case a large cavity fills the lateral lobe of the cerebellum, and a round nodule of red-brown tumour (top) is present in the wall of the cyst. Small cysts are also present within the nodule. A further diffuse mass of necrotic growth in the adjacent cyst wall (bottom) shows brownish discolouration. Histologically the tumour was composed of fine capillary channels interspersed with clear lipid-laden stromal cells. Haemangioblastomas account for between 1 and 2% of all intracranial tumours. Some are associated with the von Hippel-Lindau syndrome or polycythaemia.
9.74 Microgliomatosis: brain. Microgliomatosis is a rare tumour of the phagocytic microglial cell which usually involves the cerebrum and may be multifocal. It is generally a lesion of elderly subjects. The usual form is a pinkish-grey, granular mass which tends to blur the normal anatomical markings. This one is greyish-white and is destroying the right temporal lobe and extending into the basal ganglia and lentiform nucleus. **9.75–9.80 Secondary carcinoma: brain and spinal cord.** It has been estimated that metastatic tumours form up to 30% of all intracranial tumours, carcinomas being by far the commonest. In about half the cases in the United Kingdom, the primary is a bronchial carcinoma. The secondary deposits usually appear circumscribed and spheroidal and are often attached to the dura. The smallest deposits are often located

near the junction of cortex and white matter. **9.75** This patient had a squamous carcinoma of bronchus which has given rise to a large secondary deposit in the left occipital pole (lower right). A portion of dura and falx is attached to the mass. The brain is swollen and the gyri of the left hemisphere are flattened. **9.76** This coronal section of the frontal region shows large necrotic secondary deposits in the central white matter of both cerebral hemispheres. Multiple small haemorrhagic deposits are also present in the cortex of both parietal lobes. The primary was in the breast. After bronchus, breast carcinoma is the next commonest primary tumour, other sites being kidney, skin (melanoma), gastrointestinal tract and prostate. **9.77** A feature here is the severe oedema of the affected part of the brain. A necrotic pinkish-grey secondary deposit is situated in the parasagittal region of the left frontal lobe and the cerebral hemisphere on that side is markedly swollen. Oedema of the white matter in the vicinity of a secondary deposit is often disproportionately great in comparison with the small size of the lesion and may affect the tissues some distance away from the tumour. **9.78** A large lobulated reddish-brown secondary deposit is present in the pons. The tumour has undergone necrosis and haemorrhage which proved rapidly fatal. The patient had a primary squamous carcinoma of bronchus which had disseminated widely by the bloodstream.

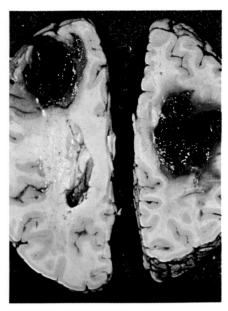

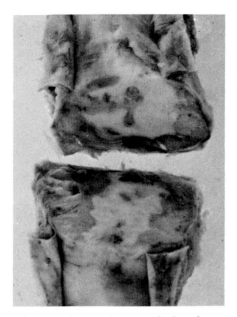

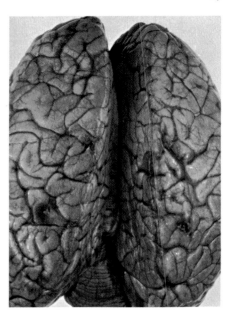

9.79 Secondary choriocarcinoma: brain   9.80 Secondary carcinoma: spinal cord   9.81 Swelling and oedema: brain

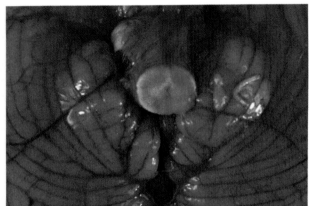

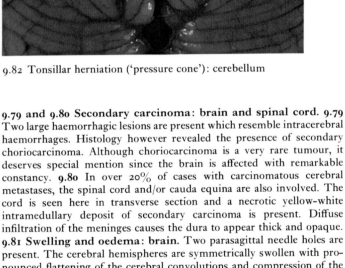

9.82 Tonsillar herniation ('pressure cone'): cerebellum

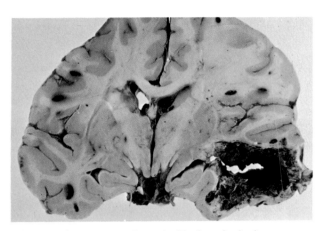

9.83 Lymphosarcoma and terminal leukaemia: brain

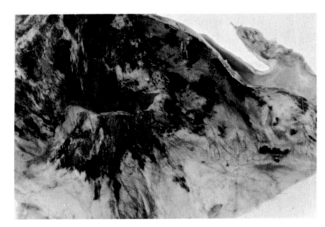

9.84 Malignant melanoma: dura

9.79 and 9.80 Secondary carcinoma: brain and spinal cord. 9.79
Two large haemorrhagic lesions are present which resemble intracerebral
haemorrhages. Histology however revealed the presence of secondary
choriocarcinoma. Although choriocarcinoma is a very rare tumour, it
deserves special mention since the brain is affected with remarkable
constancy. **9.80** In over 20% of cases with carcinomatous cerebral
metastases, the spinal cord and/or cauda equina are also involved. The
cord is seen here in transverse section and a necrotic yellow-white
intramedullary deposit of secondary carcinoma is present. Diffuse
infiltration of the meninges causes the dura to appear thick and opaque.
9.81 Swelling and oedema: brain. Two parasagittal needle holes are
present. The cerebral hemispheres are symmetrically swollen with pronounced flattening of the cerebral convolutions and compression of the
sulci. The brain swelling was due to obstructed internal hydrocephalus
and cerebral oedema, produced by a subependymal giant-cell astrocytoma.
Tentorial herniation has also occurred, with compression of the posterior
cerebral arteries and infarction of both occipital lobes. **9.82 Tonsillar
herniation ('pressure cone'): cerebellum.** The cerebellum is deeply
grooved, forming a well-marked 'pressure cone'. This has been caused by
the margins of the foramen magnum pressing on the cerebellar tonsils
displaced downwards through the foramen. The degree of impaction may
be so severe that the tips of the tonsils become necrotic. Compression of
the medulla may also occur and cause death. **9.83 Lymphosarcoma and
terminal leukaemia: brain.** There is a ragged haemorrhagic cavity in
the right temporal lobe and many small dark brown haemorrhagic
deposits of tumour are scattered throughout the subcortical white matter
of both hemispheres. Microscopy revealed the presence of lymphosarcoma.

The central white matter is swollen and the brain displaced and elongated.
The patient, who suffered from lymphosarcoma, developed a terminal
lymphocytic leukaemia. Meningeal infiltration occurs in 30% of cases of
acute leukaemia. **9.84 Malignant melanoma: dura.** The dura is
extensively infiltrated by black metastatic melanoma. The patient, a
61-year-old man, had a large congenital naevus over the occipital region
of the scalp and neck, and malignant melanoma arose at this site 9 years
prior to death. At necropsy widely-disseminated melanoma was found.

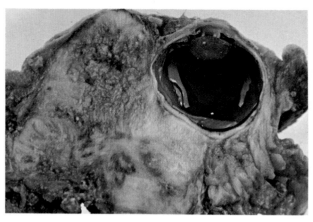

9.85 Histiocytic lymphoma: orbit

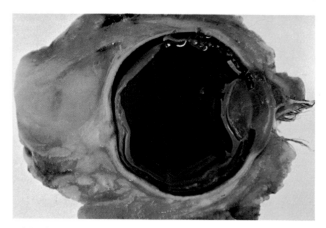

9.86 Rhabdomyosarcoma: orbit

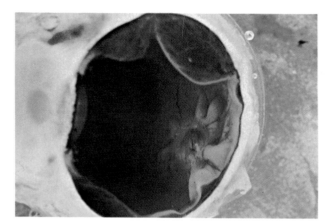

9.87 Haemangioma of retina: eye

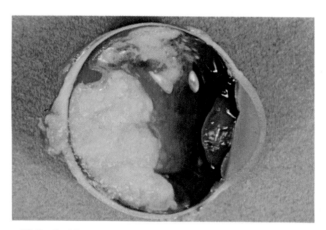

9.88 Retinoblastoma: eye

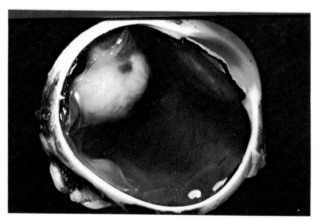

9.89 Melanoma of choroid: eye

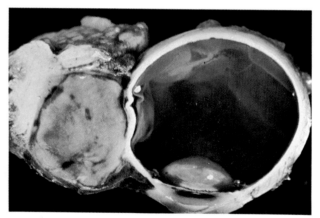

9.90 Melanoma of choroid: eye

9.85 Histiocytic lymphoma (reticulum cell sarcoma): orbit.
Orbital tumours mainly comprise lymphomas and lymphoid hyperplasias
(20%), inflammatory pseudotumours (30%), and epithelial tumours of
the lachrymal gland (50%). This lymphomatous lesion consisted of sheets
of undifferentiated cells resembling histiocytes. It forms a variegated
necrotic pinkish-brown mass which is expanding the orbital cavity widely.
9.86 Rhabdomyosarcoma: orbit. The retro-orbital tissues are
infiltrated by a pale yellowish-white tumour which is displacing the
extra-ocular muscles and partially encircling the globe. Rhabdomyosarcoma is probably the commonest primary malignant mesenchymal orbital
tumour in children. It is usually of the embryonal type, growing rapidly
and frequently disseminating by the blood stream. The prognosis is very
poor. The patient here was a 2-year-old girl. **9.87 Haemangioma of
retina (von Hippel-Lindau's disease): eye.** This shows a round
brown-coloured cystic angioma (3 mm diameter) of the retina situated
close to the macula (left). Microscopy of the retina showed microcystic
degeneration. The patient, a man of 59, presented with loss of vision in
the right eye. Benign capillary haemangioblastoma of the cerebellum is
sometimes associated with Lindau's syndrome, a condition in which
angiomatosis retinae (von Hippel's disease) is associated with non-
neoplastic congenital cysts of the pancreas and kidneys and tumours of
the kidneys and adrenals. This syndrome is familial and inherited on a
genetic basis. **9.88 Retinoblastoma: eye.** The vitreous is extremely
infiltrated by a gelatinous greyish-white mass and there is extra-ocular

extension down the optic nerve (left). Retinoblastoma is a malignant
anaplastic tumour of the retinal cells which affects young children almost
exclusively and is often present at birth. Some cases are genetically
determined and both eyes may be affected. Invasion of the optic nerve,
with intracranial spread, is common. **9.89 and 9.90 Melanoma of
choroid: eye.** Malignant melanoma of the uvea is the most common of
all intra-ocular tumours. It tends to be slow-growing and late in spreading
and has a much better prognosis than malignant melanoma of the skin.
The following are two examples of malignant melanoma of the choroid.
8.89 A white non-pigmented tumour measuring 1.2 x 1.3 cm is situated
near the equator of the eye and it bulges into the vitreous over a distance
of 1.1 cm. This type of melanoma typically grows towards the vitreous
producing first an elevation and then a retinal detachment. An inferior
retinal detachment was present here. The patient, a 48-year-old woman,
presented with myopia and flashes of light for 3 weeks. **9.90** In this
example a small well-encapsulated melanoma is present in the nasal and
inferior aspects of the left eye in an 85-year-old man. The intra-ocular
lesion is small. A large extra-ocular extension of largely necrotic yellowish-
white tumour (left) is present. It is probable that this tumour arose from
a pre-existing naevus. Melanomas arising in the choroid and ciliary body
often attain a large size before detection. The 10-year survival following
removal of the eye is 60%. The spindle cell variant has an 80% 10-year
survival.

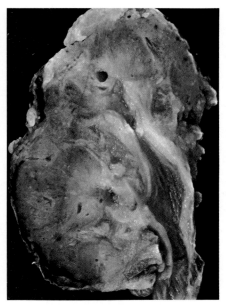

10.1 Focal dysplasia: kidney

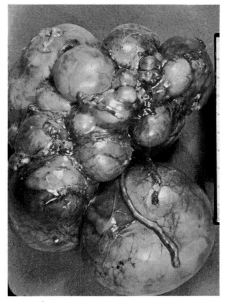

10.2 Dysplasia: kidney

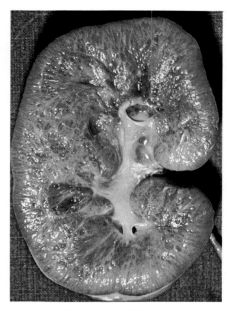

10.3 Infantile polycystic kidneys

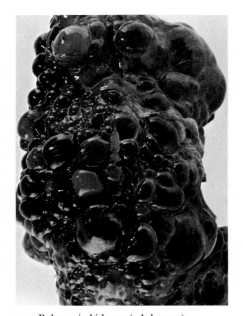

10.4 Polycystic kidneys (adult type)

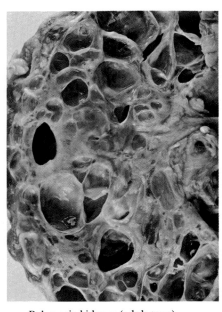

10.5 Polycystic kidneys (adult type)

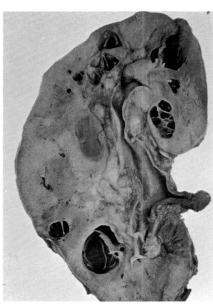

10.6 Medullary cystic disease: kidney

10.1 and 10.2 Dysplasia: kidney. Renal dysplasia is a disturbed differentiation of nephrogenic tissue, with persistence of primitive structures inappropriate to the age of the patient. The lesion may be unilateral or bilateral, and within the kidney it may be total, segmental or focal. **10.1** This shrunken distorted kidney (measuring 4 x 2 x 0.5 cm) is an example of focal dysplasia. Histology showed small cysts lined by cuboidal epithelium and dilated ducts and tubules surrounded by primitive mesenchymal tissue. It is a very rare anomaly. **10.2** This is a unilateral lesion (multi-cystic type). The kidney consists of a disorderly mass of cysts which resembles a bunch of grapes. The size of the cysts varies from a few mm to several cm (lower right). No normal parenchyma is recognisable between the white fibrous tissue septa. The calyces and pelvis are absent. The ureter is hypoplastic. Unilateral renal dysplasia is the commonest cystic disorder of the kidneys in newborn and young children. It affects both sexes equally. **10.3-10.6 Polycystic kidneys.** **10.3** This is an example of infantile polycystic kidneys (type I), a bilateral defect which is found only in newborn infants and which is incompatible with life. The kidney is enlarged and its cut surface is sponge-like from the presence of large numbers of small cysts which are located predominantly in the medulla. The cysts are saccular or cylindrically enlarged collecting tubules, apparently formed as a result of hyperplasia of the interstitial portions of the collecting tubules which develop from the ureteral buds. **10.4** This shows the adult type of polycystic kidney (type III) which is usually bilateral and is the common form in adults. The incidence of the

condition is about 1 in 500 necropsies. The organ is very large and apparently consists of numerous small and large cysts bulging through the capsule. The dark bluish-black cysts contain altered blood and the lighter ones urine. Histologically there was an irregular mixture of normal and abnormal tubules and nephrons, the cysts being derived from collecting tubules, proximal tubules and Bowman's capsule. The enlargement of the kidneys may reach massive proportions in cases presenting in middle age. In advanced cases progressive chronic renal failure ensues. In some cases there are also cysts in the liver and pancreas. There is often a family history and the mode of inheritance is thought to be dominant with variable expression. **10.5** This shows the cut surface of an adult (type III) polycystic kidney. Distortion and destruction of the renal parenchyma by the many large and small cysts is extreme. Some cysts appear to be multilocular and most have thin fibrous walls. Connective tissue is increased between the cysts. **10.6 Medullary cystic disease: kidney.** Medullary cystic disease is related to polycystic disease and two forms are recognised, medullary sponge kidney and uraemic medullary cystic disease. This is an example of the former. Scattered large and small multilocular cysts are present in the medulla or junctional region. Medullary sponge kidney is a benign asymptomatic cystic dilatation of collecting ducts of the renal medulla. It may be an incidental X-ray finding in adults, especially if associated with calculus formation. In contrast, uraemic medullary cystic disease is a fatal condition of children.

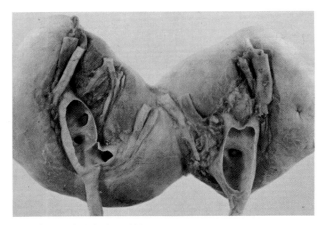

10.7 Congenital fusion: kidneys

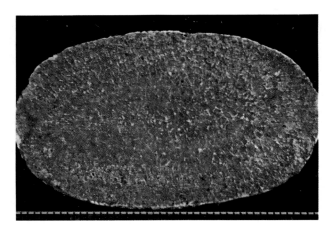

10.8 Cystine calculus

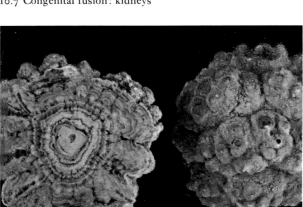

10.9 Oxalate calculus

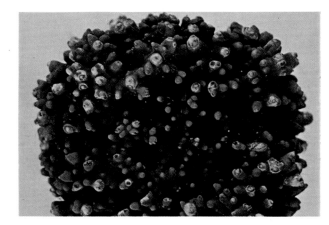

10.10 Oxalate calculus

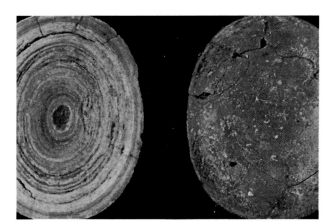

10.11 Uric acid calculus

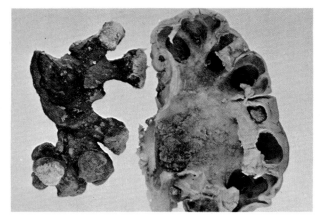

10.12 Phosphate calculus

10.7 Congenital fusion: kidneys. In congenital fusion of the kidneys, the lower poles of the organs are connected by a fibrous band or by renal tissue. In this example fusion of the lower poles has given rise to a 'horseshoe' kidney. Each kidney has a separate pelvis and the ureter passes anteriorly across the lower pole of the kidney. Fused kidneys are generally caudally displaced. **10.8 Cystine calculus.** This is a cross-section of the stone. It is large (4.8 cm long) and ovoid, and the cut surface is flecked with tiny white dots. The external surface is fairly smooth. Cystine stones are among the rarest of renal calculi. They may consist of cystine alone or of a mixture of cystine with phosphate and uric acid. Cystine stones are found in the Fanconi syndrome which is characterised by aminoaciduria, glycosuria and phosphaturia, often with acidosis and dwarfism. **10.9 and 10.10 Oxalate calculus.** Calcium oxalate stones account for about 13% of renal stones. Oxalosis is a rare primary disturbance of oxalate metabolism in children, with hyperoxaluria and deposition of calcium oxalate in the kidneys and progressive formation of oxalate calculi. Progressive renal damage, with recurrent bouts of urinary infection, eventually leads to death from renal failure. **10.9** This is a bisected oxalate stone. The external surface (right) is dark grey-brown and has multiple projections. The cut surface (left) shows typical concentric dark-coloured laminations. **10.10** The stone is large and

spherical. The colour and rough spiny surface are typical of this type of calculus. The consistence is also very hard. **10.11 Uric acid calculus.** Uric acid stones are smooth-surfaced (right) and often egg-shaped. The colour is light brown. On section (left) the structure is laminated, with regular layers around a central nucleus of dark brown material. Uric acid calculi are moderately hard. They may be found in patients with gout; and in patients with leukaemia, excessive breakdown of nucleoprotein produces hyperuricuria and sometimes stone formation. **10.12 and 10.13 Phosphate calculus.** The commonest renal stones are composed of a mixture of calcium phosphate or ammonium-magnesium phsophate and calcium oxalate. Phosphate stones are soft, smooth, white and friable. **10.12** A large 'staghorn' branching phosphate calculus (left) has been removed from the kidney where it formed a cast of the dilated pelvis and calyceal system. The kidney (right) shows extensive secondary destruction, with advanced hydronephrosis and extreme atrophy of the renal parenchyma. The cortex is very thin and the corticomedullary demarcation is blurred. Greyish-green calculous debris is present within some of the calyces. There is also a sessile papilliferous tumour in the pelvis which proved to be an adenocarcinoma of the renal pelvis, probably as a result of glandular metaplasia secondary to chronic pyelonephritis and the presence of calculi.

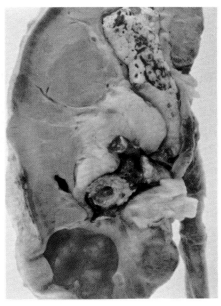

10.13 Phosphate calculus

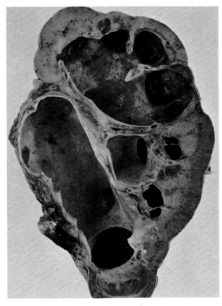

10.14 Hydronephrosis

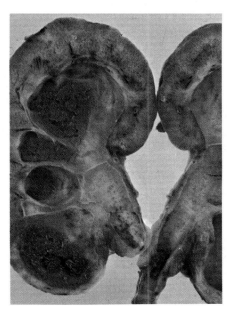

10.15 Hydronephrosis

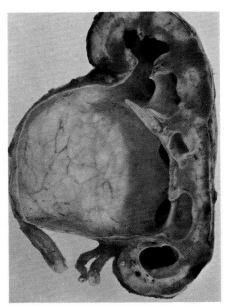

10.16 Hydronephrosis

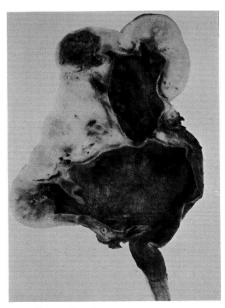

10.17 Pyonephrosis

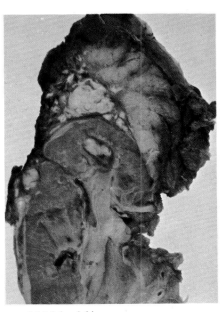

10.18 Malakoplakia

10.13 Phosphate calculus. The pelvis and calyces are distended by a branching yellowish-white stone, the surface of which shows golden-brown areas. The lower part of the kidney (bottom left) is hydronephrotic and there is an increased amount of fat in the pelvis and calyceal regions. **10.14-10.16 Hydronephrosis.** Hydronephrosis is a dilatation of the renal pelvis with atrophy of the renal parenchyma, as a result of obstruction to the outflow of urine. Including the minor and severe forms, it is one of the commonest renal lesions. **10.14** This shows severe hydronephrosis. There is extreme dilatation of the calyces and pelvis, with secondary atrophy of the renal substance. The scattered focal haemorrhages in the pelvi-calyceal mucosa are evidence of the acute-on-chronic pyelonephritis which was present. **10.15** This is a 'gravelly' kidney with masses of soft granular greenish-brown calculous debris filling the dilated and blunted calyces. Calculi are believed to form through a process of encrustation of crystalline material onto bacteria, necrotic tissue or shed epithelium in the region of the papillae. When near the surface, the calcified plaques ulcerate and further episodes of crystallisation of urinary salts may lead to the formation of granular calculous debris. This kidney is also hydronephrotic, following obstruction of the first part of the ureter by a calculus (bottom). **10.16** This bisected kidney shows a large hydronephrotic sac involving the extrarenal pelvis and upper ureter, the

lower ureter being normal. The intrarenal pelvis and calyces are dilated and the calyces flattened. The renal parenchyma is atrophied. An accessory renal artery to the lower pole (lower centre), by pressing upon and obstructing the upper end of the ureter, has caused the lesion. **10.17 Pyonephrosis.** When obstruction complicates pyelonephritis, hydronephrosis and renal atrophy are usually present. The distended hydronephrotic kidney may fill with pus to produce pyonephrosis. The renal parenchyma shows marked pallor. The dilated pelvis and calyces contained turbid pus and the pelvi-calyceal mucosa is red and intensely injected. A subcapsular abscess (2 cm diameter) is present in the upper pole. Histology showed severe acute and chronic pyelonephritis. **10.18 Malakoplakia.** Malakoplakia, meaning 'soft plaque', is a rare condition of unknown aetiology in which circumscribed, slightly elevated plaques or nodules ranging in size from 1 mm to 5 cm or more form in the bladder, ureter or renal pelvis. In this case, multiple discrete yellowish-white plaques are present within the calyces and beneath the renal capsule and, somewhat unusually, the process has extended (above) into the perinephric fat. The lesions in malakoplakia may be single or multiple and histologically they consist of vacuolated histiocytes with characteristic cytoplasmic Michaelis-Gutmann 'inclusions'. The condition is usually found in women over the age of 30. This patient was a 58-year-old woman.

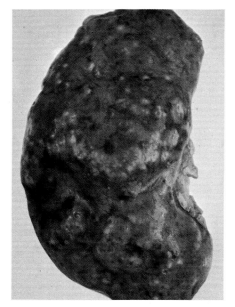

10.19 Acute suppurative pyelonephritis

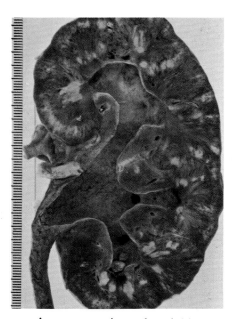

10.20 Acute suppurative pyelonephritis

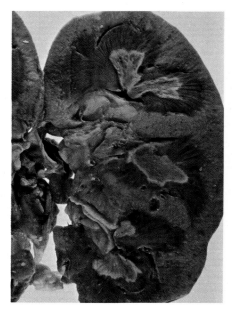

10.21 Acute pyelonephritis and papillary necrosis

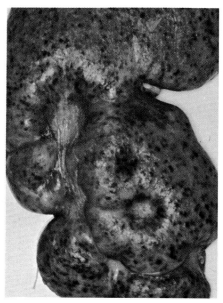

10.22 Chronic pyelonephritis

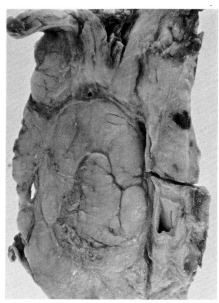

10.23 Lipomatosis: kidney

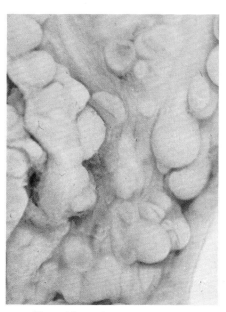

10.24 Ureteritis cystica

10.19-10.21 Acute suppurative pyelonephritis. 10.19 This is the capsular surface of the kidney. Multiple discrete slightly depressed yellowish-white abscesses are present. The blood vessels around them are engorged. There is also a broad shallow scar (centre left), evidence of chronic pyelonephritis. The kidney is acute pyelonephritis is usually enlarged. The more severe forms are usually associated with obstruction and in this patient, a man of 68, both ureters were obstructed by a large carcinoma of the bladder. **10.20** This is a hemi-section of the kidney. The organ is swollen and very congested. Multiple yellowish absesses are present, mainly in the cortex but also in the medulla. In suppurative pyelonephritis the abscesses in the cortex tend to have a wedge shape similar to that of small infarcts. The straight yellowish streaks within the medulla represent pus within dilated collecting tubules. The calyces are dilated and 'blunted'. The pelvis is also dilated. The mucosa of the pelvis and calyces is intensely hyperaemic and focal haemorrhages are present. Two small phosphate calculi are located in the lower pole calyx (bottom). **10.21 Acute pyelonephritis and papillary necrosis.** The kidney is of normal size. The cortex is of normal width and the corticomedullary differentiation is well-preserved. The distal part of each papilla is greyish-white and necrotic, with a congested border. The incidence of necrotising papillitis varies in different countries from 0.2% to 3.7% of routine necropsies. The main predisposing conditions are acute pyelonephritis, urinary tract obstruction, diabetes mellitus and excessive consumption of analgesic, especially phenacetin-containing, drugs.

10.22 Chronic pyelonephritis. The capsular surface shows broad depressed scars, each with a greyish-white centre. Typically the scarred areas in chronic pyelonephritis are located over dilated calyces. The scarring of the cortical tissue may be more diffuse than in this instance, the surface of the kidney then showing a fine nodularity. The parenchyma is often considerably reduced but in a patchy way. One kidney is often more affected than the other, or one alone may be affected, and this often serves to distinguish the condition from other forms of 'contracted kidneys'. The patient had a terminal phase of malignant hypertension, with necrosis of glomeruli and arterioles, giving rise to the multiple haemorrhages visible over the surface of the kidney. **10.23 Lipomatosis: kidney.** A marked xanthogranulomatous reaction with the presence of many fat-containing histiocytes is sometimes found in the kidneys in chronic pyelonephritis, and the lesion illustrated here is thought to represent a severe form of chronic xanthogranulomatous pyelonephritis rather than a renal lipoma. As the section through the organ shows, the renal parenchyma has been more or less replaced by a lobulated fatty mass. **10.24 Ureteritis cystica.** This is a close-up view of the mucosal surface of the ureter. Many small thin-walled cysts are present in the submucosa. Ureteritis cystica may occur at any age but it is commoner in the elderly. It may be unilateral or bilateral. It occurs most frequently in the upper third of the ureter and at the uretero-pelvic junction and is frequently associated with similar cysts in the pelvis and bladder.

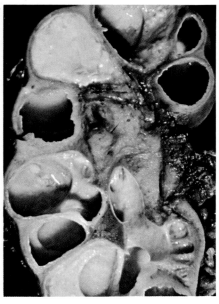

10.25 Tuberculous pyonephrosis

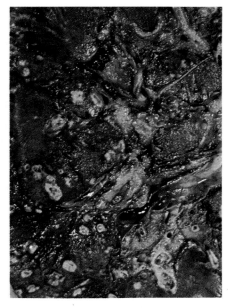

10.26 Nocardiosis: kidney

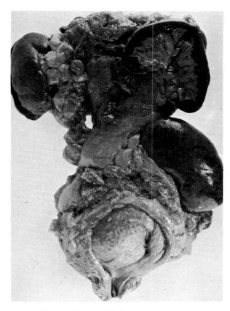

10.27 Transplanted kidney

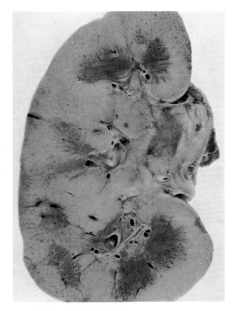

10.28 Transplanted kidney

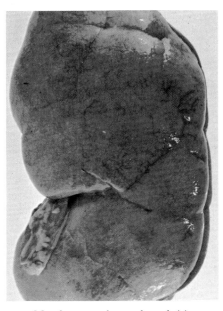

10.29 Membranous glomerulonephritis

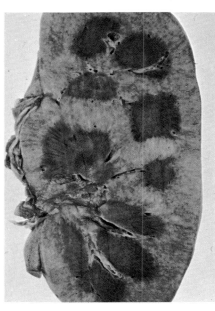

10.30 Membranous glomerulonephritis

10.25 Tuberculous pyonephrosis. There is gross destruction of renal tissue, the parenchyma being reduced to a thin shell surrounding dilated calyces. The calyces (top) are filled with inspissated caseous material. The tuberculous process usually starts in the medulla with ulceration of the papilla and extends into the pelvis and ureter. Obstruction of the ureter as a result of stricture formation generally plays a part in the development of tuberculous pyonephrosis. Caseous ulcerative renal tuberculosis is bilateral in about 75% of cases and about half the cases also have pulmonary tuberculosis. **10.26 Nocardiosis: kidney.** Nocardiosis is caused by *Nocardia asteroides*, a branching gram-positive filamentous organism which may produce lesions in the lungs, brain and kidneys. It sets up a chronic suppurative process, and the cut surface of this kidney shows multiple focal yellow-white abscesses, many of which have undergone central necrosis and suppuration. Infection may occur in patients with tuberculosis, lymphomas or in patients on immunosuppressive therapy. **10.27 and 10.28 Transplanted kidney.** In each of the following two cases, the transplanted kidney had been obtained from a cadaver. **10.27** The patient, a 46-year-old man, had chronic glomerulonephritis and renal failure. The transplanted kidney, swollen and plum-coloured, is situated above the opened bladder. The patient's own kidneys are shrunken, with a striking reduction in cortical thickness and a marked increase in pelvic and calyceal fat. The patient died from fungal endocarditis two months after the transplant. The kidney had failed to function

and histology confirmed the presence of the vascular lesions of chronic rejection. **10.28** This patient survived for six months after the renal transplant and several rejection episodes were controlled by immuno-suppressants. This is the cut surface of the donor kidney. It is pale and swollen and the surface bulges. The corticomedullary differentiation is indistinct and the medullary pyramids bulge into the compressed calyces. The vessels appear thick-walled. The mucosa of the pelvis and calyces is granular, opaque and yellowish-green. **10.29 and 10.30 Membranous glomerulonephritis.** In membranous glomerulonephritis the kidneys may be enlarged, normal or reduced in size depending on the stage at which the disease is seen. The proximal convoluted tubules contain lipid in the early stages and lipid-containing cells may sometimes be seen in the glomeruli. Collections of foamy macrophages are also commonly found in the interstitium and may be associated with cholesterol granulomas. All these changes are accentuated when the nephrotic syndrome is present. **10.29** The kidney is swollen and pale, and the capsular surface is smooth, apart from persistent fetal lobulation. The colour is yellowish-brown from the presence of lipid in the tubular epithelium. The appearances shown here are typical of the earlier stages of membranous glomerulo-nephritis, and the patient, a man of 58, died from acute haemorrhagic pancreatitis. The kidneys weighed 290 g. **10.30** In this case the patient suffered from the nephrotic syndrome. The kidney is large and pale and the yellow colour of the lipid-rich cortex contrasts with that of the medulla.

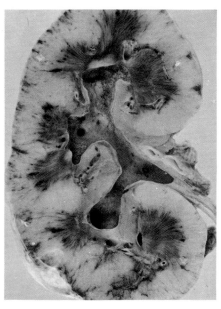

10.31 Amyloidosis: kidney

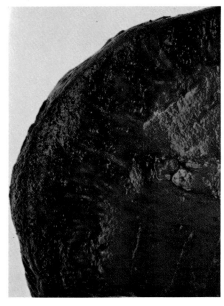

10.32 Amyloidosis: kidney

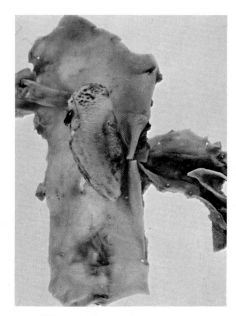

10.33 Thrombosis: renal veins

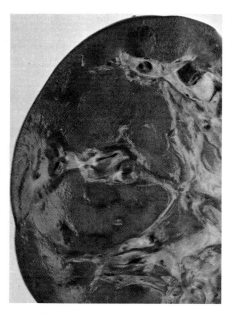

10.34 Systemic lupus erythematosus and
sickle cell anaemia: kidney

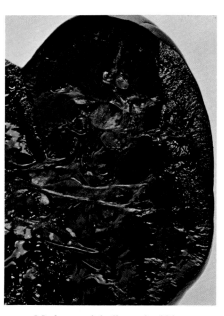

10.35 Methaemoglobulinaemia: kidney

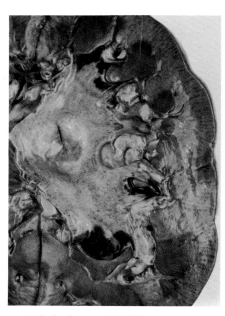

10.36 Aplastic anaemia: kidney

10.31 and 10.32 Amyloidosis: kidney. The kidney is involved with great frequency in the secondary forms of amyloidosis (80%) and in the primary form in about 35% of cases. Grossly the kidneys are equally increased in size and are pale and firm. The cut surface may feel 'greasy'. The total weight may exceed 600 g but in the later stages they may be contracted and granular. The amyloid is deposited in relation to basement membrane of capillaries and tubules. **10.31** This is a very advanced stage of renal amyloidosis. The organ is greatly enlarged and the broadened cortex is yellowish-white and waxy-looking. Small focal subcapsular haemorrhages are present. In the early stage of renal amyloidosis the proximal tubules contain lipid but as the disease progresses, secondary tubular atrophy results. **10.32** Iodine stains amyloid a mahogany-brown colour. A slice of the kidney shown on 10.31 has been placed in Lugol's solution and the amyloid in the glomeruli causes the glomeruli to stand out as brown dots in the cortex. The patient had bilateral renal vein thrombosis. **10.33 Thrombosis: renal veins.** An ovoid pale grey thrombus is situated within the vena cava and grey-brown thrombus extends into both renal veins. Bilateral renal vein thrombosis in adults may produce the nephrotic syndrome and microscopy of the kidneys often shows a membraneous nephropathy associated with marked tubular atrophy. Renal vein thrombosis is often associated with vena caval thrombosis, as here. **10.34 Systemic lupus erythematosus and sickle cell anaemia: kidney.** The kidneys are involved in 80 to 90% of cases of systemic lupus erythematosus coming to necropsy. There are no gross characteristic appearances in the kidneys, and their size may be normal,

increased or moderately reduced. The cortex of this kidney is pale and the corticomedullary junction is blurred. The patient, a 39-year-old West Indian woman, sustained an acute sickle cell crisis a few days before death, and microscopy showed widespread plugging of the vasa recta by sickle-shaped red cells and patchy necrosis of cortical tissue. Necrosis of occasional papillae is evident macroscopically (top). **10.35 Methaemoglobulinaemia: kidney.** The patient ingested a large quantity of weed-killer, sodium chlorate. This caused acute methaemoglobulinaemia. The kidney is a dark chocolate-brown colour and the skin and mucous membranes were a similar colour. Toxic methaemoglobulinaemia is produced by a number of chemical substances which increase the rate of auto-oxidation of the haemoglobin in the red cells and so induce the formation of methaemoglobin. The majority of cases of chronic methaemoglobulinaemia are due to prolonged self-medication with analgesic tablets containing phenacetin. **10.36 Aplastic anaemia: kidney.** In this condition thrombocytopenia frequently leads to troublesome bleeding which may be fatal. This patient, a 27-year-old woman, was found to have aplastic anaemia during her second pregnancy and she died six months later from septicaemia associated with recurrent haemorrhages. No cause for the aplastic anaemia was ascertained clinically. The kidney is enlarged and pale, and petechial haemorrhages are present throughout the cortex. More extensive recent haemorrhages are present in the calyces. Small pinpoint haemorrhages are visible in the pelvic mucosa.

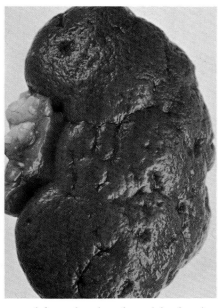

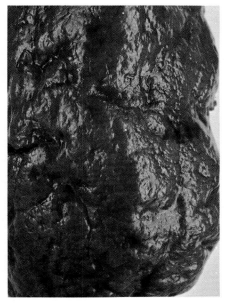

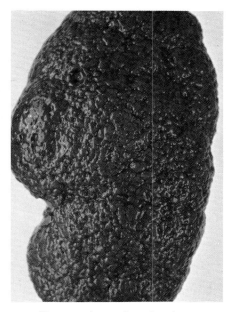

10.37 Atherosclerosis and arteriolosclerosis: kidney

10.38 Atherosclerosis: kidney

10.39 Hypertensive nephrosclerosis

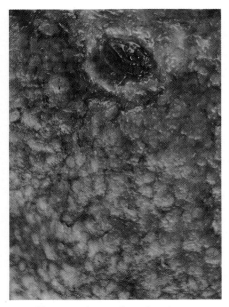

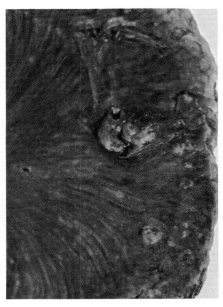

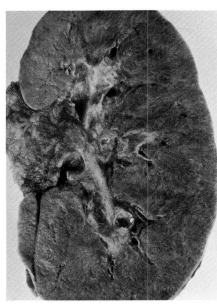

10.40 Hypertensive nephrosclerosis

10.41 Hypertensive nephrosclerosis

10.42 Malignant hypertension: kidney

10.37 and 10.38 Atherosclerosis and arteriolosclerosis: kidney. In patients with advanced atherosclerosis the kidneys are usually reduced in size and scarred due to the slow ischaemia resulting from atherosclerotic narrowing of the larger renal arteries. **10.37** The scars are often large and coarse, as shown here, where they form punctate circular depressions. Some of the scars are connected by thin fissuring scars. The intervening surface is granular, as a result of arteriolosclerosis. **10.38** This is a more extreme example of the coarse subcapsular scars found in atherosclerosis and hypertension. The kidney is irregularly contracted and the many shallow depressed broad scars give it a distinctly 'lobular' appearance. Scarring of this severity may be difficult to distinguish from pyelonephritic scarring. An important distinguishing feature is that hypertensive scars are not accompanied by the deformity of the underlying calyx which is found in chronic pyelonephritis. **10.39-10.43 Hypertensive nephrosclerosis. 10.39** This patient, a 74-year-old woman, had diabetes mellitus but the renal lesion is that of generalised arteriolosclerosis and atherosclerosis. The surface of the organ shows a diffuse fine nodularity. Both kidneys were equally affected and weighed 200 g. Histology showed focal subcapsular ischaemic scars. A small simple retention cyst is present (upper left). In diabetes there may be a variety of glomerular lesions and the renal arteries tend to be atherosclerotic. **10.40** The patient suffered from essential hypertension and left ventricular

failure. This is a close-up view of the finely granular surface of the kidney. A shallow coarser pit is seen (top right) close to a subcapsular cyst. Typically both kidneys were affected and equally but moderately reduced in size. The capsule was adherent to the cortical surface. **10.41** This is the cut surface of the contracted kidney shown in 10.40. There is considerable thinning of the cortex and the coarser subcapsular pits appear as shallow V-shaped scars (right). The arcuate and interlobular arteries (centre) stand out prominently, being thick-walled as a result of medial hypertrophy and atherosclerosis. The surface of the kidney was firm in consistence, with a detectable increase in resistance on sectioning from interstitial fibrosis. **10.42** The patient, a 23-year-old man, had malignant hypertension, and died from an intracerebral haemorrhage. The cut surface of the kidney has a blotchy mottled red colour, due to petechial haemorrhages throughout the cortex and medulla. The small arteries appear dilated. There are haemorrhages in the mucosa of the pelvis and calyces and the pelvic fat is increased and haemorrhagic. The kidney is of normal size. The size of the kidneys in malignant hypertension varies greatly, depending on the length of the clinical course and the presence of a pre-existing benign phase. In rapidly progressive disease the kidneys are often of normal size. In this case they weighed 360 g. Histologically there was fibrinoid necrosis of the glomeruler tufts and afferent arterioles (necrotising arteriolitis) and haemorrhage.

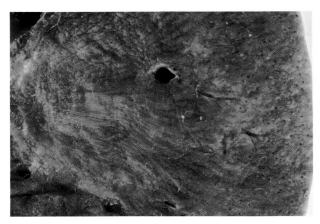

10.43 Malignant hypertension: kidney

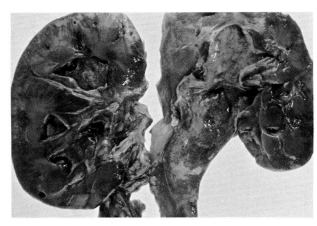

10.44 Waldenström's macroglobulinaemia: kidneys

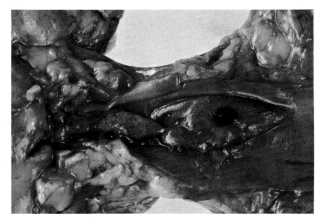

10.45 Renal vein thrombosis

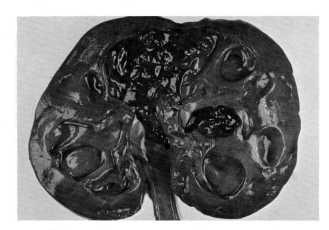

10.46 Christmas disease: kidney

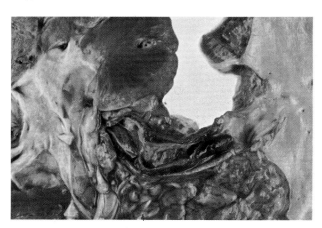

10.47 Dissecting aneurysm: renal artery

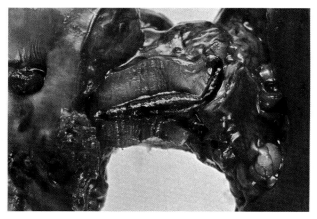

10.48 Embolus: renal artery

10.43 Malignant hypertension: kidney. This is a close-up of the cut surface of the kidney shown in 10.42. Within the cortex the pinpoint haemorrhagic glomeruli are clearly visible and thin longitudinally-running haemorrhagic streaks are present within the medulla. **10.44 Waldenström's macroglobulinaemia: kidneys.** The patient was treated with cyclophosphamide and as a result developed an inflamed contracted bladder that necessitated transplantation of the ureters into a 'rectal bladder'. The kidneys are enlarged (combined weight 500 g). The calyces and pelves are dilated and the mucosal surface is covered with a purulent exudate. The ureters also are dilated and the mucosal surface inflamed. Microscopy of the kidneys revealed diffuse infiltration by lymphocytes and plasmacytoid cells, with associated changes of acute pyelonephritis. **10.45 Renal vein thrombosis.** One renal vein is occluded by an adherent pale red-brown thrombus, the surface of which shows fine striations. Both veins were similarly affected. The kidney (left) is pale. The nephrotic syndrome was present clinically. In renal vein thrombosis the kidneys may be normal or increased in size. They are usually pale and soft. The thrombus is generally located within the main renal veins and its larger branches and is usually organised. **10.46 Christmas disease: kidney.** Christmas disease (haemophilia B) is a rare haemorrhagic disorder due to a deficiency of plasma thromboplastin component (factor IX). It is inherited as a sex-linked recessive character.

The patient, a 23-year-old man, presented with intractable haematuria. The upper pole calyx and pelvis of the kidney are distended with recent blood clot and occasional haemorrhages are present in the cortex. Haematuria is not uncommon in patients with severe haemophilia in whom it often occurs spontaneously. It may be accompanied by ureteric colic. **10.47 Dissecting aneurysm: renal artery.** This shows the renal artery and hilum of the kidney. The proximal part (right) of the renal artery is normal but there is a chronic dissection of the wall of the distal two-thirds of the vessel, with formation of a double channel which extends into the hilar region. The tip of the adjacent papilla is necrotic (left). Dissecting aneurysm of the renal artery is rare and in the few cases described the aorta was not similarly affected. The patient, a 61-year-old man with systemic hypertension, died from uraemia due to chronic glomerulonephritis. **10.48 Embolus: renal artery.** A pale red embolus occludes the left renal artery at its origin (left). The opened artery also contains red-brown propagated thrombus (right). The embolus originated from the left atrium, the patient, a 74-year-old man, having chronic rheumatic heart disease. The left kidney was acutely congested but no gross infarction was visible. The right kidney (weight 30 g) was shrunken and fibrotic as a result of a previous episode of infarction. Old organised thrombus occluded the orifice of the right renal artery. The patient died from acute renal failure.

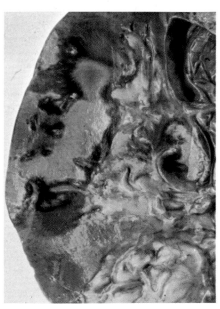

10.49 Infarction: kidney

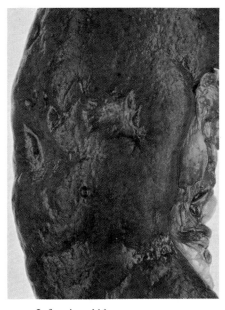

10.50 Infarction: kidney

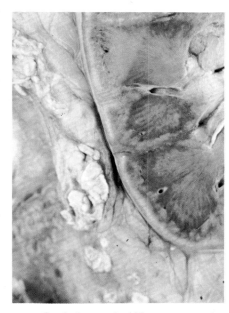

10.51 Cortical necrosis: kidney

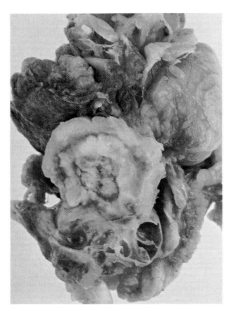

10.52 Angiomyolipoma: kidney

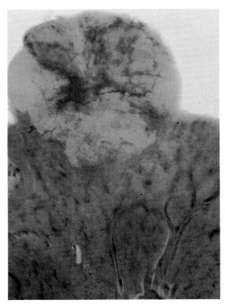

10.53 Adenoma: kidney

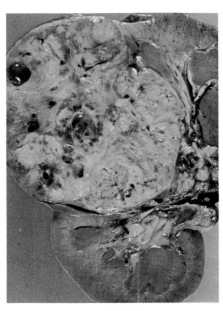

10.54 Adenocarcinoma: kidney

10.49 and 10.50 Infarction: kidney. Most infarcts of kidney are embolic in origin, the embolus coming from the heart. The underlying lesion in the heart may be valvular disease (chronic rheumatic endocarditis) with atrial fibrillation, myocardial infarction or subacute bacterial endocarditis. **10.49** This recent infarct forms an irregular yellowish-white mass bordered by a dark-red haemorrhagic zone. The infarct involves the cortex and extends into the medulla. The subcapsular cortex is swollen and there is no depression of the infarcted zone. **10.50** The patient had chronic rheumatic heart disease, with thrombus formation in the left atrium, and had sustained repeated minor episodes of renal infarction. These are the fibrosed remnants of the old infarcts. They form four irregular deeply depressed areas on the capsular surface. The base of each is greenish-white, the colour being due to the underlying contracted fibrous tissue. The scars of old infarcts tend to form deep V-shaped depressions on the cut surface which contrast with the shallower broad U-shaped pyelonephritic scars. **10.51 Cortical necrosis: kidney.** The kidney is swollen and pale. Apart from a thin subcapsular zone (appearing red), the whole of the cortex is necrotic and yellow. The columns of Bertin are similarly affected. The adjacent perinephric fat shows yellowish-white foci of necrosis. Necrosis of the whole cortex is rare, and the medulla, juxtamedullary cortex and a rim of subcapsular cortex are usually spared even in the severe bilateral forms. Most cases occur in pregnancy and are associated with antepartum haemorrhage and/or

toxaemia. In this case the lesion was a complication of the severe shock and hypotension which followed a bout of acute pancreatitis. **10.52 Angiomyolipoma: kidney.** Small hamartomas are occasionally found in the medulla or cortex, appearing as solitary grey nodules. They usually consist of smooth muscle, connective tissue, blood vessels and fat. This one is relatively large (3 x 2 x 1.5 cm) and forms a complex lobulated cystic yellowish-white mass. Similar tumour-like nodules found in cases of tuberose sclerosis may attain a size of several cm but almost invariably remain benign. **10.53 Adenoma: kidney.** Renal adenomas are commonly seen in the outer cortex, and this one forms a small (1 cm diameter) solid rounded mass which projects from the surface of the kidney. A fibrous capsule separates it from the cortical tissue. Its colour is yellow, with a central area of brownish haemorrhage. Adenomas vary in size from a few mm up to 3 cm and two forms are described: small grey tumours with a papillary cystadenomatous pattern on histological examination; and small solid yellow nodules (as here) composed of sheets or cords of granular or clear (lipid-rich) cells similar in structure to clear-cell carcinomas. Some authorities suggest that adenomas represent the early stage of renal carcinomas. **10.54 Adenocarcinoma: kidney.** The tumour forms a large (7 cm diameter) smooth rounded mass in the upper pole of the kidney which has extended into the hilum and infiltrated the renal vein. The cut surface is a pale yellow but grey fibrous septa traverse it and there are areas of haemorrhage and cystic necrosis.

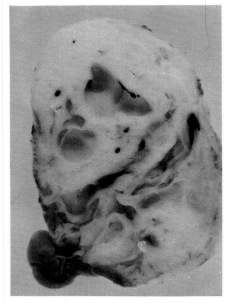

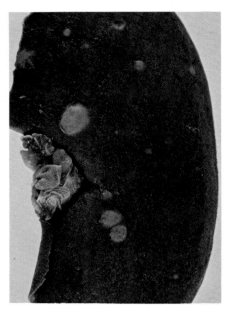

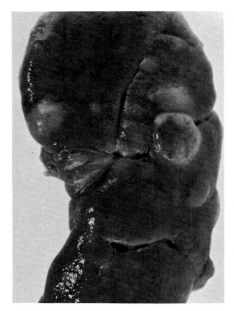

10.55 Wilms' tumour (nephroblastoma): kidney

10.56 Secondary carcinoma: kidney

10.57 Lymphocytic leukaemia: kidney

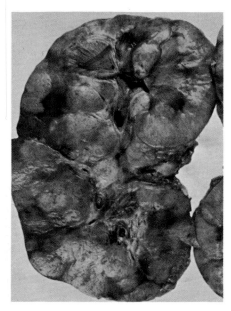

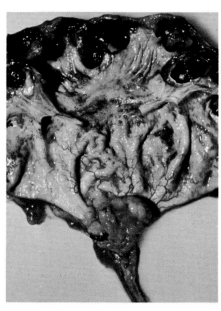

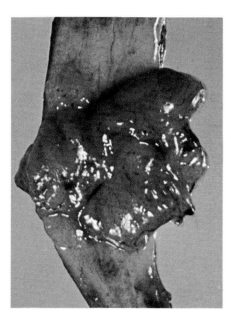

10.58 Histiocytic lymphoma: kidney

10.59 Transitional cell carcinoma: renal pelvis

10.60 Papilloma: ureter

10.55 Wilms' tumour (nephroblastoma): kidney. A large creamy-white tumour has largely replaced the kidney, a small portion of which is visible at the lower left. Numerous cysts and focal haemorrhages are present within the growth. Wilms' tumour is a mixed tumour which consists of malignant connective tissue intermingled with glandular tubules and primitive glomeruli. It accounts for about 20% of childhood tumours, the average age of the subjects being 3 years. Initially the lesion is encapsulated but extension and haematogenous dissemination soon occur. **10.56 Secondary carcinoma: kidney.** The capsular surface is studded with discrete white secondary deposits. The primary tumour was an undifferentiated carcinoma of bronchus. Renal metastases are found in about 8% of patients dying from malignant disease, the common primary sites being breast, lung, skin and thyroid. Incidentally the unaffected surface of this kidney also shows finely granularity, as a result of essential hypertension and arteriolosclerosis. **10.57 Lymphocytic leukaemia: kidney.** Leukaemic infiltrates are frequently found in the kidneys, where they begin as small perivascular aggregates which grow into discrete deposits resembling metastatic carcinoma. This patient was a 17-year-old girl with acute lymphocytic leukaemia who died from a pontine haemorrhage. The capsular and cut surface of the kidney is studded with elevated pale spherical nodules 0.5 to 1.5 cm in diameter. **10.58 Histiocytic lymphoma (reticulum cell sarcoma): kidney.**

The patient, a 62-year-old man, died from disseminated histiocytic lymphoma. The kidneys weighed 1055 g and this shows one in section. The renal tissue, both cortical and medullary, is almost completely replaced by large rounded yellow deposits which in places are confluent. **10.59 Transitional cell carcinoma: renal pelvis.** A sessile papillary yellowish-grey tumour is growing at the pelvi-ureteric junction. By blocking the ureter it has produced intrarenal hydronephrosis, with marked loss of renal substance. There is extensive calyceal haemorrhage and the blood vessels of the pelvic mucosa are congested. The commonest tumours of the renal pelvis are transitional cell papillomas and papillary carcinomas. Squamous carcinoma is rare; it may be infiltrative or papillary, metastasises early and has a poor prognosis. Mucus-secreting adenocarcinoma is very rare and is always associated with 'colonic' metaplasia secondary to chronic calculous pyelonephritis (see 10.12). **10.60 Papilloma: ureter.** The ureter has been opened to show the lumen filled at one point by a large sessile papillomatous growth. Histologically this was a well-differentiated transitional cell papilloma but the large majority of primary tumours of the ureter are transitional cell carcinomas. Squamous and adenocarcinomas also occur. About 75% of the primary tumours are located in the lower third of the ureter. They spread early and more extensively than bladder tumours, with lymphatic permeation, and consequently have a poor prognosis.

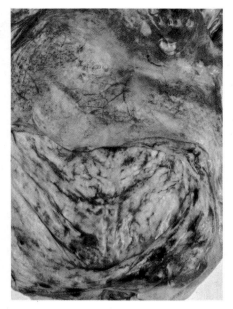

10.61 Acute (haemorrhagic) cystitis

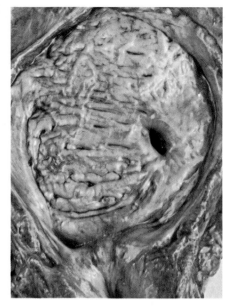

10.62 Hypertrophy and diverticulum: bladder

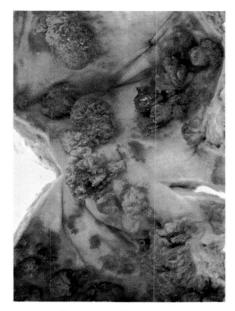

10.63 Papillomas: bladder

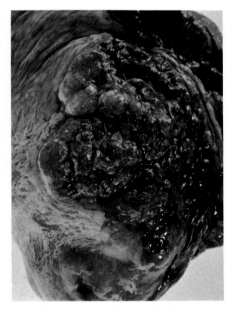

10.64 Squamous carcinoma: bladder

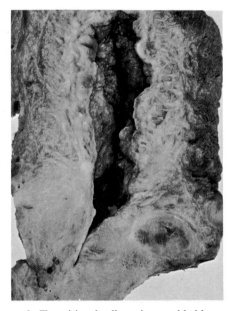

10.65 Transitional cell carcinoma: bladder

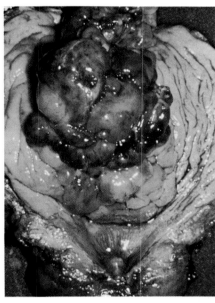

10.66 Rhabdomyosarcoma: bladder

10.61 Acute (haemorrhagic) cystitis. The patient was an 80-year-old woman with a carcinoma of pancreas who developed a klebsiella urinary tract infection. The bladder mucosa is swollen and oedematous, with patchy areas of haemorrhage. Acute cystitis varies greatly in severity. When severe, congestion is marked and ulceration and haemorrhage may occur, so-called haemorrhagic cystitis. Haemorrhagic cystitis may also follow infection and trauma secondary to an indwelling urinary catheter. **10.62 Hypertrophy and diverticulum: bladder.** The muscle coat of the bladder is hypertrophied as shown in the increase in the thickness of the bladder wall and the prominence of the muscle trabeculae. Hypertrophy followed obstruction to the outflow of urine by an enlarged prostate. There is also a smooth-mouthed diverticulum on the posterior wall. Stasis of urine within a diverticulum predisposes to infection and calculus formation. **10.63 Papillomas: bladder.** The patient worked for many years in the rubber industry. Multiple small sessile papillomas are present on the posterior wall of the bladder. Papillomas are the commonest epithelial tumours of the bladder. They are best regarded as potentially malignant growths, since 50% recur within one year and about 25% develop into invasive carcinomas in five years. Histologically they consist of fronds of fibrovascular tissue covered with a layer of transitional epithelium that varies in its degree of differentiation. Rupture of the delicate stromal blood vessels often leads to haematuria. The papillomas are often multiple, as in this case, and may cover large areas of the bladder (papillomatosis). **10.64 Squamous carcinoma: bladder.** A large fleshy red and ulcerated tumour almost completely fills the bladder lumen. Histologically it was a squamous carcinoma. Squamous carcinoma accounts for 7% of all bladder carcinomas and it has a poor prognosis. **10.65 Transitional cell carcinoma: bladder.** The tumour is a nodular brownish mass which has infiltrated the muscle coat of the bladder very extensively. The bladder is thick-walled and contracted, a change which is also partly due to irradiation fibrosis. Histology showed the tumour to be a poorly-differentiated transitional cell tumour with areas of squamous differentiation. Transitional cell tumours account for 90% of bladder neoplasms and are commonly located in the trigone, lateral walls and around the ureteral orifices. They are four times as frequent in males. **10.66 Rhabdomyosarcoma: bladder.** A lobulated grape-like (botryoid) mass of gelatinous pinkish-white tumour is located on the posterior bladder wall. The botryoid form of rhabdomyosarcoma (sarcoma botryoides) accounts for about 46% of all rhabdomyosarcomas and consists mainly of oedematous myxomatous tissue. It occurs predominantly in the genito-urinary tract of infants and has a very poor prognosis, repeatedly recurring locally and then disseminating by lymphatics and bloodstream.

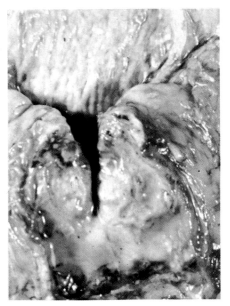

11.1 Purulent prostatitis

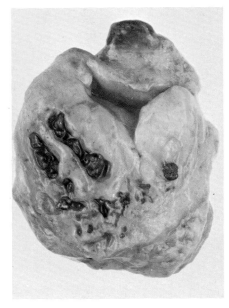

11.2 Calculi: prostrate

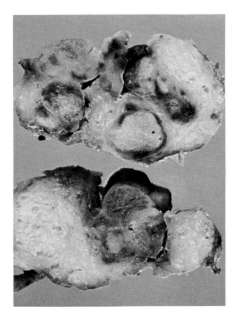

11.3 Infarction: prostrate

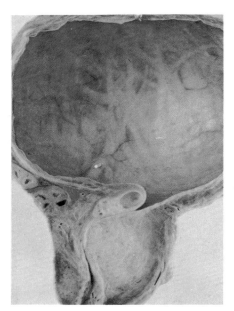

11.4 Adenomatous hyperplasia: prostrate

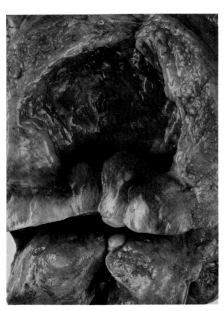

11.5 Adenomatous hyperplasia: prostrate

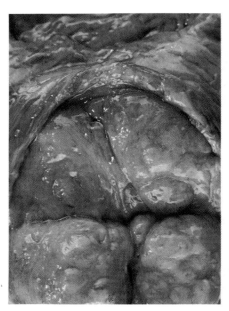

11.6 Adenomatous hyperplasia: prostrate

11.1 Purulent prostatitis. The prostate is enlarged and oedematous and a large abscess cavity within it is filled with thick green pus. Acute prostatitis is linked with infections of the urethra or bladder and is often a complication of urethral catheterisation. The commonest organisms are staphylococci, streptococci, gonococci and coliforms. Multiple abscesses are often present. **11.2 Calculi: prostate.** Calculi are found in the prostates of 20-30% of men over the age of 50. The calculi may be endogenous (true) or exogenous (false). Endogenous calculi form around organic material, are often multiple, and vary in size from 1 mm up to 5 cm. Exogenous calculi are rarer and form around a nucleus of phosphates and urates. This shows multiple endogenous calculi, within an enlarged cystic prostate. The dark greenish-brown calculi, triangular and facetted, lie within dilated ducts. **11.3 Infarction: prostate.** Two slices of nodular enlarged prostate are shown. A large brownish recent infarct is present in the lower one and there are three older yellowish-white infarcts, surrounded by a haemorrhagic border, in the upper one. Infarction results from vascular insufficiency in an enlarged gland and is found in 25% of adenomatous prostates. Local trauma following instrumentation may be a precipitating factor. Atherosclerosis and hypertension predispose and occasionally polyarteritis nodosa is responsible. Embolic infarction can occur in bacterial endocarditis. Histological examination often shows squamous metaplasia in the prostatic acini adjacent to the infarct. **11.4-11.6 Adenomatous hyperplasia: prostate.** Adenomatous hyper-plasia rarely occurs before the age of 50 years. The gland generally weighs between 40 and 100 g and grossly is smooth or nodular with a rubbery consistence. The appearance of the cut surface depends on whether the hyperplasia is mainly glandular or fibro-muscular. When it is predominantly glandular, well-circumscribed nodules are present, surrounded by pearly-white tissue. Cysts are common. In the fibro-muscular type of hyperplasia, the cut surface is a homogeneous pale colour. The chief complication of an enlarged prostate is urethral obstruction, with secondary effects on the bladder, ureters and kidneys. **11.4** In this sagittal section of the prostate, the greyish-white anterior lobe is uniformly enlarged and the posterior urethra elongated, tortuous and compressed. The urinary outlet is elevated above the floor of the bladder by the enlarged middle lobe. The bladder is distended and its wall is thinned. Stretching of the bladder wall has rendered the ureteric orifice (probe) incompetent. **11.5** A greatly enlarged prostate comprising two nodular lateral lobes and a prominent medial lobe projects into the bladder neck. The bladder mucosa is acutely inflamed (haemorrhagic cystitis). The bladder wall is hypertrophic, thick and contracted. **11.6** This shows the cut surface of both lateral lobes of a very nodular prostate. The creamy-white nodules vary in size and are separated by delicate greyish-white septa. Occasional small cysts are present. The spongy hyperplastic nodules have compressed the surrounding gland into a 'capsule' (top).

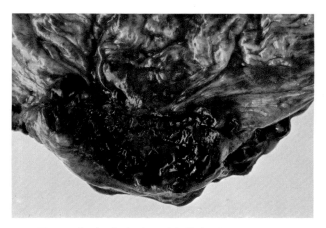

11.7 Haemorrhagic diathesis and defibrination state: prostrate and bladder

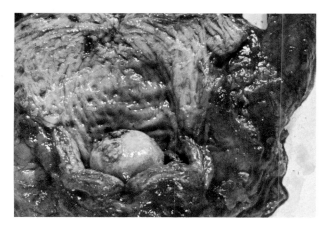

11.8 Adenocarcinoma: prostrate

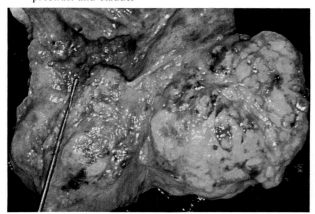

11.9 Adenocarcinoma: prostrate

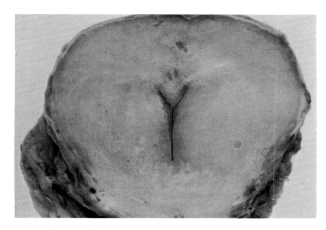

11.10 Adenocarcinoma: prostrate

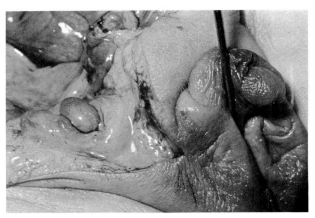

11.11 Undescended testis

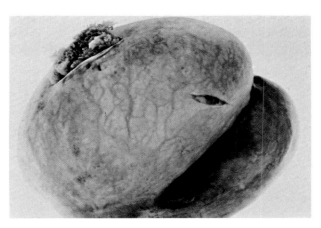

11.12 Torsion: testis

11.7 Haemorrhagic diathesis and defibrination state: prostate and bladder. The patient had a prostatectomy and developed a severe transfusion reaction. This was followed by widespread destruction of fibrin and platelets within the bloodstream, and a defibrination and haemorrhagic diathesis developed. Bleeding into the prostatic bed has been extensive and much blood clot is present. There was also bleeding from many other sites. **11.8-11.10 Adenocarcinoma: prostate.** Carcinoma of the prostate may be clinically symptomatic or occult. The occult form is found incidentally during histological examination and is much the commoner, 15-20% of nodular hyperplastic prostates containing foci of carcinoma. About 75% of carcinomas of the prostate are located in the posterior lobe and 95% seem to begin in the subcapsular region. The following three cases are examples of clinically significant lesions. **11.8** A large ovoid white tumour with an ulcerated surface projects into a hypertrophied trabeculated bladder from the region of the posterior and middle lobes. The yellowish-brown anterior and lateral lobes are enlarged. **11.9** In this sagittal section, a probe is seen within the prostatic urethra. A large craggy white growth occupies the posterior and lateral lobes of the prostate. Within it there are foci of haemorrhage. Nodular

tumour extends onto the base of the bladder neck. **11.10** This is a transverse section of a diffusely enlarged malignant prostate. The absence of nodularity should be noted. The cut surface is a pale buff colour, with yellowish areas of necrosis and thin fibrous strands. Grossly carcinomas are hard in consistence. Between 70 and 80% of clinical cases metastasise to bone. **11.11 Undescended testis.** Cryptorchidism is the congenital malposition of the testis anywhere along its route of descent. The incidence is about 4% in boys under 15 years of age and about 0.2% in adults. The testis is situated within the commencement of the inguinal canal at the pelvic brim. After puberty the cryptorchid testis is always smaller than normal, and is more liable than a normal testis to develop a tumour. **11.12 Torsion: testis.** Torsion can occur at any age, and the sudden twisting of the spermatic cord produces strangulation of the testicular and epididymal blood vessels. Congestion and haemorrhage result, but later necrosis and infarction are produced. In this case the lesion is advanced and the testis is swollen and a slate-blue colour as a result of gangrenous infarction. The predisposing causes of torsion are undue mobility and abnormal attachments of the testis. Most examples occur in undescended testes.

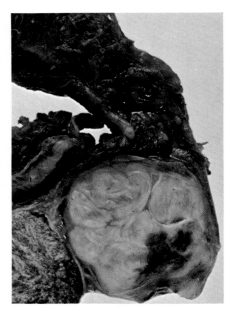

11.13 Paratesticular leiomyosarcoma

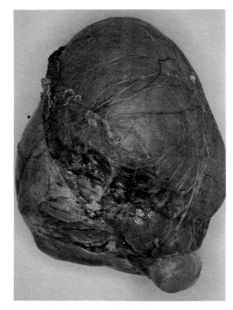

11.14 Simple cyst: epididymis

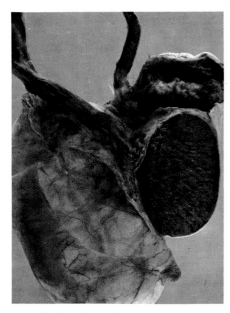

11.15 Hydrocele: testis

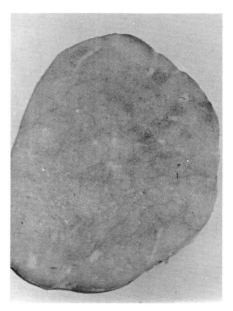

11.16 Granulomatous orchitis

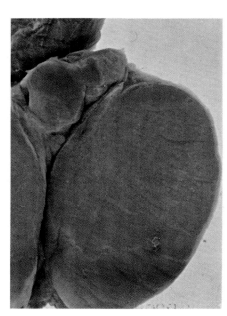

11.17 Diffuse syphilitic orchitis

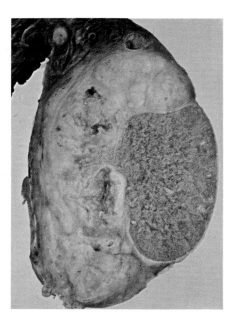

11.18 Tuberculosis: epididymis

11.13 Paratesticular leiomyosarcoma. A 52-year-old man noted a hard painless swelling in the scrotum which proved to be a large ovoid tumour closely related to the upper portion of the epididymis. This shows the cut surface of the neoplasm. It appears fleshy, whorled and greyish-white, with an area of haemorrhage (lower right). Histology showed it to be a leiomyosarcoma. Paratesticular leiomyosarcoma is a very rare lesion. **11.14 Simple cyst: epididymis.** The cyst is large and thin-walled. Thick bands of fibrous tissue are stretched over the wall. Epididymal cysts may be congenital or acquired, the latter being the commoner. They usually result from obstruction, and if they contain spermatozoa they are known as spermatoceles. Haemorrhage within the cyst results in cholesterol crystal formation and fibrosis of the wall. **11.15 Hydrocele: testis.** A hydrocele is an abnormal accumulation of serous fluid in the sac of the tunica vaginalis. In this example the sac, which has been opened, is large and unilocular with a thin fibrous tissue wall in which there are numerous delicate blood vessels. About 25 to 50% of acute hydroceles are due to trauma. Others may complicate acute infections or tumours. They usually contain straw-coloured fluid. In chronic hydrocele the wall may be thickened and the testis compressed and atrophic. **11.16 Granulomatous orchitis.** The body of the testis was swollen and had a firm rubbery consistence. On section, the testicular tissue has been replaced by a buff-coloured tissue in which a nodular pattern is detectable. Granulomatous orchitis is a chronic non-specific inflam-

matory lesion of uncertain aetiology which produces a hard swelling of the testis that may simulate a tumour. It predominantly affects middle-aged men and is frequently associated with trauma. Infection and auto-immune disease have been postulated as possible factors. Histology shows a tuberculoid appearance consisting of tubular structures lined by epithelioid cells, lymphocytes, plasma cells and giant cells. **11.17 Diffuse syphilitic orchitis.** Syphilitic orchitis, which can occur in congenital or acquired syphilis, may take the form of either a diffuse interstitial fibrosis or of one or more gummas. In this case the lesion is diffuse, and the testis is small and has a uniform tan colour. The consistence of the organ was hard and on histology increase in fibrous tissue was very marked. In contrast the gummatous testis is enlarged, globular and smooth, with yellowish-white or grey necrotic areas. In contrast to tuberculosis, syphilis typically involves the testis before the epididymis. **11.18 Tuberculosis: epididymis.** The epididymis (top and bottom) is greatly enlarged and replaced by a yellowish-white caseous mass which in parts is undergoing cystic degeneration. It is usual for the testis to remain uninvolved even in the presence of extensive epididymal involvement, and the tunica vaginalis is intact and forms a thick white capsule around the body of the testis. Tuberculous epididymitis is often unilateral and may occur at any age. It frequently complicates pulmonary or genito-urinary tract tuberculosis.

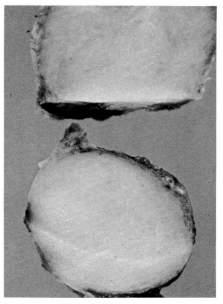

11.19 Adenomatoid tumour: testis

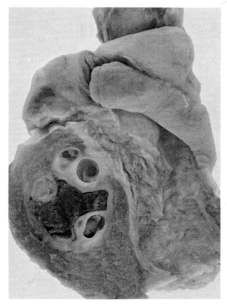

11.20 Teratoma: testis

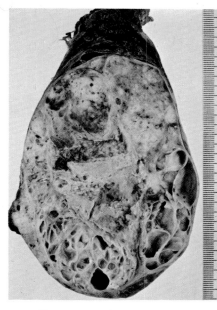

11.21 Teratoma: testis

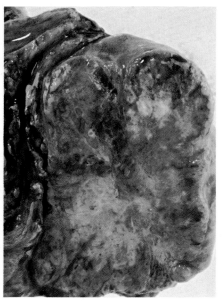

11.22 Teratoma: testis

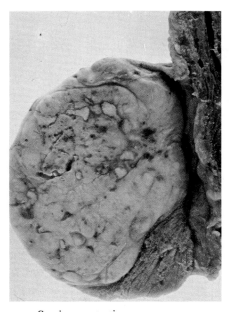

11.23 Seminoma: testis

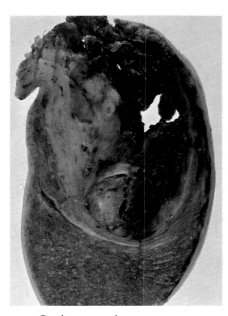

11.24 Seminoma: testis

11.19 Adenomatoid tumour: testis. The tumour formed a discrete round mass (5 x 5 cm) in the epididymis. Its cut surface is grey-white and has an indistinct whorled pattern. The adenomatoid tumour is the commonest tumour of the epididymis. It is generally a painless solitary firm nodule, in patients between 20 and 60 years of age. The histogenesis is controversial but most authorities regard it as Mullerian in origin. The lesion may be found occasionally on the surface of the testis or in the tunica or spermatic cord; and in women on the posterior aspect of the uterus, Fallopian tubes, or ovary. **11.20-11.22 Teratoma: testis.** About 30% of testicular tumours are teratomas. Most of them are partly solid and partly cystic. The solid areas often undergo necrosis and cysts of all sizes form which contain serous or blood-stained fluid. The best-differentiated lesions tend to be almost entirely cystic, and the poorly-differentiated highly malignant ones more solid, with areas of haemorrhage and necrosis. **11.20** This teratoma is an oval cystic mass 1.5 cm in diameter situated in the body of the testis. The cysts are lined by thick greyish-white fibrous tissue, but the tissue in the centre is necrotic and haemorrhagic. Histology showed that a choriocarcinoma, one of the rarest and most malignant complications of teratoma, had developed, and the patient, aged 36, died from multiple lung secondaries. **11.21** This lesion is a mixture of teratoma and seminoma. The testicular tissue has been replaced by a large ovoid tumour of a mixed cystic and solid pattern. The lower pole of the testis (bottom) is almost entirely cystic tumour but the central mass is solid and yellowish-white, with areas of haemorrhage and necrosis. The term 'combined tumour' describes this type of lesion in which seminomatous and teratomatous components can be identified. **11.22** This is a highly malignant, poorly-differentiated teratoma. It was a solid mass, measuring 6 x 4 cm in a man aged 44. Its cut surface is pinkish-white with yellow areas of necrosis and haemorrhage. No cysts are present. Histology revealed that the tumour was an undifferentiated teratoma with occasional gland spaces (teratocarcinoma). **11.23 and 11.24 Seminoma: testis.** Seminoma is the commonest testicular tumour, accounting for 40% of the total. The larger tumours may replace the entire testis whereas the small tumours are circumscribed and lobulated. **11.23** The cut surface of this lesion shows a lobulated pale-grey opaque mass with small areas of yellowish necrosis and haemorrhage. **11.24** An ovoid partly-circumscribed yellowish-grey neoplasm occupies the upper two-thirds of the body of the testis. The tunica albuginea is thickened and haemorrhagic (right). The growth has extended into the epididymis (top left). A large portion of the tumour has undergone haemorrhagic necrosis. Most 'pure' seminomas have a homogeneous appearance and extensive haemorrhage as shown here is rare. Histology of this tumour showed it to be spermatocytic in type. Lymphatic and vascular invasion is present in 60% of seminomas.

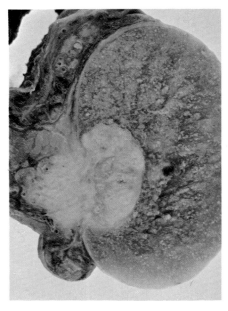

11.25 Undifferentiated tumour: testis

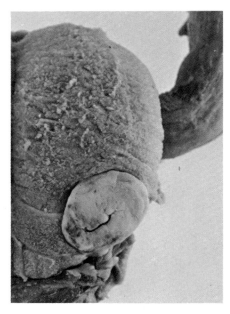

11.26 Sertoli cell tumour: testis

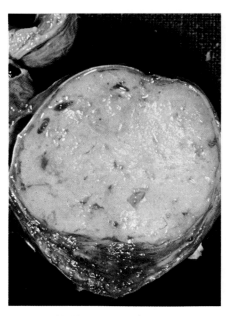

11.27 Orchioblastoma: testis

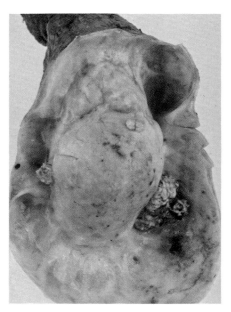

11.28 Hydrocele and teratoma: testis

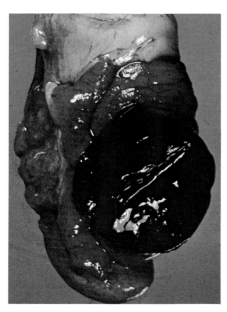

11.29 Interstitial cell tumour: testis

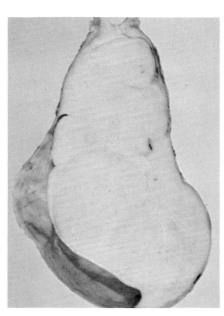

11.30 Lymphosarcoma: testis

11.25 Undifferentiated tumour: testis. A small ovoid tumour in the hilum of the testis is extending into the testis and epididymis. Its cut surface is very pale and has a whorled pattern. Histologically the lesion was an undifferentiated carcinoma. The undifferentiated tumours are assumed to be anaplastic teratomas but because of their carcinomatous structure they are sometimes called embryonal carcinomas. Although they are among the smallest tumours they often show invasion of the capsule and epididymis. **11.26 Sertoli cell tumour: testis.** The patient was a 35-year-old man with gynaecomastia. A small ovoid (1 cm diameter) tumour is located within the lower pole of the testis. It is well-encapsulated and the cut surface is solid and a uniform grey-white colour. Tiny areas of haemorrhage are visible. Sertoli cell tumours are very rare and do not normally invade the substance of the testis. **11.27 Orchioblastoma: testis.** This is a rare rapidly-growing tumour of the infantile testis. It consists of papillary adenocarcinomatous tissue which forms mantles around blood vessels, an appearance that has led some to regard it as an endodermal sinus tumour. The average age of the patient is 1½ years and that was the age in this case. The tumour grows rapidly and has usually replaced the testis by the time of orchidectomy, and in this example the testis has been replaced by a round non-encapsulated yellowish-white tumour within which there are tiny cystic areas. **11.28 Hydrocele and**

teratoma: testis. Hydrocele is a rare complication of testicular neoplasms. This shows an opened, thick-walled creamy-white hydrocele sac. The body of the testis is enlarged, from the presence within it of a malignant teratoma. Small papillary projections of teratoma are present on the surface of the tunica of the testis (top), and friable papillary yellowish masses of tumour are also present within the inner surface of the tunica vaginalis of the hydrocele sac (right). **11.29 Interstitial cell tumour: testis.** This uncommon benign growth is derived from the interstitial (Leydig) cells. It accounts for about 1% of testicular tumours and typically forms a small round or ovoid yellow-brown mass which is invariably located within the substance of the testis. This specimen, from a 4-year-old boy with precocious puberty, is a dark brownish encapsulated mass which measured 1.7 x 1.8 cm. The dark colour is due to the presence of large quantities of lipofuscin. **11.30 Lymphosarcoma: testis.** The body of the testis, epididymis and cord are diffusely invaded and expanded by a cream-coloured and remarkably homogeneous tissue. There is no evidence of necrosis, though this may be present in some lesions. Malignant lymphoma constitutes 7% of all testicular tumours. Frequently it is bilateral. Most occur between the ages of 60 and 80 years. Grossly the body of the testis is usually hard and may be lobulated. Histologically the majority are poorly-differentiated lymphocytic lymphomas.

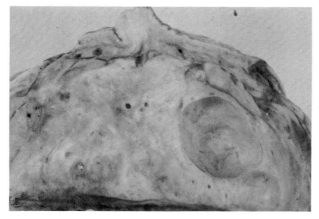

12.1 Fibroepithelial hyperplasia: breast

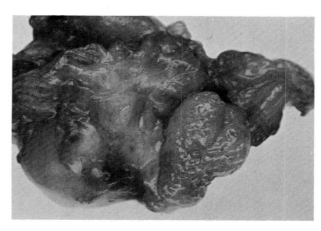

12.2 Intraduct papilloma: breast

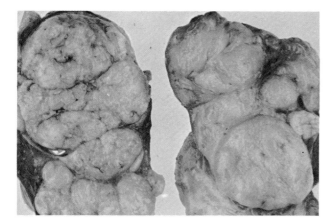

12.3 Fibroadenoma: breast

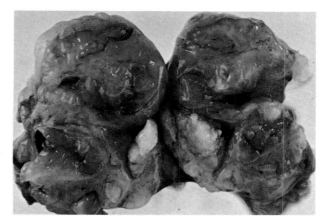

12.4 Fibroadenoma: breast

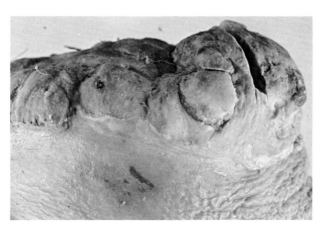

12.5 Giant fibroadenoma: breast

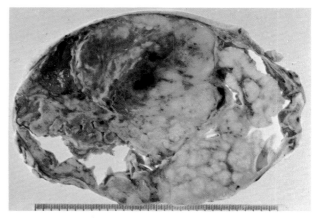

12.6 Giant fibroadenoma: breast

12.1 Fibroepithelial hyperplasia ('chronic mastitis'): breast. This condition is often bilateral and is usually found in women in the last decade of reproductive life. On palpation the breast tends to feel 'shotty' and firm. In this example, the cut surface shows replacement of the glandular tissue by greyish-white fibrous tissue within which are small and large cysts (lower right). The cysts are usually multiple and variable in size. **12.2 Intraduct papilloma: breast.** Intraduct or intracystic papillomas occur predominantly in parous pre-menopausal women and are often multiple. Most patients present with a sero-sanguineous discharge from the nipple. The papilloma is typically located within the lactiferous ducts or forms a nodule projecting into a cyst beneath the areola. In this case, a firm lobulated pale yellow papilloma (1.5 cm diameter) is present within a dilated duct (lower right). The lesion has a granular surface and forms a raspberry-like nodule. **12.3 and 12.4 Fibroadenoma: breast.** Fibroadenomas essentially consist of distorted giant lobules formed by focal uncoordinated overgrowth of the epithelial and connective tissues of the breast. They are the commonest breast tumour in women between the ages of 13 and 30 years, with a peak incidence between 20 and 25. They are usually firm, lobulated, sharply-delineated and occasionally multiple. They may be 'hard' or 'soft', the latter type tending to occur in older patients. Two histological variants of the 'hard' variety are recognised, the intracanalicular and the pericanalicular. **12.3**

Two large (6 cm in long axis) intracanalicular fibroadenomas are shown in section. Each is well-encapsulated and made up of 'lobules' of yellowish glistening connective tissue separated by clefts of red fibrous tissue septa. **12.4** Occasionally a 'soft' fibroadenoma presents a mucinous appearance on section, from the presence of large amounts of connective tissue glycosoaminoglycan. This soft gelatinous lobulated mass (measuring 6 x 5 cm) was removed from the breast of a 50-year-old woman. Histology showed a well-marked myxomatous change in the stroma. This change reaches an extreme form in the giant fibroadenoma. **12.5-12.7 Giant fibroadenoma: breast.** Giant fibroadenomas occur in older women, between 40 and 50 years of age. They are bulky growths as a rule, solid and bosselated. A minority are cystic. The connective tissue component is conspicuous and very myxomatous, and may mask the glandular structures. Most are benign though a few behave like sarcomas. In the majority of cases, the lesion has evolved from a pre-existing fibroadenoma. **12.5** This specimen is very large, filling the breast and protruding through the skin to produce a large fungating ulcer. Ulceration of the skin over a giant fibroadenoma is unusual. **12.6** This is the cut surface of another giant fibroadenoma (15 x 11 cm) from a 49-year-old woman. Most of the tumour consists of solid pinkish-white tissue, with yellow myxomatous areas, as well as recent haemorrhage (top) and cystic degeneration and necrosis (lower left). Polypoid masses project into the cystic cavities.

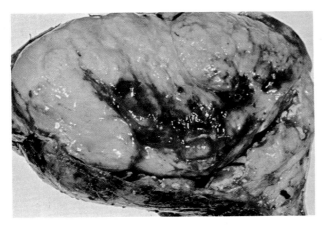

12.7 Cystosarcoma phylloides: breast

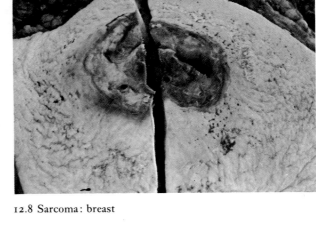

12.8 Sarcoma: breast

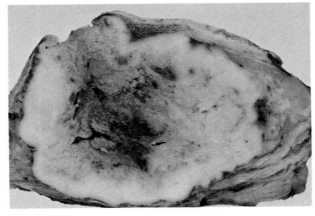

12.9 Sarcoma: breast

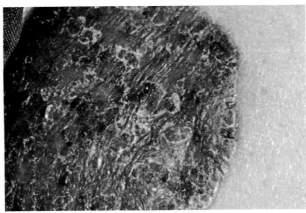

12.10 Paget's disease: breast

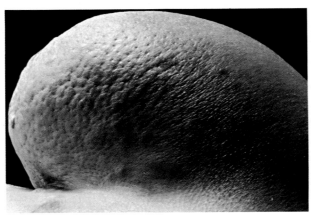

12.11 Carcinoma: breast

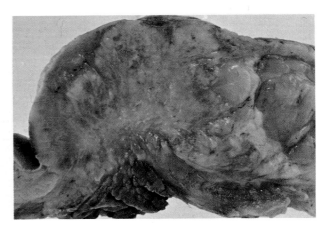

12.12 Carcinoma: breast

12.7 Cystosarcoma phylloides: breast. The term cystosarcoma phylloides is sometimes applied to giant fibroadenoma but is best reserved for giant fibroadenomas in which malignant change is definitely present. The term is derived from the macroscopic appearance of the cut surface and particularly the leaf-like pattern. This shows the cut surface of a markedly myxomatous tumour with extensive recent haemorrhage. **12.8 and 12.9 Sarcoma: breast.** Sarcoma of the breast is a rare tumour and probably represents less than 1% of all malignant breast tumours. It is usually a fibrosarcoma, but liposarcoma, leiomyosarcoma and rhabdomyosarcoma have been described. It is more malignant than the malignant giant fibroadenoma and tends to metastasise by the bloodstream. **12.8** This shows a depressed ulcer in the skin overlying a sarcoma. **12.9** This is a section of the breast shown in 12.8. The tumour underlying the ulcer is a large (10 x 7 cm) ovoid white mass with a central area of necrosis and haemorrhage. **12.10 Paget's disease: breast.** The nipple is indrawn and the areola replaced by a red, granular, ulcerated area, the surface of which is covered with dry greyish-white scales. Paget's disease typically has a long duration and is nearly always associated with an

intraduct carcinoma. It usually affects women 50 to 60 years of age. The histogenesis is still debatable but intra-epidermal spread from an intraduct carcinoma is more likely than a primary origin from the epidermis of the nipple or areola. **12.11-12.18 Carcinoma: breast.** Local spread of breast carcinoma with involvement of the subareolar lymphatic plexus is common, and retrograde spread to the skin via the periductal lymphatics and lymphatics of Cooper's ligaments is also frequently found. **12.11** This shows the 'peau d'orange' appearance which may follow such spread. The skin over the breast is yellowish-brown, with raised nodules and many pitted areas. The peau d'orange appearance is produced by bulging of severely oedematous skin around the hair follicles and sweat glands. The oedema is caused by occlusion of the deep lymphatics. **12.12** The tumour is a large lobulated pinkish-white mass in the centre of which there are tiny yellowish-white necrotic foci. The underlying pectoral muscles are deeply invaded and the nipple and adjacent skin are also infiltrated and ulcerated. Skin involvement results from lymphatic permeation and direct spread. About 40% of carcinomas are located in the upper outer quadrant of the breast.

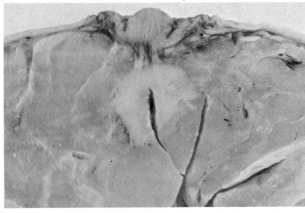

12.13 Scirrhous carcinoma: breast

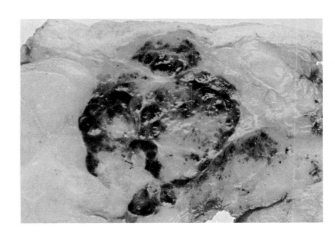

12.14 Mucinous carcinoma: breast

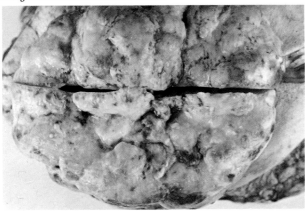

12.15 Medullary carcinoma: breast

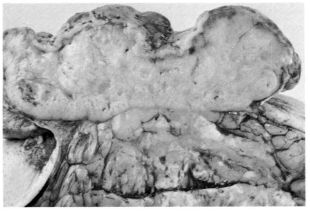

12.16 Medullary carcinoma: breast

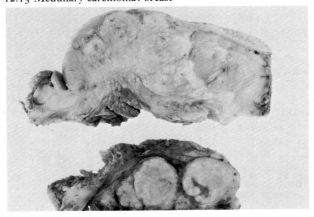

12.17 Scirrhous carcinoma: breast

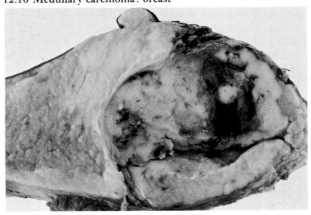

12.18 'Lactational' carcinoma: breast

12.13-12.18 Carcinoma: breast. 12.13 This is a scirrhous type of carcinoma. It forms a small white mass beneath the nipple, but radiating claw-like processes extend from its edge into the adjacent fat. Extension into the nipple ducts has also occurred, with characteristic indrawing of the nipple. The tumour was hard and gritty on section. The average age of occurrence is 50 years. **12.14** This is mucinous carcinoma, an uncommon lesion. The term mucinous (or colloid) carcinoma is reserved for those neoplasms in which the growth is largely replaced by a mucinous substance. This lesion is a translucent lobulated jelly-like mass with areas of recent haemorrhage and traversed by fibrous septa. Mucinous carcinomas tend to be large and bulky. The prognosis is variable. A few have a very poor prognosis but most grow slowly and spread is relatively late. The latter are associated with a more favourable outcome than the other types of breast carcinoma. **12.15** Medullary carcinoma constitutes about 5-10% of all breast cancers. It is usually a large soft tumour, situated deep within the breast, and on section appears as a soft opaque grey-white mass flecked with haemorrhage and necrosis. The lesion is often well-circumscribed, with a well-defined growing edge. Skin ulceration is rare but it has occurred on a very extensive scale in this example. The tumour has penetrated the skin to form a large irregular polypoid ulcerated mass, the surface of which is covered with a necrotic greenish slough. **12.16** This is the lesion shown in 12.15. Section reveals a large ovoid solid creamy-white growth with an apparently smooth regular outline. **12.17** The breast (top) contains a large irregular lobulated pinkish-white scirrhous carcinoma which is flecked with yellowish foci of necrosis. In the portion of axillary fat (below) there are two enlarged lymph nodes extensively replaced by yellowish-white secondary tumour. About 60% of patients with breast carcinoma have axillary metastases at the time of removal. **12.18** This is a 'lactational' carcinoma. Clinically such a tumour resembles an acute inflammatory lesion of the breast and is therefore a special type by virtue of the clinical presentation. It pursues a rapidly malignant course. This specimen is a large greyish-white tumour and extensive central necrosis and haemorrhage are prominent features. Acute inflammatory or lactational carcinoma comprises about 1% of all mammary carcinomas and usually occurs in young women, particularly during lactation. This patient, a 30-year-old woman, was lactating following childbirth and hyperplastic lobules are visible on the left.

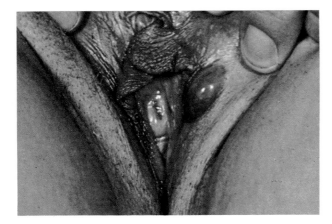

12.19 Hidradenoma: vulva

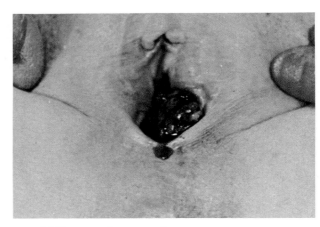

12.20 Malignant melanoma: vulva

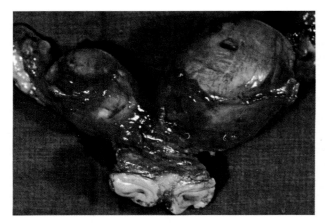

12.21 Bicornuate uterus and bicollis

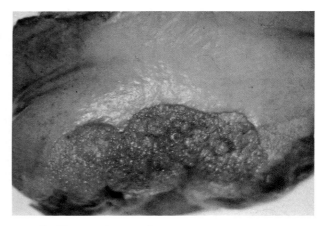

12.22 Papillary erosion: cervix

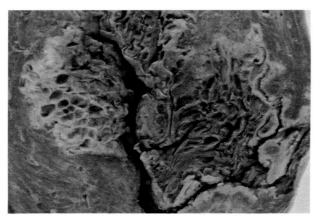

12.23 Gas-gangrene: uterus

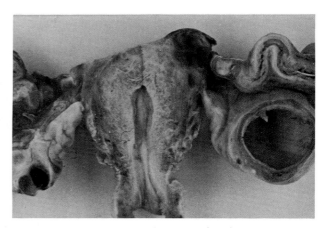

12.24 Bilateral pyosalpinx and tubo-ovarian abscesses

12.19 Hidradenoma: vulva. The lesion forms a raised bluish-black nodule on the labium major. The vulva is the most frequent site for hidradenoma, but hidradenoma comprises less than 3% of all vulval cysts and tumours. It is usually small (1-2 cm) and cystic and situated on the labia majora. It may project above the surface but more commonly it is subcutaneous. It usually occurs between the ages of 30 and 50. **12.20 Malignant melanoma: vulva.** The tumour is an irregular polypoid black mass growing just at and protruding through the introitus. Malignant melanoma constitutes about 2% of malignant vulval tumours, whereas melanoma of the vagina is the rarest of the malignant vaginal tumours and is usually located just within the introitus. The lesion tends to ulcerate and bleed. It can occur at all ages. **12.21 Bicornuate uterus and bicollis.** Congenital anomalies of the uterus, vagina and vulva follow failure of fusion of the midline portions of the Mullerian ducts at various levels and to varying degrees. All grades between complete and minimal failure of fusion occur. In this case, the body of the uterus has two 'horns' (bicornuate uterus) of somewhat unequal size, and two cervices are also present (bicollis). **12.22 Papillary erosion: cervix.** The term erosion is a clinical description for a reddened area around the external os, and this example forms a granular, velvety reddish papillary area on the surface of the cervix. It is not an ulcer, however, and

histological examination of the affected area showed only the presence of endocervical columnar epithelium within papillae, crypts and glandular formations. Different histological patterns of the columnar epithelium give rise to several types of erosion, namely the flat, papillary, adenomatous and follicular. An erosion may be large or small, or asymmetrical. **12.23 Gas-gangrene: uterus.** The myometrium of the fundus is extensively replaced by a honeycomb of necrotic tissue and cysts containing greenish-brown pus. The endometrium is also covered by a thick purulent exudate. In pyometria, anaerobic organisms are frequently present, alone or in combination with aerobic organisms. In this case the causative organism was *Clostridium welchii*. Usually the lesion results from induced abortion, curettage or interruption of pregnancy. This patient had an abortion. **12.24 Bilateral pyosalpinx and tubo-ovarian abscesses.** The patient was a 33-year-old woman with gonococcal infection. Such an infection tends to produce extensive fibrous adhesions, pyosalpinx, and tubo-ovarian abscesses. The endometrium is covered with a greenish exudate. The Fallopian tubes are thickened and retort-shaped, as a result of inflammatory adhesions and contain opaque greenish-yellow pus. Their serosal surface is hyperaemic. The ovary on the left contains a corpus luteum and some simple follicular cysts.

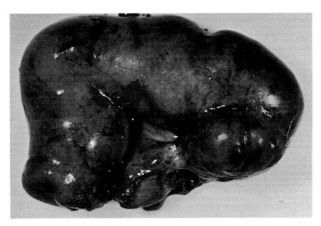

12.25 Tuberculous pyosalpinx

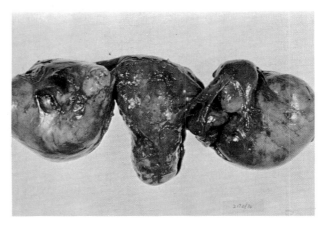

12.26 Endometriosis: ovaries

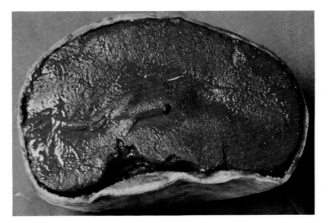

12.27 Endometriosis: ovary

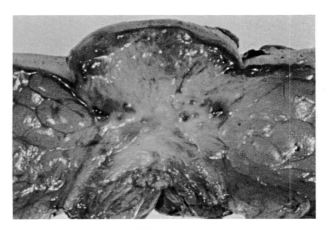

12.28 Endometriosis: umbilicus

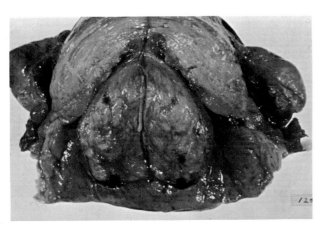

12.29 Stromal endometriosis: uterus

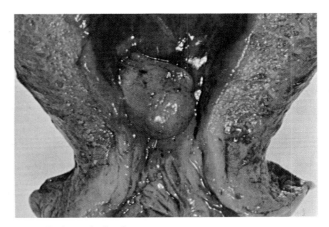

12.30 Endocervical polyp: uterus

12.25 Tuberculous pyosalpinx. In the United Kingdom pelvic tuberculosis is found in about 5% of infertile patients between 20 and 40 years of age. The method of spread to the pelvis is by the bloodstream from a focus elsewhere. This Fallopian tube is thickened, dilated, tortuous and flask-shaped. The serosal aspect is hyperaemic and fine fibrous adhesions are visible. Tuberculosis usually starts in the distal part of the tube, which gradually thickens and becomes tortuous but soft in consistence. In the later stages the lumen contains caseous material, as did this tube. **12.26-12.29 Endometriosis.** Endometriosis is the presence of functioning endometrium in ectopic sites. The ovary is the commonest site and in about half the cases both ovaries are affected. **12.26** Bilateral multilocular ovarian cysts are present. The one on the right is a shiny blue thin-walled cyst, the colour resulting from the contained blood. The serosal surface of the ovaries and uterus shows haemorrhagic tags and is irregularly puckered by fibrous adhesions, particularly well seen (centre right) linking the ovary to the lateral aspect of the body of the uterus. **12.27** This is a 'chocolate cyst' of ovary, a thin-walled cyst filled with altered blood. The term tarry cyst is sometimes also used. The lining of the cyst is fairly thin but sometimes it is thick and granular. The nature and colour of the cyst depend on the menstrual phase, the amount of recent haemorrhage, the duration of the process, and the reaction to extravasated blood. In earlier lesions there may be multiple cysts but later there is just one. The endometrium may be destroyed by the haemorrhage and replaced by collections of haemo-

siderin-laden macrophages. **12.28** This is a section through the umbilicus. The ectopic endometrial tissue has caused the formation of a raised greyish-white mass within which there are several small blood-filled cysts. Umbilical endometriosis is rare but extension of endometriosis within the pelvis is common. Involvement of operation wounds is thought to result from implantation of endometrial tissue at operation and a similar mechanism may have been responsible in this case. **12.29** This is another rare form of 'endometriosis', namely stromal endometriosis. The uterus is bulky and a large fleshy tongue-shaped mass of tissue fills the cavity and projects through the cervical os. The wall of the uterus is thickened and yellowish-white polypoid nodules of the tissue may be seen in the myometrium. Microscopically the tissue is composed of endometrial stromal cells which may invade the lymphatic channels and blood vessels in the myometrium, and most authorities regard stromal endometriosis as a localised low-grade stromal sarcoma which remains confined to the uterus. It usually occurs between the ages of 30 and 50 years. **12.30 Endocervical polyp: uterus.** A rounded gelatinous polyp fills the endocervical canal. It is a benign lesion. Endocervical polyps are usually multiple, small and pedunculated. They are soft in consistence and covered with mucus. The larger ones may protrude through the external os. Histologically such a polyp is composed of a fibrous tissue stroma covered by mucin-secreting columnar epithelium of the type that normally lines the endocervix.

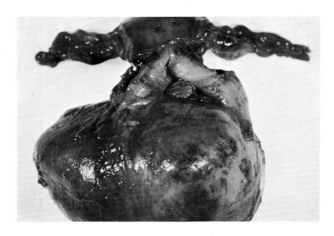

12.31 Leiomyoma: uterus

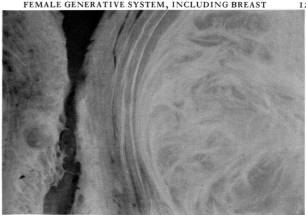

12.32 Leiomyoma: uterus

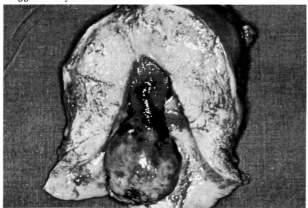

12.33 Leiomyomas: uterus

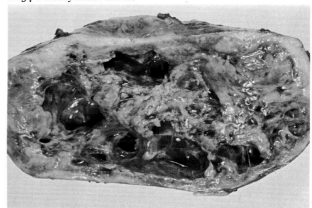

12.34 Leiomyomas: uterus

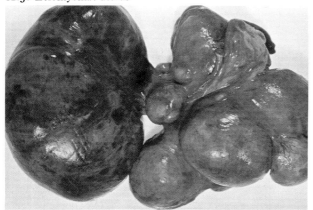

12.35 Leiomyoma: uterus

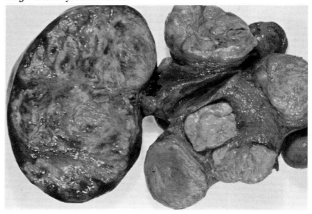

12.36 Leiomyoma: uterus

12.31-12.37 Leiomyoma: uterus. Leiomyomas are usually multiple. About 60% are located within the myometrium (intramural), about 20% are submucous, and about 20% are subserous. **12.31** This one is cervical in origin. Cervical leiomyomas are usually solitary and two types are described: those that lie within the cervix and are surrounded by it (true cervical), and those that are embedded in the outer part of the wall of the cervix (paracervical). This one is paracervical. It forms a large smooth ovoid mass which expands and displaces the cervix. The serosal surface is haemorrhagic. The body of the uterus sits on top of the tumour. **12.32** This shows in close-up the cut surface of part of a large round intramural leiomyoma. It demonstrates the shiny pinkish-white whorled appearance of the lesion. There is a well-developed false capsule of greyish-brown fibrous tissue and compressed muscle around the tumour. This patient was pregnant and during pregnancy a large tumour like this may undergo a form of necrosis called 'red degeneration'. **12.33** This shows multiple subserous and intramural leiomyomas. The largest of these (left) is subserous and pedunculated. It is a dusky red colour as a result of intense vascular engorgement following torsion of the pedicle.

Torsion of submucosal or subserous leiomyomas, with twisting of the pedicle, is an unusual complication. **12.34** This is the cut surface of the leiomyoma shown in 12.33. The large tumour (left) which had undergone torsion has a haemorrhagic appearance which contrasts with the pallor of the other tumours (right) in the wall of the uterus. The latter shows clearly the characteristic shiny whorled pattern of leiomyomas. **12.35** This is a pedunculated submucous leiomyoma. Arising from the fundus of the uterus it now protrudes through the cervical os. It is ovoid and suspended on a broad elongated stalk. The pedicle is haemorrhagic as a result of torsion and impairment of the blood supply, and the tumour is in consequence necrotic and gangrenous. Its colour is yellow-green and there is evidence of recent haemorrhage. The tip of the tumour is ulcerated and infected. **12.36** This leiomyoma, on section, shows extensive cystic and hyaline degeneration, the usual greyish-white tissue being replaced by gelatinous pink tissue. Irregular strands of tissue traverse the cystic cavities (centre). Hyaline degeneration is very common and present to a variable degree in most leiomyomas. The hyalinised areas appear translucent and may liquefy to produce the cystic areas.

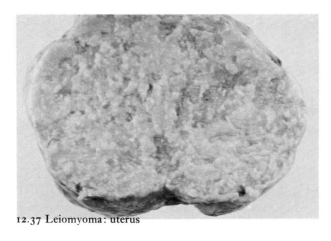

12.37 Leiomyoma: uterus

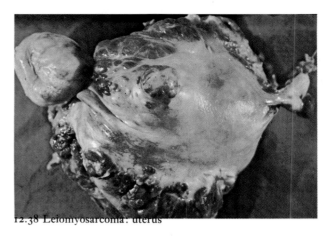

12.38 Leiomyosarcoma: uterus

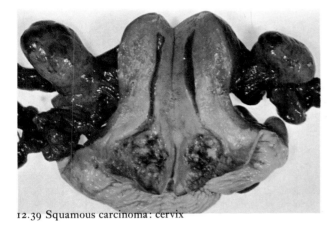

12.39 Squamous carcinoma: cervix

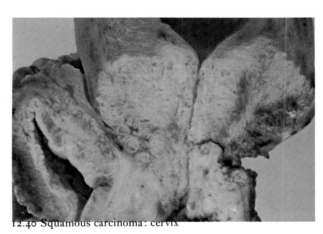

12.40 Squamous carcinoma: cervix

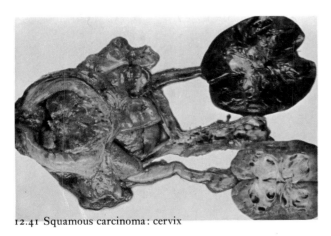

12.41 Squamous carcinoma: cervix

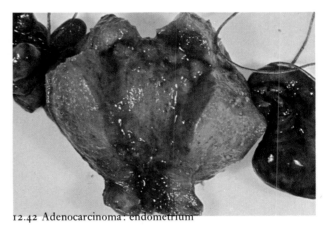

12.42 Adenocarcinoma: endometrium

12.37 Leiomyoma: uterus. The cut surface of this leiomyoma has a speckled white colour due to widespread granular calcification. Calcification is often found in leiomyomas in post-menopausal women and usually follows necrosis. Two forms of calcification occur. In one form (as shown here), granular masses of calcium salts are deposited throughout the tumour; in the other, they are laid down in layers mainly at the periphery. **12.38 Leiomyosarcoma: uterus.** This shows the fundus of a very bulky uterus. Multiple nodules of reddish-brown lobulated tumour (upper and lower centre) protrude through the serosal surface, and on section extensive invasion of the uterine wall and cavity by similar tumour was found. Leiomyosarcomas comprise 50% to 75% of various series of uterine sarcomas. Most arise *de novo* and only very rarely does a leiomyoma progress to sarcoma. Typically a leiomyosarcoma tends to be a soft haemorrhagic type of growth. **12.39-12.41 Squamous carcinoma: cervix.** Squamous carcinoma of the cervix constitutes 11% of all malignant tumours in women, second only to breast carcinoma in frequency. Macroscopically three types are recognised; the excavating ulcerating, the nodular papillary, and the flat infiltrating. **12.39** This lesion forms an irregular, ulcerating and partly papillary growth which involves the ectocervix and extends over the posterior wall of the endocervix. **12.40** This is an advanced lesion. The uterus, cervix, bladder and upper vagina are shown in sagittal section. The cervix is expanded

by a diffuse yellowish-white infiltrating tumour, the surface of which is finely cystic in parts. There is invasion of the upper vaginal vault and posterior wall of the bladder. The vagina is the most frequent site of direct spread in carcinoma of the cervix and extension onto the vault and down the vaginal wall is almost always present in advanced disease. **12.41** Parametrial, paracervical and paravaginal spread frequently occurs early with carcinoma of the cervix and direct infiltration of the bladder and ureters is common. Urinary tract obstruction with infection and impaired renal function inevitably follow. Terminal uraemia is the usual mode of death and this illustrates such an event. Both kidneys, ureters and bladder are shown. Bilateral hydronephrosis and hydroureter have developed, secondary to intrapelvic spread of the tumour. In addition the mucosa of the opened bladder is infiltrated by red-brown friable polypoid tumour. **12.42-12.45 Adenocarcinoma: endometrium.** Macroscopically, endometrial carcinoma may be diffuse or discrete. The diffuse variety may be confined to the endometrial layer and appear as pale friable polypoid growth. Discrete tumours are commoner in the upper posterior wall of the fundus and they may be polypoid or papillary. They frequently show myometrial invasion. **12.42** This is the discrete type of lesion. Irregular pale nodules of growth are present in the fundus of the opened uterus, adjacent to both cornua. The Fallopian tubes are distended and dark-coloured from haemorrhage into them.

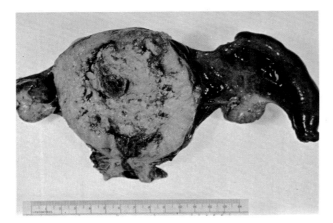

12.43 Adenocarcinoma: endometrium

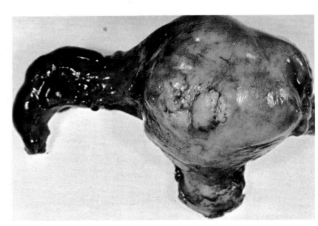

12.44 Adenocarcinoma: endometrium

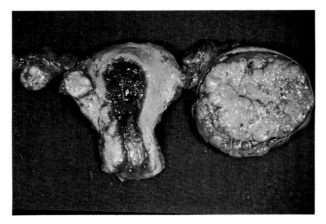

12.45 Adenocarcinoma: endometrium

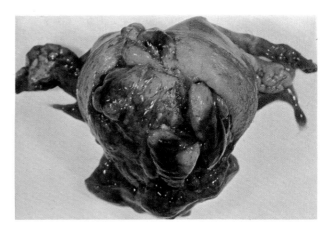

12.46 Mesodermal mixed tumour: uterus

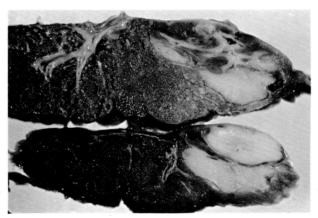

12.47 Chorioangioma: placenta

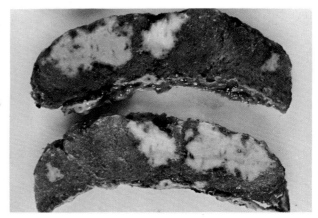

12.48 Infarction: placenta

12.43-12.45 Adenocarcinoma: endometrium. 12.43 This is the diffuse pattern of growth. The cavity of the uterus is enlarged and filled with a pinkish-white sessile polypoid tumour in which there are areas of haemorrhagic necrosis (top left). The right Fallopian tube is distended and blue-black from haemorrhage within it. Spread to the uterine portion of the tube occurs directly from tumour growing in the region of the cornu. Further spread within the tube is usually by lymphatics or along the mucous membrane to involve the greater part of the tube. **12.44** Endometrial carcinoma tends to spread outside the uterus late in the course of the disease compared with carcinoma of the cervix. This is the serosal surface of the uterus from 12.43. Extensive infiltration of the myometrium is present, producing multiple peritoneal nodules (left) and a greyish-white mass (centre). **12.45** The carcinomatous tissue forms a haemorrhagic polypoid mass confined to the fundus of the uterus. However the right ovary (right) contains a large spherical coarsely-lobulated pinkish-white metastasis. The ovary is one of the principal sites of secondary deposits from endometrial carcinoma, and one or both may be affected. The incidence of ovarian involvement varies between 5% in surgical specimens to 15% at necropsy. In some cases, it may be impossible to exclude the possibility that the ovarian tumour is a coincidental carcinoma. A small intramural leiomyoma is present (left) and the left ovary is slightly enlarged. **12.46 Mesodermal mixed tumour: uterus.** The cavity of the uterus is distended by a gelatinous

pinkish-white lobulated and polypoid mass in which there is evidence of recent haemorrhage. The cut surface appeared fleshy and sarcomatous. Mesodermal mixed tumour occurs almost exclusively in the body of the uterus, cervix or vagina. It may occur at all ages but in older patients it is commonest in the corpus. It appears to grow from the mucosal stroma. The prognosis is poor. **12.47 Chorioangioma: placenta.** Chorioangioma is the commonest placental tumour, with an incidence of about 0.8% of all placentas examined. Multiple lesions are present in about 10% of cases. It is frequently situated on the fetal aspect. Macroscopically it is a sharply-defined rounded or lobulated lesion, usually red in colour but sometimes much paler, as in this example, which forms a sharply-defined smooth white mass within the placenta. Histologically it consists of fibrous connective tissue and small blood vessels. **12.48 Infarction: placenta.** Several infarcts are present in each of the two sections of this placenta. They are yellowish-white and of very irregular shape. Some are surrounded by a dark haemorrhagic border. Placental infarction is due to interference with the maternal circulation and occlusion of spiral arteriolar sinusoids. The infarcts are continuous with the maternal surface, often sharply circumscribed, and vary in size. Recent infarcts are red in colour, but when the lesions occur some time before delivery, the haemoglobin is broken down and the area appears yellowish-white. They are commonly seen in toxaemia of pregnancy.

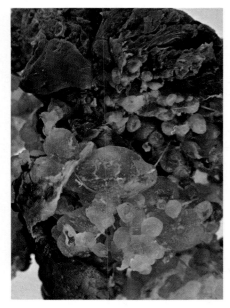

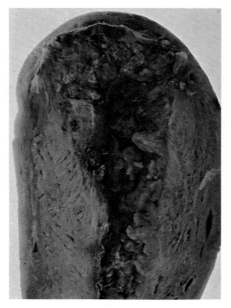

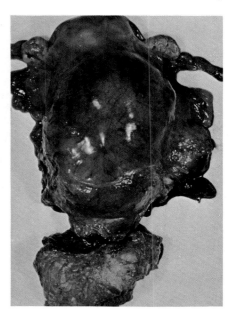

12.49 Hydatidiform mole   12.50 Hydatidiform mole: uterus   12.51 Choriocarcinoma: uterus

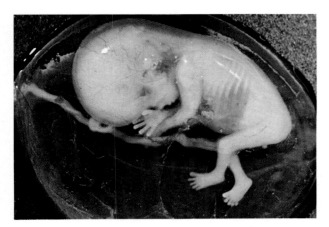

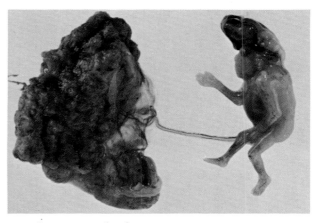

12.52 Spontaneous abortion   12.53 Spontaneous abortion

12.49 and 12.50 Hydatidiform mole. Hydatidiform mole is a rare complication of pregnancy, developing in about 1 to 2000 pregnancies in the United States. It is characterised by the progressive swelling of the stroma of the chorionic villi associated with either loss of or failure of development of the fetal vascular system and accompanied by a variable degree of trophoblastic proliferation. The common pathogenetic factor is absence or death of the early embryo with disappearance of embryonic vessels. In other words it may be a temporarily missed abortion of a 'blighted' ovum, whose chorionic villi continue to enlarge to form grape-like vesicles during the additional weeks they are retained in the uterus. **12.49** This shows a mass of such cystic villi, in the form of discrete rounded translucent vesicles. Greyish-white foci of trophoblastic proliferation are visible over the vesicles (centre). **12.50** This is a sagittal section of a uterus containing a hydatidiform mole. The cavity of the uterus contains grape-like vesicles and there is extensive local invasion of the myometrium by molar villi as a consequence of the proliferating trophoblastic activity. Some moles are particularly aggressive and show invasive properties, with vascular permeation (chorioadenoma destruens). Such a lesion may cause uterine perforation but only rarely do moles behave in a truly malignant fashion. **12.51 Choriocarcinoma: uterus.** Choriocarcinoma is a malignant tumour of trophoblast. Its incidence varies from 1 to 40,000 to 1 in 100,000 pregnancies. It is preceded by a hydatidiform mole in 40 to 50% of cases and in about 25% of cases it follows an abortion or ectopic pregnancy. Grossly it is a bulky haemorrhagic necrotic tumour which tends to metastasise to the lung, vagina, brain and liver. In this case, the tumour forms a large mass which has expanded the lower part of the body of the uterus and invaded the cervix and upper vagina. **12.52-12.54 Spontaneous abortion.** It is probable that about one half of all early ova develop abnormally and most of these abort, often before the mother recognises that she is pregnant. Of clinically apparent pregnancies, 10 to 15% terminate spontaneously.

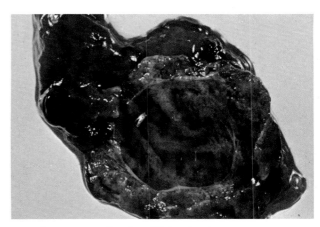

12.54 Spontaneous abortion: blighted ovum

12.52 This shows an early fetus with intact membranes but no placenta. The age of gestation is approximately 10-12 weeks. **12.53** This fetus shows a gross malformation of the central nervous system with exteriorisation of the brain as a result of failure of the neural tube to close. Congenital malformations of the central nervous system are the commonest group of abnormalities in the newborn, the most frequent being anencephaly which occurs in about 1 in 500 births. **12.54 Blighted ovum.** A complete spontaneously aborted pregnancy of about 12 weeks' gestation is shown. The sac has been opened. There is no embryo or evidence of vessels in the chorionic plate (centre circular area), the sac containing only mucoid fluid. Blighted ova are common in early spontaneous abortions and many have an abnormal chromosomal constitution.

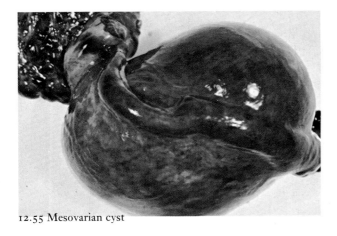

12.55 Mesovarian cyst

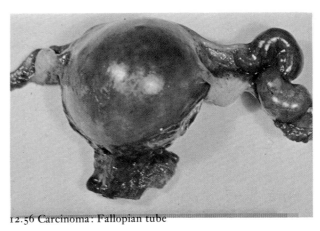

12.56 Carcinoma: Fallopian tube

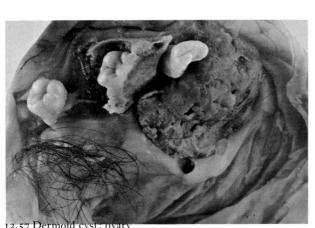

12.57 Dermoid cyst: ovary

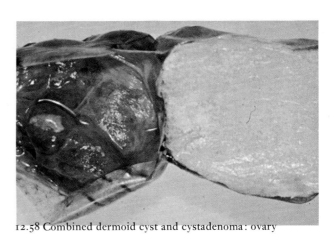

12.58 Combined dermoid cyst and cystadenoma: ovary

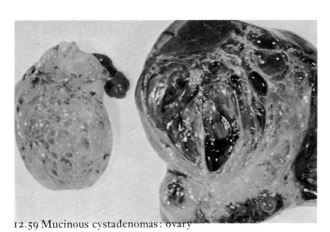

12.59 Mucinous cystadenomas: ovary

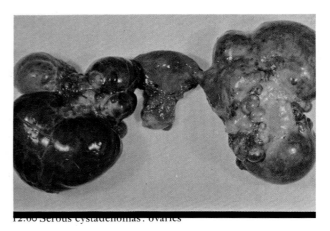

12.60 Serous cystadenomas: ovaries

12.55 Mesovarian cyst. Mesovarian cysts are separate from the ovary and tube and may develop from mesonephric or paramesonephric remnants. Large laterally-placed paraovarian cysts may arise from the rete ovarii. This specimen, in the mesovarium, is large, red-brown and typically smooth-surfaced. The Fallopian tube is displaced over its surface. The cyst contained watery fluid and its wall was composed of a thin layer of fibrous tissue lined by cuboidal epithelium. The term 'broad ligament cyst' is frequently used when the histogenesis is uncertain. **12.56 Carcinoma: Fallopian tube.** Carcinoma of the Fallopian tube is very rare, constituting less than 1% of genital cancer. In about a quarter of the cases it is bilateral. In this case the right tube is affected. It is dilated and tortuous and the middle portion is bluish-black from the presence of a haemosalpinx. The tumour usually involves the distal third of the tube and is papillary in type. There is often an associated hydrosalpinx or pyosalpinx on the affected side. **12.57 Dermoid cyst: ovary.** A dermoid cyst is a benign cystic teratoma and although sebaceous material and hair are prominent among the contents, the solid areas usually present may contain tissues derived from ectoderm, endoderm or mesoderm, such as skin, epithelium, bone, cartilage and teeth. This one is typically thin-walled and unilocular. It contains hair (bottom left) and yellowish-brown sebaceous material (centre). Three well-formed teeth are present on a raised solid area. Dermoid cysts constitute about 25% of all ovarian tumours. They are bilateral in about 10% of cases and can occur at all ages. **12.58 Combined dermoid cyst and cystadenoma: ovary.**

Mucinous cysts and dermoid cysts in some instances occur together in an ovary. In this bilocular cyst the cyst on the left is a mucinous cystadenoma and the thin-walled cyst on the right is a dermoid cyst filled as usual with inspissated yellowish-white sebaceous material. Alimentary-type epithelium occurs in ovarian teratomas and the mucinous cyst may represent overgrowth of this type of epithelium in the teratoma. **12.59 Mucinous cystadenomas: ovary.** Bilateral multilocular cysts are present. The smaller, on the left, is a yellowish-white mass containing many small cysts. The larger, on the right, is also multiloculated, the cysts containing yellowish-brown watery mucinous fluid (top). Areas of haemorrhage are present. Mucinous cystadenomas constitute between 20% and 25% of ovarian tumours. They tend to be bilateral and are often very large. They are found in the age group 20 to 50 years. Malignant change is rare. **12.60 to 12.62 Serous cystadenoma and cystadenocarcinoma: ovary.** Serous cystadenoma is one of the commonest primary ovarian tumours, constituting 30% of all ovarian tumours, and serous cystadenocarcinoma comprises more than half of ovarian carcinomas. Benign serous cystadenomas are usually multilocular, thin-walled cysts with a smooth outer wall. About 20% of the simple cysts are bilateral and about half of the malignant ones are bilateral. The malignant varieties usually occur from 30 to 60 years of age. They tend to be large, usually being over 15 cm in diameter. **12.60** This shows bilateral benign cystadenomas. They are large irregularly-lobulated masses replacing both ovaries. The bluish discolouration is due to haemorrhage into the cyst.

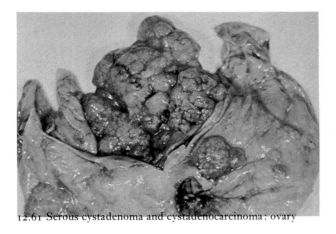

12.61 Serous cystadenoma and cystadenocarcinoma: ovary

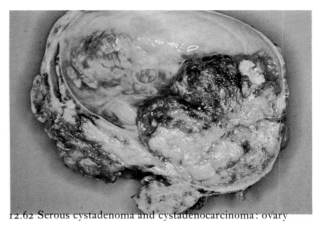

12.62 Serous cystadenoma and cystadenocarcinoma: ovary

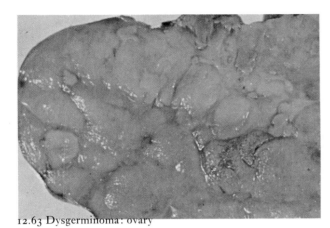

12.63 Dysgerminoma: ovary

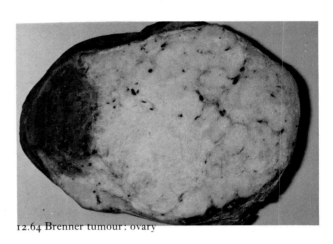

12.64 Brenner tumour: ovary

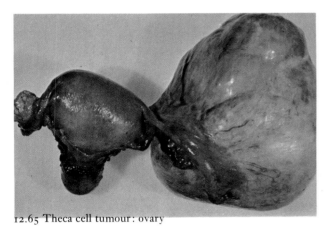

12.65 Theca cell tumour: ovary

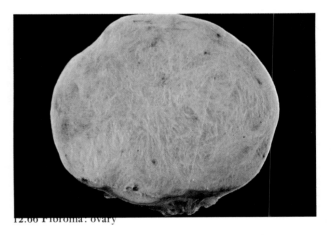

12.66 Fibroma: ovary

12.61 and 12.62 Serous cystadenoma and cystadenocarcinoma: ovary. 12.61 The presence of papillary structures lining the cyst, with solid nodules of tissue, is highly suggestive of malignancy, and these features are evident in this opened serous cystadenoma. The wall of the cyst is thin but the inner surface contains solid masses of pale pink friable papillary tissue. The external surface of a cyst like this often has crumbly excrescences of solid tumour growing on it which may spread into the peritoneum. **12.62** This cyst is frankly carcinomatous. A mass of haemorrhagic necrotic pinkish-white tissue (lower right) projects into the cyst cavity and in addition solid nodules of tumour project from the external surface of the cyst. **12.63 Dysgerminoma: ovary.** Dysgerminoma is an epithelial tumour of primordial germ cells of the embryonic gonad. It constitutes 4 to 5% of malignant tumours and 1% of all ovarian tumours, being commonest between the ages of 10 and 30 years. 50% occur on the right side, 35% on the left, and the remainder are bilateral. The cut surface of this one shows it to be a solid lobulated pinkish-grey encapsulated lesion with foci of whitish necrosis (left). **12.64 Brenner tumour: ovary.** The Brenner tumour comprises about 2% of all ovarian

tumours. It occurs usually between the ages of 40 and 70 and is nearly always unilateral. It may be solid or cystic, and about 20% are associated with mucinous cystadenomas. This one is a smooth ovoid solid tumour. The colour of the cut surface is a pale creamy-white, with brown areas of old haemorrhage (left). Fibrous septa traverse the mass and give it an indistinct lobular appearance. **12.65 Theca cell tumour: ovary.** Theca cell tumour is a rare lesion. It is usually benign, unilateral, and commonly occurs in post-menopausal women. This one is a large, smooth, faintly-lobulated solid grey-pink mass, with large veins running over its surface. The cut surface had the fibrous texture of a fibroma but was bright yellow from the presence of lipid. **12.66 Fibroma: ovary.** Ovarian fibroma constitutes about 2% to 5% of ovarian tumours and usually occurs in middle-aged-to-elderly patients. In about 10% of cases the lesion is bilateral and in about a third ascites is present. Typically the tumour is well-defined, tough and fibrous with a whorled pattern on section. These features are evident in this example. It is a smooth-surfaced, spherical mass, and fibrous trabeculae are prominent in the glistening white cut surface.

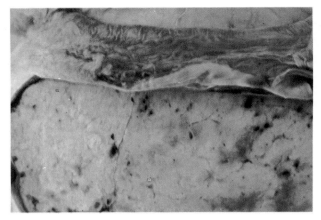

12.67 Granulosa cell tumour: ovary

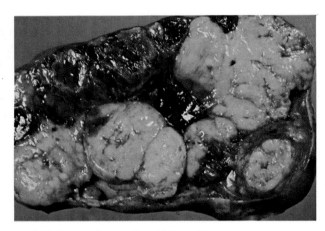

12.68 Malignant theca cell and hilar cell tumour: ovary

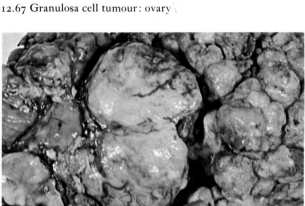

12.69 Mesonephroid carcinoma: ovary

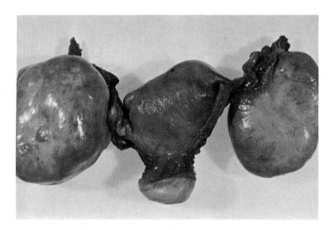

12.70 Krukenberg tumours: ovaries

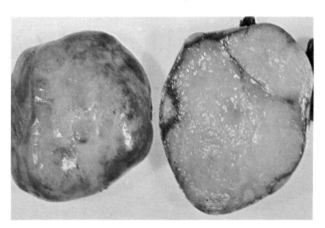

12.71 Krukenberg tumours: ovaries

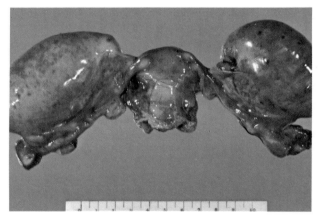

12.72 Burkitt's (African) lymphoma: ovaries

12.67 Granulosa cell tumour: ovary. This is part of the cut surface of the solid tumour. It is pale yellow and flecked with foci of haemorrhage. A smooth white capsule (top) is present. Granulosa cell tumour is the commonest 'special' ovarian tumour and constitutes between 4 and 9% of ovarian tumours. It is almost always unilateral and may occur at any age, although about two-thirds occur in post-menopausal women. It is usually associated with excessive production of oestrogen. About one third behave as malignant tumours. Granulosa cell and theca cell tumours are commonly mixed. **12.68 Malignant theca cell and hilar cell tumour: ovary.** Malignant theca cell tumours are very rare. Hilar cell tumours are extremely rare and probably arise from cells indistinguishable from Leydig cells in the testis. They are usually associated with masculinisation, although occasionally feminisation has been reported. The cut surface of this ovoid tumour shows solid nodules of pale yellowish-white tissue and necrotic haemorrhagic brown tumour (top). **12.69 Mesonephroid carcinoma: ovary.** This is a rare type of ovarian carcinoma of uncertain histogenesis found in older patients. It is usually partly cystic and partly solid. This example is coarsely-lobulated pinkish-brown mass which in places is cystic (left) and in others solid papillary (lower right). Histologically it was composed predominantly of clear cells. The histological

pattern varies in mesonephroid carcinoma, however, and the lesion has to be distinguished from endodermal sinus tumour, endometrioid tumour and serous papillary cystadenoma. **12.70 and 12.71 Krukenberg tumours: ovaries.** Krukenberg tumours characteristically are solid bilateral growths which tend to retain the shape of the ovaries. The outer surface may be smooth but is more often coarsely lobulated. They are metastatic carcinomas, the commonest primary tumours being in stomach, colon and breasts. Metastatic carcinoma accounts for about 20% of all ovarian carcinomas. **12.70** Bilateral solid smooth tumours with a faintly bosselated outline (left) have replaced both ovaries. **12.71** The external surface of the tumour on the left is shown. It is smooth, glistening and coarsely lobular. The cut surface of the tumour on the right shows a mucoid or myxomatous tissue. Histologically Krukenberg tumours consist of mucin-secreting cells including 'signet-ring' forms within a fibrous stroma. **12.72 Burkitt's (African) lymphoma: ovaries.** About 40% of children with Burkitt's lymphoma present with primary abdominal involvement, and bilateral ovarian tumours are especially characteristic. This shows large (9 x 5 cm and 7 x 5 cm) ovarian tumours on each side of an infantile uterus. The surfaces of the tumours are uniformly smooth and dusky-pink in colour.

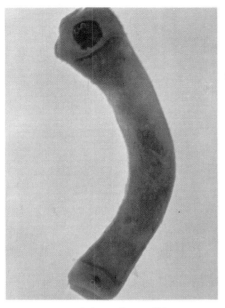

13.1 Osteogenesis imperfecta: tibia

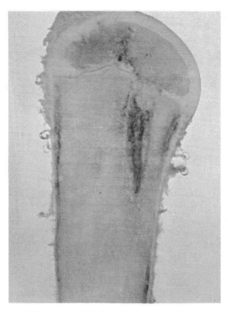

13.2 Osteopetrosis: humerus

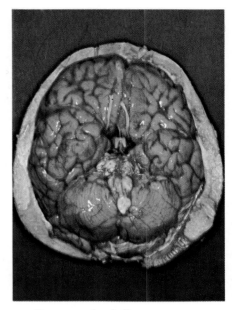

13.3 Osteopetrosis: skull

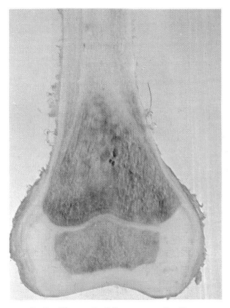

13.4 Infantile cortical hyperostosis: femur

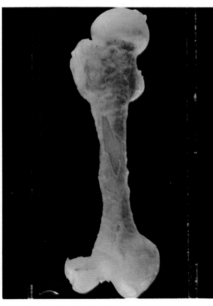

13.5 Achondroplasia: femur

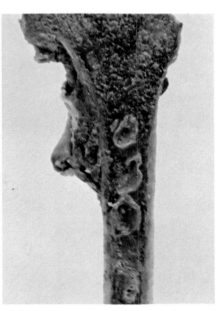

13.6 Acute pyogenic osteomyelitis: femur

13.1 Osteogenesis imperfecta: tibia. This is the tibia from a young child, the epiphyses at both ends of the bone being prominent but normal. The shaft of the bone is slender and markedly bowed. The cortex is much thinner than normal. Osteogenesis imperfecta is a generalised skeletal abnormality which results from an autosomal dominant gene defect. It may be present at birth (osteogenesis imperfecta congenita) or become manifest during childhood (osteogenesis imperfecta tarda). The bones are both slender and brittle, and deformities and fractures are common. 13.2 and 13.3 Osteopetrosis. In this disease which is the result of an autosomal recessive gene defect, there is a failure in the removal of calcified cartilage and bone trabeculae from the metaphyseal region of bones formed from cartilage (endochondral ossification). The bones become thickened, hard and brittle, and the marrow cavity is largely replaced by calcified cartilage and dense lamellar bone. The metaphyses are frequently expanded and the cut surface may show striations. 13.2 Most of these features are visible in this longitudinal section of the upper end of a child's humerus, the most notable change however being the complete replacement of the medullary cavity of the shaft by dense bone. 13.3 The marrow cavity of the cranial vault is obliterated by dense yellowish-white bone (marble bone disease). The increased density appears to be mainly confined to the bones formed in cartilage, and 'membranous' bones such as the flat bones of the skull are only rarely involved. Changes in the bones of the skull cause stenosis of

foramina and compression of cranial nerves. 13.4 Infantile cortical hyperostosis: femur. This is a rare condition of unknown aetiology in which symmetrical periostitis affects the long bones, scapulae, clavicles and mandibles. The lower end of this femur is thickened, from abnormal and excessive periosteal bone formation. These appearances may be confused with syphilitic periostitis. 13.5 Achondroplasia: femur. The femoral shaft is shorter than normal and the upper and lower epiphyses appear relatively expanded. In achondroplasia, which results from a specific dominant gene defect, there is a quantitative decrease in the rate of endochondral ossification which in conjunction with normal periosteal (membranous) bone formation results in the tubular long bones appearing short and squat. 13.6 Acute pyogenic osteomyelitis: femur. The bone has been sectioned longitudinally, and this shows the upper end. A number of thick-walled abscesses are present within the medullary cavity. The abscesses contain greenish-yellow purulent exudate. Acute pyogenic osteomyelitis mostly affects infants and young children. The commonest organism is the *Staphylococcus aureus* but streptococci, pneumococci and meningococci are also encountered. Most infections are haematogenous in origin and the process typically begins in the metaphyseal region of the shaft of the long bones. Osteomyelitis of the upper femoral shaft may extend to involve the hip joint, the affected metaphysis being located within the joint capsule.

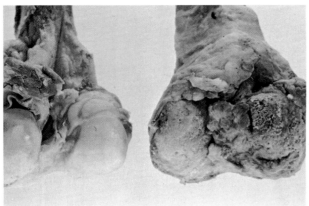

13.7 Suppurative arthritis: knee-joints

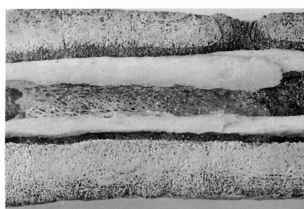

13.8 Chronic osteomyelitis: tibia

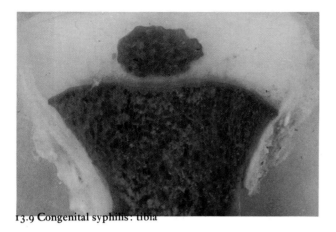

13.9 Congenital syphilis: tibia

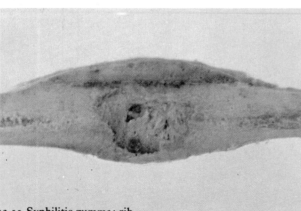

13.10 Syphilitic periostitis: femur

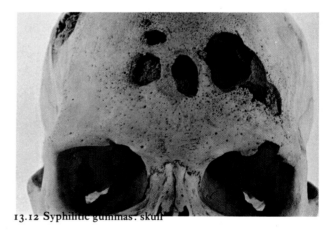

13.11 Syphilitic gumma: rib

13.12 Syphilitic gummas: skull

13.7 Suppurative arthritis: knee-joints. The patient was a 58-year-old woman with bacterial endocarditis who developed acute osteomyelitis of the femur and suppurative arthritis of the left hip-joint and both knee-joints. This shows the lower end of both femurs. The epicondyles (right) are covered with a greenish fibrino-purulent exudate. The capsule is thickened and discoloured (top right). The organism was a group C, beta-haemolytic streptococcus. In suppurative arthritis, the infection may localise in the synovial tissues from the bloodstream or the joint may be involved by direct extension from an adjacent focus. The hip, knee, elbow, shoulder and ankle are the joints most frequently affected. **13.8 Chronic osteomyelitis: tibia.** This is a dried specimen of tibia. The central sclerotic and dense white bone is the original shaft of the tibia. It is completely necrotic and forms the sequestrum. It is surrounded by a new 'shaft' composed of spongy bone, the involucrum, formed by the periosteum after it was stripped off the original shaft. A sinus opening ('cloaca') (top right) penetrates the involucrum. This advanced form of the disease with sequestration and involucrum formation is now rare compared with the pre-antibiotic era. **13.9 Congenital syphilis: tibia.** Congenital syphilis produces osteochondritis in the long bones and a diffuse periostitis. This longitudinal section of the upper part of an infant's tibia shows the epiphyseal line to be irregular and thicker than normal, from the presence of an excess of unresorbed cartilage on the growing surface of the epiphyseal cartilage. The adjacent metaphysis also shows greyish-white thickening of the spongy cancellous trabeculae and

the periosteum is thickened. **13.10 Syphilitic periostitis: femur.** In adults the characteristic changes in bone in tertiary syphilis take the form of a diffuse periostitis. This leads to excessive periosteal, and endosteal, new bone formation and the bones become typically thickened and dense. This is a longitudinal section of a macerated dried femur. The cortical bone is thickened, very dense and chalky. The tibia, clavicle and skull are also particularly susceptible to this lesion. The tibia may be bowed and sabre-shaped. These proliferative reactions are in marked contrast to the essentially destructive nature of tuberculous lesions. **13.11 and 13.12 Syphilitic gumma.** In addition to the proliferative reactions which lead to the formation of much new bone, syphilitic infection often leads to extensive destruction of tissue through gummatous necrosis. **13.11** This is a longitudinal section of a rib. There is a fusiform swelling which has been produced by diffuse periostitis, with excessive new bone formation between the raised periosteum and the cortical bone. There is also a central yellowish-brown area of gummatous necrosis within the medullary cavity. A gross appearance like this may be mistaken for osteosarcoma. **13.12** In the flat bones of the skull, syphilitic lesions tend to be destructive in nature and subperiosteal overgrowth is generally relatively slight. This fact is illustrated by this dried skull which shows the presence of a number of large ragged cavities in both frontal bones and in the right parietal bone. There is also considerable thickening of the surrounding bone as a result of the accompanying periostitis.

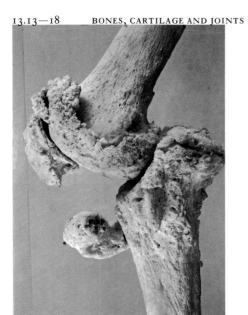

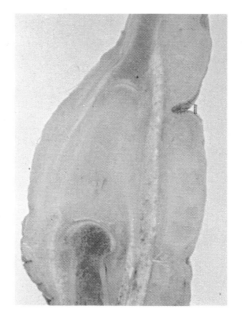

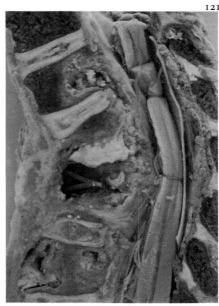

13.13 Charcot's joint: knee

13.14 Tuberculous osteomyelitis: finger

13.15 Tuberculous osteomyelitis: vertebrae

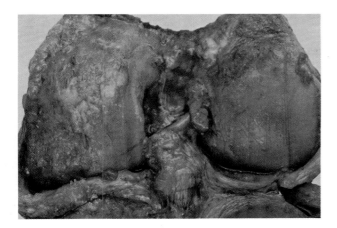
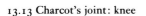

13.16 Osteoarthritis: knee-joint

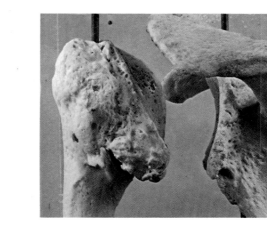

13.17 Osteoarthritis: shoulder-joint

13.13 Charcot's joint: knee. In a Charcot's (neuropathic) joint there is extreme destruction of cartilage and bone with marked osteophyte formation and mechanical disorganisation. These features are evident in this lateral view of a dried specimen of knee-joint. Destruction and disorganisation of the joint are extreme, with osteophytic overgrowth of the femoral condyles, patella and articular surface of the tibia. A large pedunculated osteophyte is present on the tibia. The degenerative and destructive changes are probably secondary to sensory disturbances. About 5–10% of tabetic patients develop Charcot's joints. **13.14 and 13.15 Tuberculous osteomyelitis.** Tuberculous osteomyelitis is usually caused by haematogenous spread from an active focus elsewhere. Children are more often affected than adults. The disease tends to affect the spinal column (Pott's disease) or the ends of long bones. In the latter the epiphyseal region is usually involved and the infection may extend into an adjacent joint. **13.14** In this instance, the disease has destroyed the middle phalanx of a finger, and the bone has been replaced by yellowish-white caseous material which has spread into the adjacent soft tissues to form a soft-tissue swelling. **13.15** This is a median sagittal section of the thoracic spine. Four adjacent vertebral bodies have been largely destroyed by caseous abscesses which have eroded into the periosteum and intervertebral disc. Collapse of the two central bodies has led to anterior spinal angulation (kyphosis) and moderate compression of the spinal cord. Extension of vertebral tuberculosis into the soft tissues may lead to the formation of a paravertebral 'cold abscess'. **13.16–13.19 Osteoarthritis.** Osteoarthritis is a very common degenerative joint disease, occurring to some degree in everyone over the age of 40. It tends to affect the large weight-bearing joints. **13.16** This is the articular surface of the femoral condyles in a severely arthritic knee-joint. The articular cartilage is whitish-yellow (left). Over the lateral aspects (left) the cartilage is nodular and thinned. There is nodularity and pitting, with irregular lipping of the margin. 'Scoring' is present over the medial condyle. **13.17** In osteoarthritis the degeneration of the articular cartilage is often accompanied by proliferation of the perichondrial tissues of the articular margins and formation of fibrocartilage and bone. This process

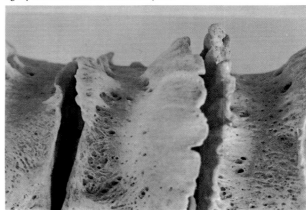

13.18 Osteoarthritis: spinal osteophytosis

is referred to as marginal lipping, and the nodular projections are termed marginal osteophytes. These changes are obvious in this dried specimen of the shoulder-joint, showing the head and neck of humerus (left) and the scapula (right). The head of the humerus is markedly distorted, with irregular projecting outgrowths of new bone (marginal osteophytes). **13.18** True osteoarthritis of the spine involves the articular cartilages of the posterior spinal joints but sometimes the lesion is confined to the formation of marginal osteophytes on the vertebral border. This is a common abnormality, known as spinal osteophytosis or spondylitis deformans, which is frequently confused with true osteoarthritis. In this dried specimen of three thoracic bodies, there is excessive marginal lipping and irregular overgrowths around the margins of the disc spaces on the anterior surfaces of the vertebrae. The condition is often accompanied by degeneration of the intervertebral discs.

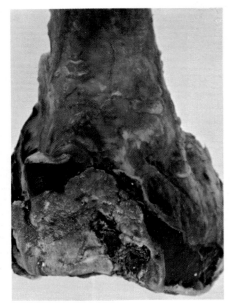

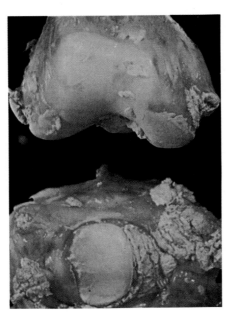

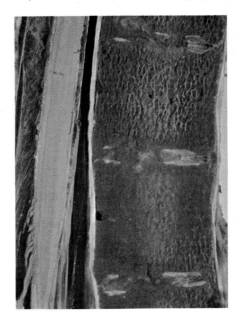

13.19 Osteoarthritis and ochronosis: femur   13.20 Gout: knee-joint   13.21 Ankylosing spondylitis: vertebrae

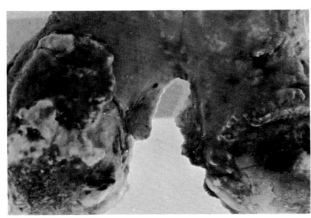

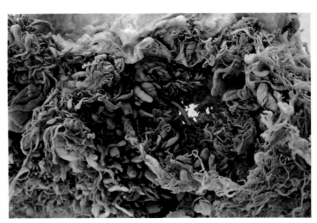

13.22 Rheumatoid arthritis: knee-joint   13.23 Villo-nodular synovitis: knee-joint

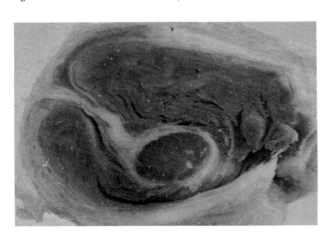

13.24 Xanthoma: tendon sheath

13.19 Osteoarthritis and ochronosis. Ochronosis is a rare genetic defect of phenylalanine and tyrosine metabolism which leads to the accumulation of excessive amounts of homogentisic acid, which tends to localise selectively in cartilage. In the later stages a severe degenerative arthritis occurs and the lower end of this femur shows distortion and destruction of the articular cartilage, the surrounding cartilage being stained black. The unstained tissue covering the articular surface of the femur is proliferated bone resulting from secondary osteoarthritis. **13.20 Gout: knee-joint.** Gout is a familial disorder of purine metabolism, characterised by recurrent attacks of arthritis in which sodium urate is deposited in the articular cartilages, synovial tissues and peri-articular tissues. Chronic inflammation leads to destruction of the articular tissues. Both articular surfaces of the knee-joint are displayed, the femoral at the top and the tibial at the bottom. Chalky-white deposits have formed over the articular cartilage and in the peri-articular tissues. About 2 to 5% of

chronic joint disease is due to gouty arthritis. **13.21 Ankylosing spondylitis: vertebrae.** The spine may be involved solely or predominantly in rheumatoid arthritis. The condition is then referred to as ankylosing spondylitis (Strumpell-Marie spondylitis). Characteristically the posterior intervertebral, costovertebral and sacroiliac joints are affected, with ossification of the margins of the intervertebral discs and spinal ligaments. This is a median sagittal section of several lumbar vertebrae, and the spinal cord is on the left. The intervertebral joints have been largely destroyed, and bony ankylosis of the vertebral bodies has occurred as a result of ossification of the annulus fibrosis of the intervertebral discs. **13.22 Rheumatoid arthritis: knee-joint.** The initial joint abnormality in this disease is an inflammatory change affecting the synovium. As this progresses, a pannus of vascular granulation tissue forms which spreads over the articular cartilage. The pannus may eventually replace the articular cartilage and so produce fibrous or bony union. This shows the articular surface of the lower end of femur. Both articular cartilages are destroyed and replaced by dark brown pannus. Joint involvement in rheumatoid arthritis is usually multiple and often symmetrical. The knee-joints and the joints of the hands and feet are most commonly involved. **13.23 Villo-nodular synovitis: knee-joint.** Pigmented villo-nodular synovitis comprises a group of lesions characterised by villous and nodular proliferation of synovial tissues. This shows replacement of the synovial membrane of an affected knee-joint by a brown mass of such tissue. Histologically it consisted of synovial cells, multinucleate osteoclasts, macrophages with fat and haemosiderin, and collections of chronic inflammatory cells. The lesion usually affects young adults and the knee-joints is the one most often involved. **13.24 Xanthoma: tendon sheath.** Xanthoma is a lesion similar to villo-nodular synovitis which may occur in tendon sheaths and bursae. Although it has been called giant-cell tumour or benign synovioma, xanthoma and villo-nodular synovitis are probably variants of a single process of a reactive rather than a neoplastic nature. This shows an affected tendon in cross-section. The tendon sheath is distended with reddish-brown tissue. The lesion tends to affect the fingers.

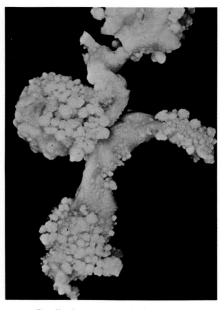

13.25 Cartilaginous metaplasia of synovium (synovial chondromatosis)

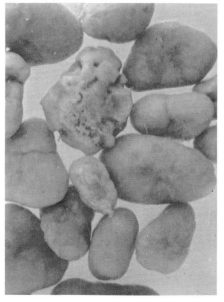

13.26 Loose bodies: knee-joint

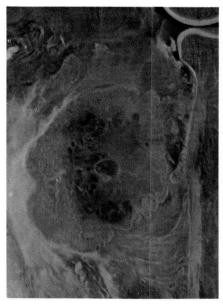

13.27 Traumatic myositis ossificans

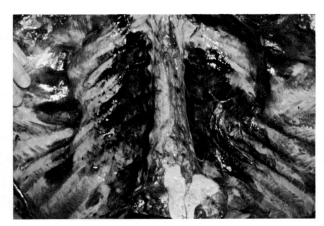

13.28 Fracture: rib

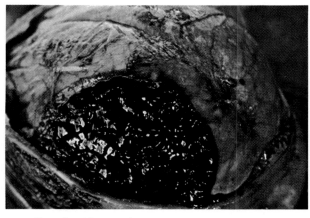

13.29 Extradural haemorrhage

13.25 Cartilaginous metaplasia of synovium (synovial chondromatosis). This is an uncommon disorder of joints which may occur as an isolated lesion or in conjunction with other forms of degenerative joint disease. Characteristically large numbers of cartilaginous bodies which tend to undergo ossification form in the synovial lining of the joint. This shows portions of excised synovial membrane from such a case. Large numbers of small rounded white masses of translucent cartilage are growing from the synovial surface. These pedunculated growths had been projecting into the joint. The cause of the condition is unknown though it probably reflects cartilaginous metaplasia of the synovium. **13.26 Loose bodies: knee-joint.** Bursal cysts occasionally form in close relation to the knee-joint. They have a thick fibrous wall and not infrequently contain rounded bodies or nodules composed of dense fibrous tissue and cartilage. These may be referred to as 'melon-seed' bodies and when they are intra-articular they are called 'joint mice'. In this case the knee-joint contained a large number of loose bodies, some of which are shown here. They are ovoid and smooth-surfaced. Two have been sectioned (above centre) and the cut surface is seen to consist of glistening lobulated cartilage. **13.27 Traumatic myositis ossificans.** Traumatic myositis ossificans is a localised lesion that usually follows one or more injuries to muscle. Oedema, haemorrhage and inflammation of the muscle progress to bone formation. In this case, a lobulated rounded mass of bone (2.5 x 3.0 cm) has formed in the muscles in front of the upper third of the radius. The adjacent bone shows subperiosteal thickening and localised intra-medullary haemorrhage. The process tends to be self-limiting. It is important to distinguish it from osteosarcoma. **13.28 Fracture: ribs.** This shows the inside of the thoracic cavity. There are multiple sym-metrical paravertebral fractures of the ribs, with extensive haemorrhage into the adjacent intercostal muscles. Fracture of ribs on this scale may produce a 'flail chest' and by preventing normal respiratory movement cause asphyxia. It is a consequence of severe impact and crush injuries, and this patient was injured in a road traffic accident. **13.29 Extradural**

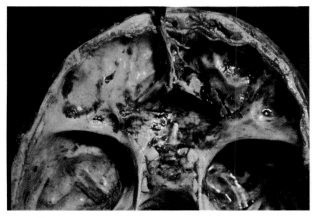

13.30 Fracture: skull

haemorrhage. Extradural haematomas are produced by blunt trauma, as a rule with fracture of the skull. Where a fracture of skull crosses the groove of the middle meningeal artery, it tends to tear the vessel which then bleeds. The temporal branch of the middle meningeal is the vessel often affected. Death is caused by compression and displacement of the brain and secondary brain-stem haemorrhages. In this case the large mass of blood clot is located in the extradural space over the fronto-temporal region of the right cerebral hemisphere. **13.30-13.32 Fracture: skull. 13.30** This shows the anterior fossa. There is a recent fracture of the cribriform plate and ethmoid bone and haemorrhage is present over the orbital roof of the ethmoid (right). The haemorrhage has extended into the right middle cranial fossa. The fracture was complicated by pneumo-coccal meningitis (see 13.32).

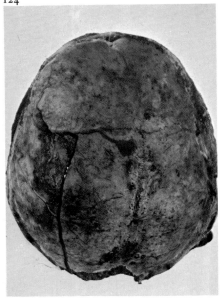

13.31 Fracture: skull

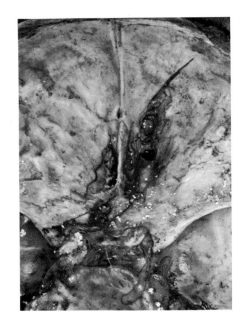

13.32 Fracture: skull

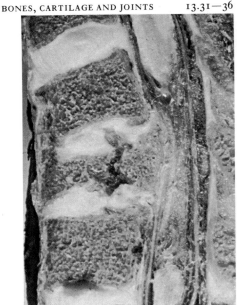

13.33 Fracture: cervical spine

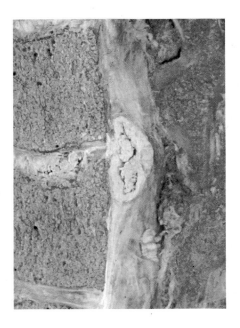

13.34 Prolapse of intervertebral disc

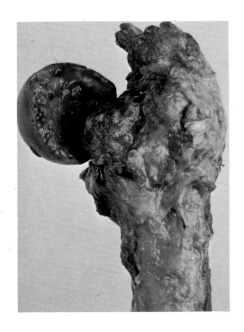

13.35 Fracture: neck of femur

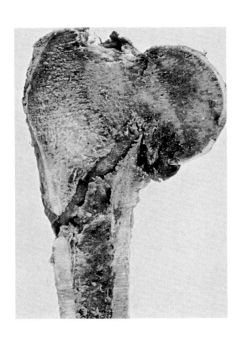

13.36 Pathological fracture: femur

13.31 and 13.32 Fracture: skull. 13.31 The inner aspect of the calvarium is shown. There is a large recent fracture involving the parieto-occipital bone. The patient, an elderly woman, sustained the fractured skull as a result of a fall. She developed a subdural haematoma which led to her death. **13.32.** A small oval craniosinus opening is present in the right cribriform plate on the ethmoid bone. The patient, a 25-year-old woman, sustained a depressed fracture of the frontal bone 5 years prior to her death. The fracture was complicated by cerebrospinal fluid rhinorrhoea for three years, but pneumococcal meningitis eventually developed and caused the patient's death. This is a well-recognised hazard of craniosinus fistula, the pneumococcus gaining access via the fracture or fistula to the subarachnoid space from an infected air sinus. **13.33 Fracture: cervical spine.** This is a median sagittal section of the cervical spine. The middle vertebral body is collapsed, with a central cystic cavity, and over two to three segments the cord has been replaced by a thin brownish scar consisting of fibrous and glial tissues. Three years before her death, the patient had sustained a fracture of the cervical spine with severe damage to the cord and paraplegia. **13.34 Prolapse of intervertebral disc.** This is a median sagittal section of lumbar vertebrae and spinal cord. Intervertebral disc material is protruding posteriorly into the spinal canal and compressing the lumbar cord. The lumbar discs are those most likely to be affected by prolapse of the nucleus pulposus, especially the discs between lumbar three and four, four and five, and lumbar five and sacral one. Protrusion of a disc is believed to be caused by trauma, usually in association with flexion or hyperextension of the spine. **13.35 Fracture: neck of femur.** This shows non-union of a subcapital fracture of the femoral neck. The shape of the pertrochanteric region of the neck is irregular, from the presence of excess of callus. The undersurface of the femoral head is nodular and a false cavity exists between the head and neck due to non-union of the fracture. Non-union may result from ischaemia of the bone ends, undue mobility, interposition of soft tissue, and infection. The bone ends become covered by fibro-cartilaginous tissue which prevents firm union by callus, and a pseudoarthrosis may result. **13.36 Pathological fracture: femur.** The patient had a carcinoma of bronchus. This is a longitudinal section of the upper end of the femur. A diagonal fracture involves the upper shaft and neck. Yellowish-brown secondary tumour occupies the medullary cavity in the region of the fracture. Pathological fracture may be the first manifestation of metastasis to bone. The fracture is often unusually painful. In the elderly, pathological fractures may also be a consequence of osteoporosis.

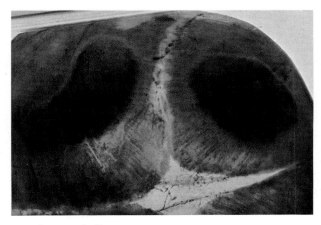

13.37 Scurvy: skull

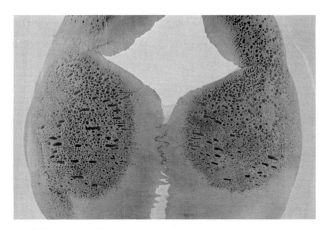

13.38 Scurvy: skull

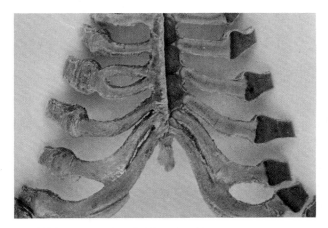

13.39 Rickets: costochondral junctions

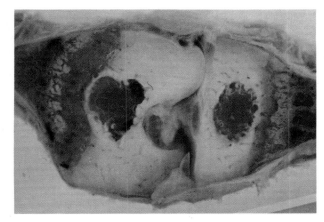

13.40 Rickets: knee-joint

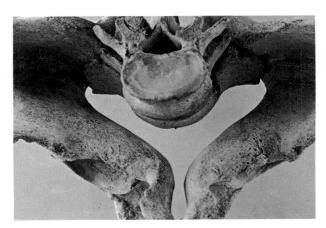

13.41 Osteomalacia: pelvis

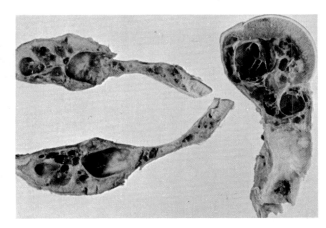

13.42 Primary hyperparathyroidism: ribs and humerus

13.37 and 13.38 Scurvy: skull. Scurvy is caused by deficiency of vitamin C. It tends to affect two age groups; children between the ages of 6 months and 2 years, and the elderly. Increased capillary fragility gives rise to haemorrhages into various tissues including the subperiosteum. Formation of connective tissues of various types is also defective. **13.37** This is the skull of a 9-month-old infant. Two flattened red bosses of spongy bone with prominent radial vascular markings are present over the parietal bones. Subperiosteal haemorrhage has been followed by organisation of the blood clot and production of the new bone. **13.38** This dried infant skull shows the bony bosses clearly. The spaces formerly occupied by blood vessels are prominent. The intervening skull bones appear porotic. In scurvy the osteoblasts are unable to form osteoid properly and bone formation and maintenance are defective. Where ossification is endochondral in type cartilage may persist and become calcified. **13.39-13.41 Rickets.** In the growing child vitamin D deficiency causes rickets. There is failure of calcification of the cartilaginous matrix in the epiphyses and osteoid also fails to calcify. The disturbance of endochondral ossification and the softness of the bones leads to skeletal deformity. **13.39** The costochondral junctions are enlarged, an appearance termed the rachitic rosary. The cut surface (right) shows that the enlargement is due to expansion of the epiphysial cartilage plates. In these there is a wide zone of abnormal osteoid and uncalcified cartilage. Rachitic rosary is often associated with a depressed sternum and indenta-

tions of the thorax at the level of the insertion of the diaphragm. **13.40** This is a coronal section through the knee-joint of an affected child, showing the lower end of the femur and the upper end of tibia. The lower femoral and upper tibial epiphyses are expanded and irregular. The cartilaginous zone (pinkish-grey) is also irregular and abnormally wide. **13.41 Osteomalacia: pelvis.** Osteomalacia is the adult counterpart of rickets. The amount of mineral in the organic matrix of bone is decreased. This is a dried specimen of 'triradiate' pelvis in which gross distortion of the pelvic outlet has followed the softening of the pelvic bones. Such an extreme degree of contracted pelvis is of obvious importance in obstetric practice. **13.42-13.44 Primary hyperparathyroidism.** Primary hyperparathyroidism implies that more parathormone is produced than normal. The usual source of the excess hormone is an adenoma, less frequently hyperplasia of all glands, and only rarely from a carcinoma of one gland. The skeletal lesions consist of generalised osteoporosis and 'osteitis fibrosa cystica'. **13.42** The changes of osteitis fibrous cystica are evident in these section of ribs and the upper end of humerus. The ribs (left) show large fusiform expansions composed of multilocular cysts. The medullary cavities are replaced by greyish-yellow fibrous tissue surrounding smaller cysts. A large multilocular brownish-coloured cyst expands the head and upper shaft of the humerus, and the adjacent medullary cavity is filled with yellowish-white fibrous tissue. The cysts of primary hyperparathyroidism are called 'brown tumours'.

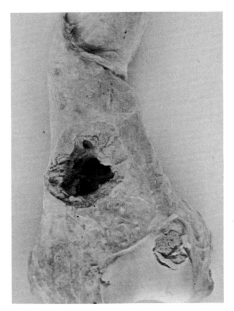

13.43 Primary hyperparathyroidism: femur

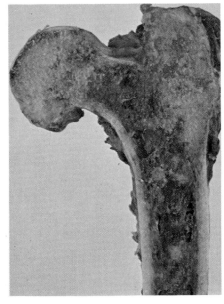

13.44 Primary hyperparathyroidism: femur

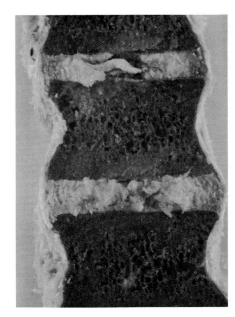

13.45 Renal rickets: vertebrae

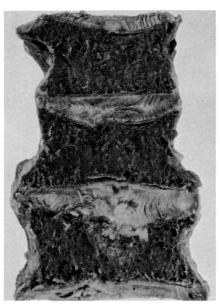

13.46 Osteoporosis: vertebrae

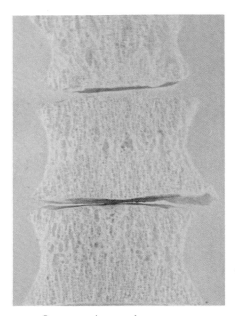

13.47 Osteoporosis: vertebrae

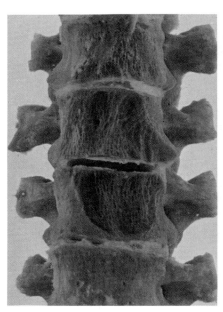

13.48 Pressure atrophy: vertebrae

13.43 and 13.44 Primary hyperparathyroidism. 13.43 This is the lower end of the femur. Severe osteoporosis has weakened the bone to such an extent that a pathological fracture of the shaft has occurred. A portion of the cortical bone has been cut away to show the very thick but soft bone. This part of the bone is occupied by a large 'brown tumour' (3 cm diameter). **13.44** This is the upper end of the right femur, bisected. The angle between the femoral neck and shaft is decreased to a right angle (coxa vara). A thin-walled cyst (1 cm diameter) is present in the base of the neck. Histology of the cyst wall showed it to consist of a thin layer of fibrous tissue but there was no evidence of active hyperparathyroidism. The patient, a 30-year-old woman who died from malignant hypertension and nephrocalcinosis, had presented at the age of 18 with hyperparathyroidism due to a parathyroid adenoma. **13.45 Renal rickets: vertebrae.** Renal insufficiency may lead to secondary hyperparathyroidism, a condition known as renal rickets. The bone changes are varied and include osteosclerosis, osteomalacia and lacunar resorption. Three lumbar vertebral bodies are shown. In each body there is a zone of increased bone density adjacent to the adjacent intervertebral discs. The bands of differing density are visible on radiographs and give rise to the appearance of 'rugger jersey' spine. **13.46 and 13.47 Osteoporosis: vertebrae.** The term osteoporosis is applied to any condition in which there is a reduction in the amount of bone tissue. It occurs most commonly

in elderly women and mainly affects the spine and pelvis. **13.46** When the vertebral bodies are porotic, disc tissue may protrude vertically into the cancellous bone of an adjacent vertebral body, to produce a Schmorl's node. The node forms a rounded mass of disc tissue deep to the end plate of the vertebral body. This is a coronal section of three lumbar vertebrae. The bodies are compressed and the trabeculae of the cancellous bone are thin due to osteoporosis. Whitish disc material protrudes from the central portion of one disc into the vertebral body below it. **13.47** This is a dried specimen of three lumbar vertebral bodies in coronal section. The trabeculae of cancellous bone are thinned. In more advanced cases, the pressure of the intervertebral discs produces concavity of the upper and lower surfaces of the bodies. **13.48 Pressure atrophy: vertebrae.** Pressure repeatedly applied to bone, from without or from within, can cause localised atrophy. In this case the pressure was exerted by an aneurysm of the thoracic aorta. The anterior aspect of three dried vertebral bodies is shown. There has been considerable loss of bony trabeculae with formation of shallow depressions. The mechanisms involved in local resorption of bone from pressure are not known but diminished blood flow may be important. It is worth noting that the avascular intervertebral discs are more resistant than the bodies themselves.

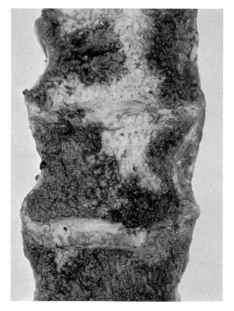

13.49 Infarction: vertebrae

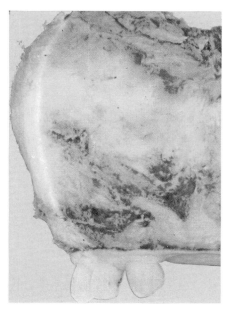

13.50 Fibrous dysplasia: maxilla

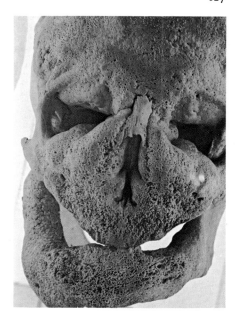

13.51 Fibrous dysplasia: skull

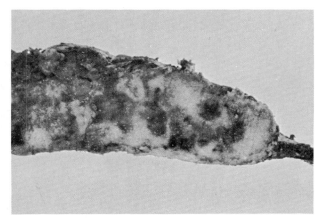

13.52 Fibrous dysplasia: rib

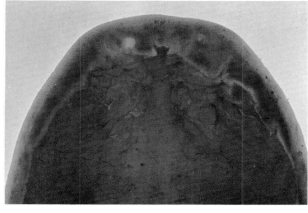

13.53 Hyperostosis frontalis interna: skull

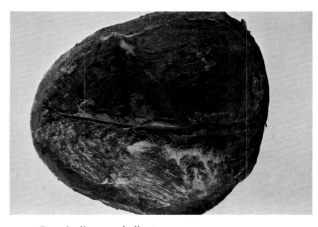

13.54 Paget's disease: skull

13.49 Infarction: vertebrae. Three lumbar vertebral bodies are shown in coronal section. Irregular yellowish-white areas of recent infarction are present. The borders of the infarcts are haemorrhagic. Infarction of bone may be seen in atherosclerosis, following some types of fracture, and in suppurative osteomyelitis. Multiple infarcts may also be found in caisson disease and sickle cell anaemia, as a result of embolic occlusion of small blood vessels. This patient developed disseminated intravascular coagulation in association with carcinomatosis. **13.50-13.52 Fibrous dysplasia.** Fibrous dysplasia is characterised by circumscribed lesions of bone in which fibrous tissue and sometimes bone trabeculae form. The lesions usually develop in childhood or adolescence. They start in the centre of the bone and expand the cortex. One bone may be affected (the monostotic form) or many (the polyostotic). The bones commonly involved are the femur, tibia, ribs and the bones of the face. **13.50** The jaw region is a common site of predilection, and this shows a greatly expanded maxilla in sagittal section. The bone has been replaced by yellowish-white fibrous tissue. Certain fibro-osseous lesions of the jaw previously described as fibrous osteomas are probably examples of monostotic fibrous dysplasia. **13.51** This dried skull is an example of leontiasis ossea, in which there is extreme fibro-osseous thickening of the cranial and facial bones and which is probably a diffuse form of fibrous dysplasia. The bone trabeculae are very coarse and the new bone correspondingly porous. **13.52** A small portion of normal rib is shown (right). The rest of the rib forms a large fusiform swelling in which thinned cortical bone encloses a mass of pale yellowish-white connective tissue which distends and replaces the marrow cavity. There are areas of haemorrhage in the connective tissue and a small cyst is present (lower left). **13.53 Hyperostosis frontalis interna: skull.** Foci of well-defined hyperostosis may be found in association with slow-growing tumours such as meningiomas, but the commonest form of hyperostosis is enostosis of the calvarium, hyperostosis frontalis interna. The patho-

genesis is unknown. In this case the frontal bones are affected. The diploe is obliterated and irregular knobs and ridges of dense bone are present on the interior surface. **13.54 Paget's disease: skull.** The calvarium is enlarged and the bones of the skull are very vascular and considerably thickened. The inner and outer tables cannot be distinguished. The diploe having been obliterated the inner surface is covered with a thick layer of fibrous tissue and the vascular markings in the bone are prominent. Paget's disease commonly affects the vertebral column, skull, pelvis and femur. Although the bones are greatly thickened, they are softer than normal in the earlier vascular stage, and even in the later heavily calcified phase the affected bones are excessively brittle. Histologically there is a very active but disorderly remodelling of the bone trabeculae.

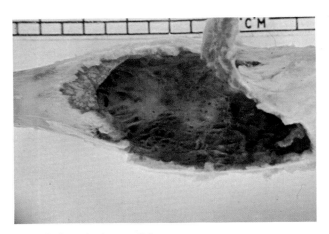

13.55 Solitary (unicameral) bone cyst

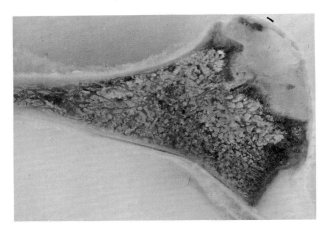

13.56 Exostosis: rib

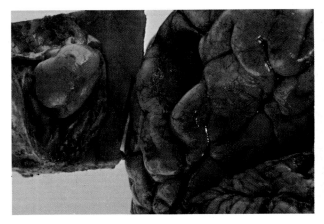

13.57 Ivory osteoma: skull

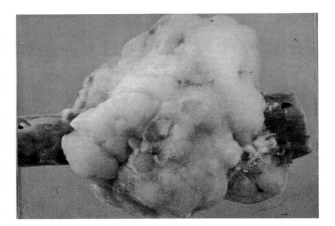

13.58 Chondroma: rib

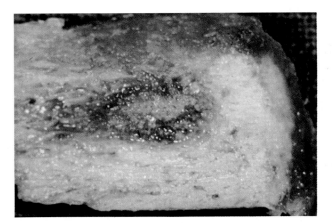

13.59 Osteoid osteoma

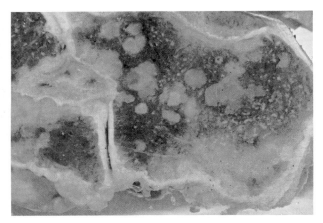

13.60 Ollier's disease

13.55 Solitary (unicameral) bone cyst. Solitary bone cyst occurs in the metaphyses of long bones in children, and in about 50% of cases the bone is the humerus, as in this example. It is a thin-walled cyst, lined with reddish-brown fibrous tissue. It contained amber-coloured fluid. The overlying cortex is expanded. Haemorrhage and fracture are common complications of this type of cyst, the aetiology of which is unknown. **13.56 Exostosis: rib.** This is the junction of rib and costal cartilage (lower right). A sessile bony mass covered with a cap of cartilage is attached to the part of the rib adjacent to the costal cartilage. The cartilage acts like an epiphysial plate and leads to formation of the cancellous bone beneath it, giving rise to a cartilage-capped mass. An exostosis of this type usually develops during childhood and it may be solitary or multiple. The commonest sites are lower end of femur and upper end of tibia. **13.57 Ivory osteoma: skull.** The osteoma has arisen from the petrous temporal bone and projects as a smooth lobulated yellowish-white mass from the floor of the middle cranial fossa. It has produced a deep depression in the temporal lobe of the brain which overlay the lesion. This type of osteoma is extremely hard. It is often regarded as a hamartoma rather than as a true neoplasm. It is almost entirely confined to the mandible and bones of the skull but sometimes grows into the paranasal sinuses. **13.58 Chondroma: rib.** The chondroma is a lobulated greyish-white mass surrounding the rib. It has the translucent appearance of cartilage. Chondroma may arise from the surface of a bone (ecchondroma) or within the bone (enchondroma). The commonest sites or origin are the short bones of the hands and feet, the ends of long bones and the pelvis, ribs, sternum and scapula. It is a benign growth and it may be solitary or multiple. **13.59 Osteoid osteoma.** Osteoid osteoma usually occurs in young adults and as a rule it is located in the shaft of a long bone, particularly the tibia and femur. There is frequently a history of pain. This is a section through the lesion. It is small (1 cm diameter), oval and reddish-yellow, and surrounded by white sclerotic bone (right). Histologically it consisted of vascular osteoblastic tissue and abundant osteoid. **13.60 Ollier's disease.** In multiple enchondromatosis there are numerous chondromas within several bones. Where the lesions are predominantly unilateral, the condition is generally referred to as Ollier's disease. In this case the many small rounded cartilaginous masses are within the os calcis and adjacent bones.

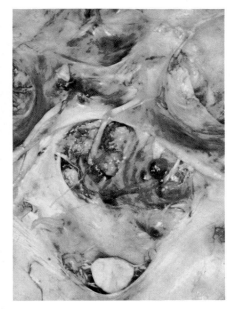

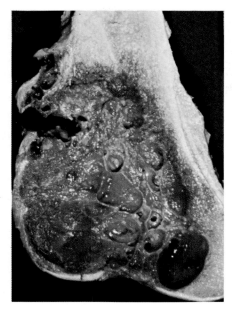

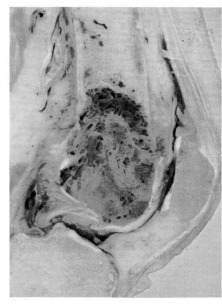

13.61 Chordoma: sphenoid

13.62 Aneurysmal bone cyst: femur

13.63 Giant-cell tumour: femur

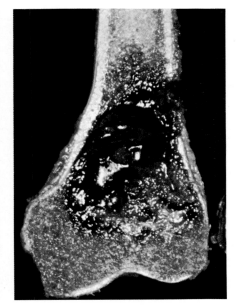

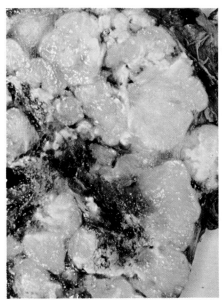

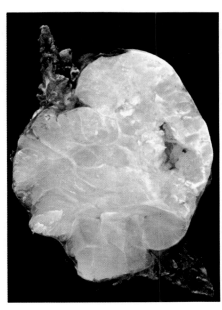

13.64 Giant-cell tumour: femur

13.65 Chondromyxosarcoma: femur

13.66 Chondrosarcoma: rib

13.61 Chordoma: sphenoid. Chordoma is a slow-growing malignant tumour arising from remnants of the notochord. It is found only in the axial skeleton, the sacral and spheno-occipital regions being the commonest site. Typically it is a lobulated tumour consisting of highly vacuolated (physaliphorous) cells in a mucoid stroma. This one forms a pinkish lobulated mass within the basi-sphenoid and basi-occiput. The right third cranial nerve is stretched over its surface. **13.62 Aneurysmal bone cyst: femur.** Most of the lower end of the femur has been destroyed by a brown-coloured multilocular cystic lesion. The adjacent cortical bone (left) is thin and expanded. Aneurysmal bone cyst is usually seen in patients under 30 and involves either the metaphyseal region of the shaft of a long bone or the vertebral column. It tends to be eccentrically placed, with ballooning of the periosteum. **13.63 and 13.64 Giant-cell tumour: femur.** Giant-cell tumour typically involves the end of a long bone and originates towards the lateral or medial aspect of the bone. The commonest sites are the lower end of femur, upper end of tibia and lower end of radius. It tends to involve the adjacent joint. The following two examples are in the lower end of the femur. **13.63** A grey-brown neoplasm has expanded the lower end of the femur. There are areas of cystic degeneration and haemorrhage. The cortical bone is expanded over the tumour and greatly thinned and destroyed. **13.64** The tumour is a circumscribed haemorrhagic mass in the distal shaft of the femur. The overlying cortex is thin but the

bone contour is not expanded. Histologically the lesion consists of numerous multinucleated giant cells lying in a well-vascularised spindle-cell stroma. About 50% recur after local curettage. Most giant-cell tumours occur in patients between 20 and 40 years of age. **13.65 Chondromyxosarcoma: femur.** The tumour which measured 7 x 4 cm was in the upper femoral shaft of a 37-year-old woman. This shows part of it in section. The tumour is coarsely lobular and bluish-white in colour, with a soft gelatinous consistence. Histological examination showed myxosarcomatous areas alternating with chondrosarcomatous areas. The tumour had previously been diagnosed both on radiographic and histological grounds as a chondromyxoid fibroma but its subsequent rapid growth with extension into muscle and the complication of a pathological fracture of the bone demonstrated its sarcomatous nature. **13.66 Chondrosarcoma: rib.** Chondrosarcoma is a malignant tumour characterised by the formation of cartilage but not of bone. It is found between the ages of 30 and 60 years and affects mainly the pelvis, ribs, scapula, humerus and femur. The appearances are variable, ranging from a bulky lobulated firm translucent tumour to a soft ill-defined myxomatous mass. This one is a firm, lobulated mass. The cut surface is bluish-white and translucent with thin white fibrous tissue septa separating nodules of cartilaginous tissue.

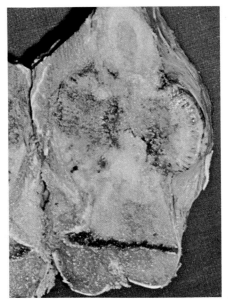

13.67 Fibrosarcoma: femur

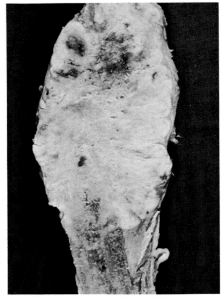

13.68 Fibrosarcoma: femur

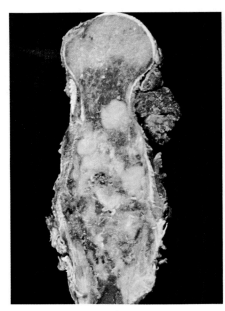

13.69 Osteosarcoma: humerus

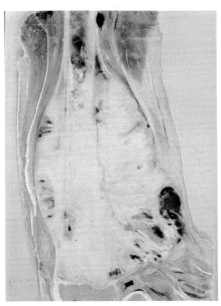

13.70 Osteosarcoma

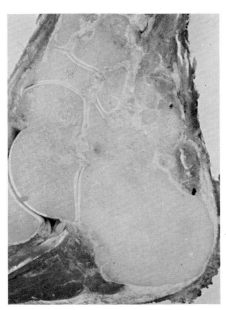

13.71 Osteosarcoma: os calcis

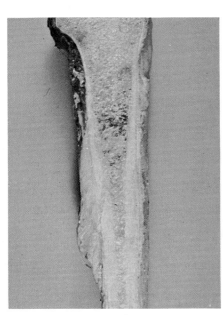

13.72 Ewing's tumour: humerus

13.67 and 13.68 Fibrosarcoma: femur. Fibrosarcoma is a rare tumour which usually involves a long bone, particularly the distal part of the femur or proximal tibia. In contrast to osteogenic sarcoma, it affects people between 20 and 60 years of age. **13.67** This lesion is a large greyish-white tumour of the lower end of the femur. There is extensive yellowish-grey necrosis and the neoplasm has broken through the cortex on each side of the shaft to form dome-shaped subperiosteal masses. **13.68** This patient suffered from Paget's disease. Between 5 and 10% of cases with generalised Paget's disease develop a sarcoma, the commonest sites being in the major long bones, pelvis and skull. Most are pleomorphic osteosarcomas but chondrosarcoma and fibrosarcoma also occur. The tumours are generally highly malignant. This fibrosarcoma has expanded the femoral shaft to form an elongated fusiform faintly-lobulated whitish tumour in which there are foci of necrosis and haemorrhage (top). The adjacent shaft (bottom) is thickened by Paget's disease. **13.69-13.71 Osteosarcoma.** Osteosarcoma is the commonest primary malignant bone tumour. It frequently shows a wide variation in histological structure but is characterised by the formation of bone and osteoid tissue by the tumour cells. The tumour cells may also form cartilage or fibrous tissue. The amount of ossified tissue varies and the terms sclerosing and osteolytic may be applied to these variants. Most tumours occur between the ages of 10 and 20 years. The lesion is highly malignant and metastasises

readily by the bloodstream. The metaphyses of long bones, lower end of femur, upper end and humerus are the commonest sites. **13.69** The central yellowish-white tumour is replacing the marrow cavity of the proximal part of the shaft of the humerus and expanding and infiltrating the overlying cortex. The cut surface shows circumscribed bluish-white cartilaginous tissue (top), mingled with ill-defined yellowish-white areas of tumour osteoid (bottom). **13.70** The end of a long bone is replaced by dense white tumour which has obliterated the medullary cavity and infiltrated through the cortex on both sides, producing marked elevation of the periosteum. The cut surface is pale yellow-white and hard-looking. Radiating vertical white spiculations of new bone ('sun-burst' appearance) are present beneath the periosteum. **13.71** This is a sclerosing type of osteosarcoma. It is a dense white tumour which has largely destroyed the os calcis. **13.72 Ewing's tumour: humerus.** Ewing's tumour usually occurs between the ages of 5 and 15 years. This one is a yellowish-white swelling in the centre of the diaphysis of the humerus. The overlying cortex and periosteum are infiltrated, producing a fusiform mass. The periosteal bone formation (right) shows the characteristic 'onion-skin' appearance. Ewing's tumour frequently metastasises to other bones. The common sites for the lesion are the shafts and metaphyses of long bones, femur, tibia, humerus and fibula.

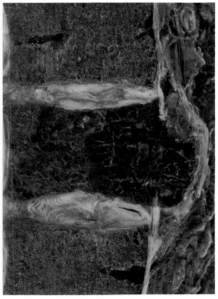

13.73 Cavernous haemangioma: spine

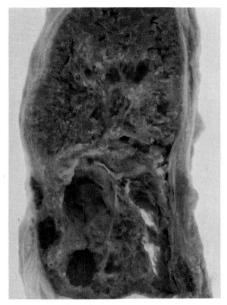

13.74 Lymphangioma: sternum

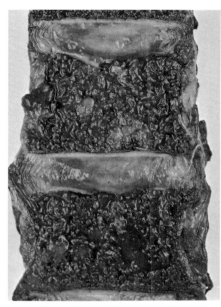

13.75 Secondary carcinoma: vertebrae

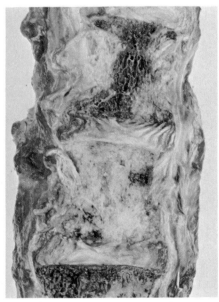

13.76 Secondary carcinoma: vertebrae

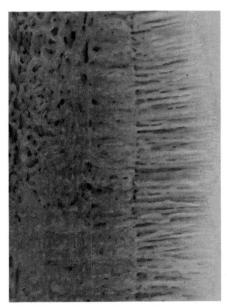

13.77 Secondary carcinoma: skull

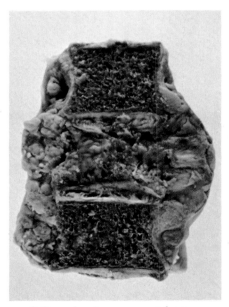

13.78 Secondary sarcoma: vertebrae

13.73 Cavernous haemangioma: spine. Three lumbar vertebrae are shown in median sagittal section. The central body is partly replaced by a brown-coloured cavernous angioma which has expanded posteriorly. Angioma of bone occurs most commonly in the vertebral bodies, and the incidence at necropsy may be as high as 10%. Most are hamartomatous malformations rather than true neoplasms. The blood vessels of which they consist may be either capillary or cavernous in type. **13.74 Lymphangioma: sternum.** The sternum has been bisected. It is distended by a brownish cystic vascular mass. Lymphangioma of bone is extremely rare. It is a benign lesion composed of lymphatic vessels some of which are dilated to form cystic spaces. The lesion may be solitary or multiple. The latter is frequently associated with soft-tissue lesions of the same type. **13.75-13.77 Secondary carcinoma: bone.** Osseous metastases are found in 15 to 30% of necropsies on patients with malignant disease. In order of frequency, the bones most often involved are the spine, pelvis, femur, skull, ribs and humerus. The deposits may be circumscribed or diffuse. The primary tumours which tend to metastasise to bone are breast, prostate, lung, kidney and stomach. **13.75** Two lumbar vertebral bodies are shown. They contain small round yellowish-white secondary

deposits. The primary tumour was a carcinoma of breast. **13.76** These two lumbar vertebral bodies have been largely replaced by secondary deposits. These are pale and sclerotic and histology showed extensive new bone formation. The intervertebral discs have been spared. Secondary deposits of carcinoma are generally destructive (osteolytic), and osteosclerotic metastases are usually prostatic in origin. In this case however the metastases were from a primary carcinoma of breast. **13.77** This is a dried specimen of the skull, and it is an extreme example of osteosclerotic secondary carcinoma. The bone of the calvarium is increased in density and large numbers of vertically orientated trabeculae of new bone have been formed by the raised periosteum, producing a striking striated appearance. Diffuse osteosclerotic skull secondaries are most commonly seen in prostatic cancer. **13.78 Secondary sarcoma: vertebrae.** One of the vertebral bodies has been extensively invaded by lobulated greyish-pink tumour, and it is showing early collapse and a compression-fracture. Extensive paravertebral spread has occurred over the surface of the two adjacent vertebrae. The tumour is a metastatic leiomyosarcoma originating from a paratesticular primary. Haematogenous spread to lungs and bones is commonly found in sarcomas (see 6.81).

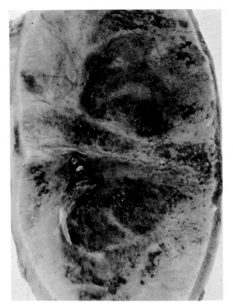

13.79 Secondary melanoma: skull

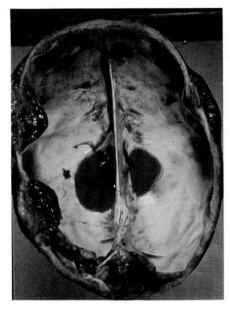

13.80 Secondary neuroblastoma: skull

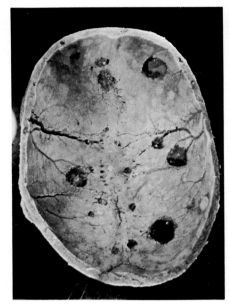

13.81 Myelomatosis: skull

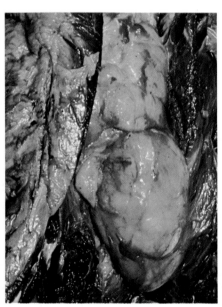

13.82 Liposarcoma

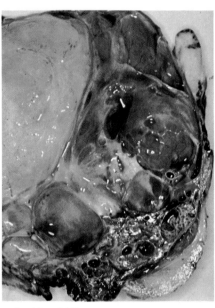

13.83 Myxoid liposarcoma

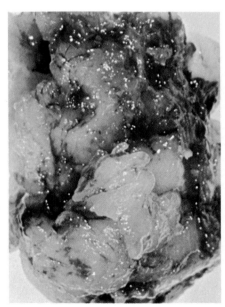

13.84 Myxoma: jaw

13.79 Secondary melanoma: skull. This shows the inner surface of part of the calvarium. Much of it appears black, as a result of extensive infiltration by heavily-pigmented malignant melanoma. Most secondary deposits in bone are haematogenous in origin, but occasionally a bone may be involved by direct extension. This patient developed a primary malignant melanoma in a blue naevus of the skin over the occiput 9 years earlier. The melanoma recurred locally and subsequently invaded the skull by direct spread. The dura was also involved. Widely disseminated deposits were found *post mortem*. **13.80 Secondary neuroblastoma: skull.** In children, neuroblastoma of the adrenal is the commonest source of bone metastases. In this case, a number of large haemorrhagic secondary deposits are destroying the diploe and inner and outer tables of the calvarium. **13.81 Myelomatosis: skull.** This is the inner surface of the vault of the skull. Numerous punched-out haemorrhagic osteolytic deposits are present. Myelomatosis is one of the most frequent malignant conditions of the skeleton. It usually occurs in patients over the age of 50. The common sites are spine, pelvis, ribs, sternum and skull. **13.82 and**

13.83 Liposarcoma. 13.82 Liposarcoma is the most common primary malignant tumour of soft tissues, making up about 20% of all soft-tissue sarcomas. It arises primarily in deeper structures, and about 50% are found in the lower limb, in the thigh or gluteal region. This one is a large deep-seated lobulated bright yellow mass situated between the muscles of the thigh. **13.83** Myxoid liposarcoma is the commonest variant of liposarcoma. The cut surface of this specimen shows a very variable pattern which ranges from smooth yellow lobulated fat (top left) to myxoid gelatinous tissue with extensive areas of cystic degeneration and haemorrhage (below). The well-differentiated form (myxoliposarcoma), which occurs between the ages of 25 and 50 years, behaves as a locally invasive lesion but about 60% show a tendency to recur repeatedly over many years. **13.84 Myxoma: jaw.** The tumour consists of soft gelatinous lobulated tissue. Myxoma of bone seems to occur exclusively in the jaw. About 60% occur in the second and third decades and the mandible and maxilla are equally involved. It is believed to arise from the dental papilla and is sometimes called an odontogenic myxoma.

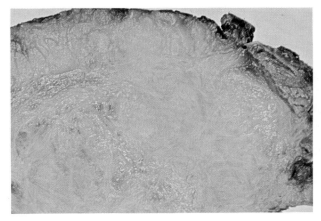

13.85 Infiltrating fibromatosis

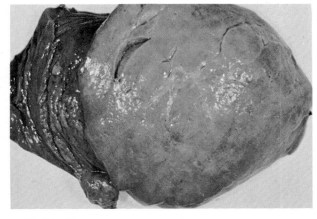

13.86 Fibrolipoma: uterus

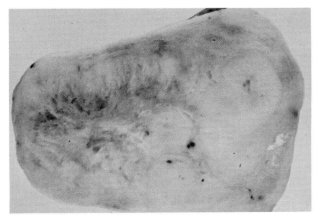

13.87 Fibrosarcoma: chest wall

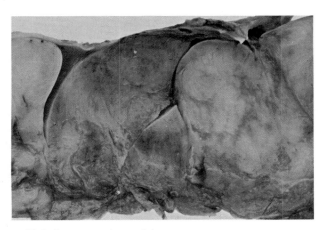

13.88 Leiomyosarcoma: pelvis

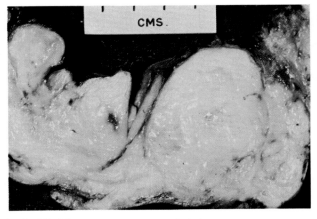

13.89 Rhabdomyosarcoma: urogenital sinus

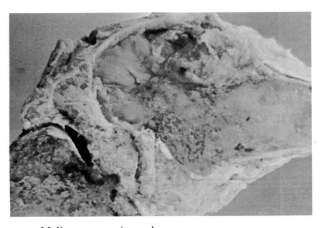

13.90 Malignant synovioma: knee

13.85 Infiltrating fibromatosis. The subcutaneous fat is widely infiltrated by an ill-defined greyish-white mass which is traversed by interweaving bundles of fibrous tissue. The aggressive infiltrating fibromatoses are a group of benign lesions of connective tissue which arise in both superficial and deep structures and microscopically closely resemble fibrosarcoma. **13.86 Fibrolipoma: uterus.** The fundus has been opened to display a large bright yellow tumour, the cut surface of which is faintly lobulated and traversed by white fibrous septa. Certain rare fatty tumours resembling leiomyoma are occasionally found in the uterus. True lipoma of the uterus has been described but it has to be differentiated from some lipomatous neoplasms which are in fact examples of extreme fatty change in a leiomyoma. **13.87 Fibrosarcoma: chest wall.** Fibrosarcoma is a malignant tumour of fibroblasts. It is a rare tumour and about 80% occur in soft tissues. Most are well-differentiated and behave as low-grade non-metastasising tumours. This one is a large smooth ovoid tumour from the chest wall of a 47-year-old woman. It had been previously excised but recurred. The cut surface is creamy-white and has a faintly whorled appearance. Cystic degeneration and haemorrhage are present (left). **13.88 Leiomyosarcoma: pelvis.** Malignant smooth muscle tumours are relatively rare and about 30% arise in soft tissues. The retroperitoneum is the commonest site (70%) and this one was located in the retroperitoneal tissues of the pelvis of a 55-year-old woman. It is a bulky irregularly-lobulated grey-white mass traversed by slit-like clefts. Leiomyosarcomas are typically nodular or lobulated with areas of haemorrhage and necrosis. They often attain a large size and tend to metastasise to the liver and lungs. **13.89 Rhabdomyosarcoma: urogenital sinus.** Rhabdomyosarcoma is the second-commonest malignant tumour of the soft tissues. There are three main types; the adult pleomorphic, the embryonal alveolar, and the embryonal botryoid. This is an example of the last type, which is the commonest of the three types. It is a lobulated pinkish-white growth arising from the region of the urogenital sinus in a neonate. Most rhabdomyosarcomas occur in infants, the two commonest sites being the head and neck and the genito-urinary tract. Botryoid rhabdomyosarcoma is typically polypoid and myxomatous. It tends to recur locally and in the later stages haematogenous spread ensues. The prognosis is very poor. **13.90 Malignant synovioma: knee.** This is a sagittal section of the knee-joint. A large pinkish-white tumour is infiltrating the lower femur (top), extending into the knee-joint, and spreading over the articular surface of the tibia (bottom). Synovial sarcoma originates in the juxta-articular soft tissues rather than in the synovial membrane of the joint (less than 5%). It occurs predominantly in young adults and the commonest site is around the knee. It is a highly malignant growth with a tendency to dissemination by the bloodstream.

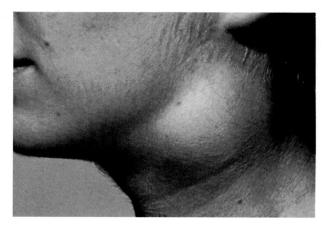

14.1 Branchial cyst

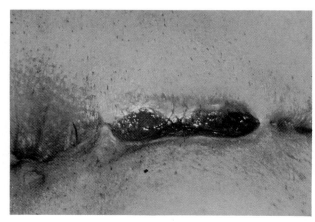

14.2 Pilonidal sinus

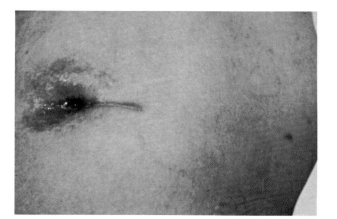

14.3 Sinus in Crohn's disease

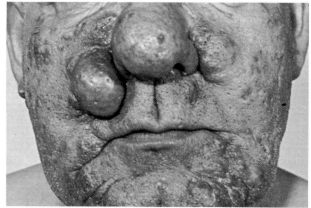

14.4 Rhinophyma

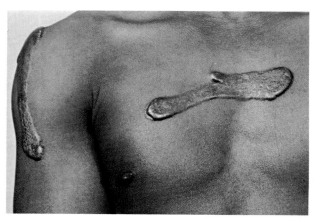

14.5 Keloid

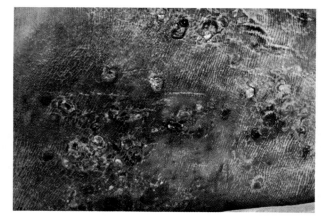

14.6 Maduromycosis (Madura foot)

14.1 Branchial cyst. A branchial cyst (lymphoepithelial or lateral cervical cyst) is thought to arise from epithelium sequestrated in cervical lymph nodes and is typically located near the angle of the jaw, anterior to the sternomastoid. Microscopically it is lined with stratified squamous or ciliated columnar epithelium, and lymphoid tissue with germinal follicles is also present. It usually becomes apparent clinically during the third decade and this one formed a large subcutaneous swelling on the side of the neck of a young woman. The swelling was fluctuant. The cyst may become acutely inflamed (see 1.3). **14.2 Pilonidal sinus.** This is the natal cleft, the anus being on the left. Multiple sinuses are present in the cleft, the large central sinus containing a tuft of hair. The adjacent subcutaneous fat is red and inflamed. Histologically a pilonidal sinus is lined with squamous epithelium and there is a foreign-body giant-cell reaction to the hair. In most cases the sinus is an acquired lesion. The primary sinus may have one or many openings all of which are strictly in the mid-line. Over 80% occur in young adults aged between 20 and 30 years, men being more often affected than women. **14.3 Sinus in Crohn's disease.** This is the right loin of a patient with Crohn's disease. There is a puckered sinus at the posterior end of a surgical scar, and the surrounding skin is reddened and excoriated. In the chronic stages of Crohn's disease, perforation of the intestinal wall with formation of fistulas may occur. External fistulas nearly always reach the skin surface through the scar of a previous operation which in this case was an appendicectomy. **14.4 Rhinophyma.** The skin of the lower part of the nose and face is nodular, with bulbous swellings of the nose and right cheek. This change in the skin is produced by hypertrophy and hyperplasia of the sebaceous glands, with dilatation and plugging of the ducts by keratinous material. Histologically the adjacent tissues show increased vascularity, chronic inflammation and progressive fibrosis. **14.5 Keloid.** A keloid represents an excessive fibroblastic response to various forms of trauma with formation of a hypertrophic cutaneous scar. Microscopically it consists of thick bands of collagen and very large active-looking fibroblasts. Keloid formation is more common in the negroid races than in the Caucasian, and in this example two large oval keloids have formed over the shoulder and upper chest of a male negro. The edge of each lesion is raised and the centre depressed. Keloids usually develop as a reaction to burns, incisions or vaccinations but may occur spontaneously as in this case. **14.6 Maduro-mycosis (Madura foot).** This lesion is a mycetoma, a chronic suppurative subcutaneous infection of the foot, caused by a variety of fungi which enter through the skin from the soil. This shows the sole of an affected foot. It is swollen and covered with sinus openings and abscesses, several of which (right) appear black. The appearance of the fungal grains determines the colour of the mycetoma.

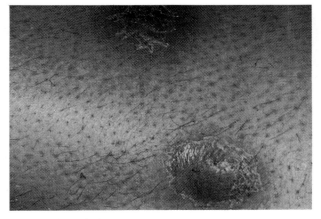

14.7 Erythema induratum

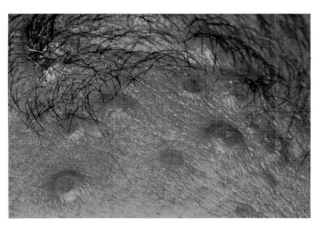

14.8 Herpes zoster

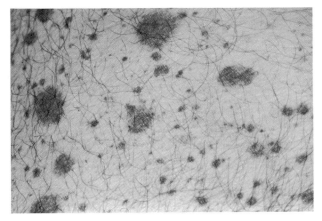

14.9 Drug rash

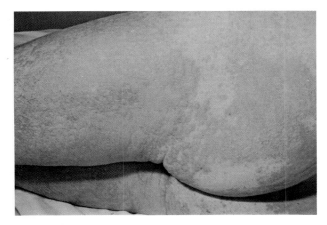

14.10 Urticaria

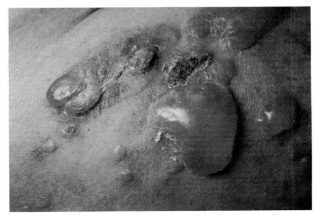

14.11 Bullous pemphigoid

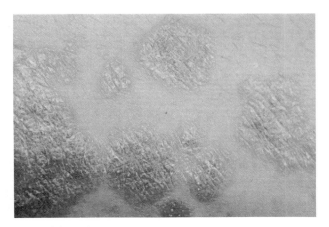

14.12 Lichen planus

14.7 Erythema induratum. This lesion occurs almost exclusively on the distal parts of the legs of young women. In this instance it takes the form of two raised dusky-brown indurated nodules covered with white scales. Histologically there was a chronic granulomatous reaction with tubercle formation, fat necrosis and endarteritis obliterans within the adipose tissue. Patients with erythema induratum usually have a tuberculous focus elsewhere but in some cases no evidence of this can be found. **14.8 Herpes zoster.** Herpes zoster is an acute infection that occurs almost exclusively in adults. The distinctive clinical features of the disease are a consequence of a virus infection of the nerve cells in the sensory ganglia of the cranial and spinal nerves. The skin lesions begin as papules which rapidly become vesicular and later pustular. These changes are visible in this close-up of affected skin at the junction of the back of the neck and the scalp. A crop of vesicles has formed and some of these have become pustular, with a flattened crater-like surface due to crust formation (right) and healing. **14.9 Drug rash.** Some of the toxic reactions to drugs are allergic in origin and skin rashes are common. The usual rash is morbilliform, resembling the rash of measles. In this case the rash is macular. Drugs which can produce allergic skin reactions include the pencillins, sulphonamides, barbiturates, analgesics and anti-epileptic drugs. **14.10 Urticaria.** This shows the left buttock and upper thigh. The skin is covered with a diffuse semi-confluent pink maculo-papular rash. The affected area is slightly raised, from the presence of subepidermal oedema. Urticaria is a very common condition which affects either sex at any age. The lesions are usually transient and subside in two or three days. There are many causes. **14.11 Bullous pemphigoid.** Bullous pemphigoid occurs mainly in the skin and mucous membranes of the elderly. The vesicles are subepidermal and contain fibrin. This shows several swollen vesicles (bullae) and their content of clear yellow fluid. Some authorities consider bullous pemphigoid to be a bullous variant of dermatitis herpetiformis but others regard it as a form of erythema multiforme. **14.12 Lichen planus.** The rash consists of rounded, glistening, flat-topped pinkish papules, the surface of which contain whitish lines (Wickham's striae). The papules tend to itch and are classically distributed over the flexor aspects of the wrists, forearms and legs. Microscopically there is hyperkeratosis, acanthosis, pointed rete pegs, liquefaction degeneration, and a dense subepidermal inflammatory zone. The condition is typically chronic and may last from months to years, with a tendency to resolve spontaneously.

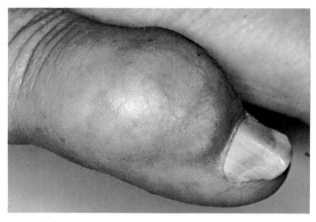

14.13 Gouty tophus

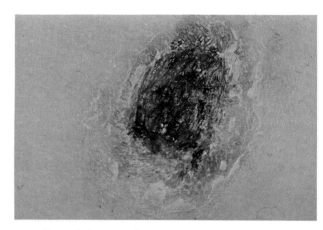

14.14 Systemic lupus erythematosus

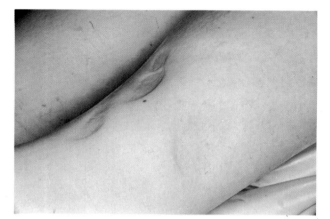

14.15 Oedema: skin

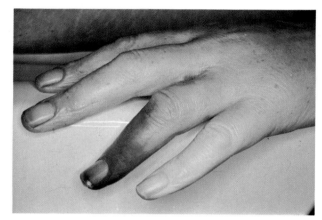

14.16 Digital gangrene

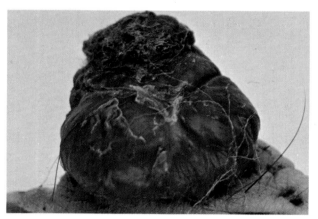

14.17 Pyogenic granuloma: skin

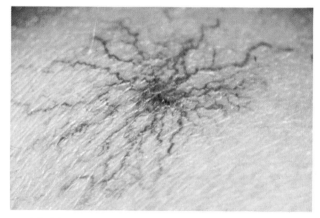

14.18 Spider naevus

14.13 Gouty tophus. In gout, urate crystals may be deposited in synovial membranes of joints, juxta-articular tissue and cartilage. The larger deposits are called tophi and the masses of urate crystals within them are surrounded by fibrous tissue and numerous foreign-body giant cells. This tophus forms a red shiny swelling over the terminal phalanx of the fifth finger. **14.14 Systemic lupus erythematosus.** The lesions is a red, moderately indurated macular patch. The skin surrounding it is red and slightly scaly. In systemic lupus erythematosus the patches are less well-defined than those of discoid lupus and merely part of a widespread disorder. The patches typically occur on the face. In the acute lesions they may be bullous or ulcerated. **14.15 Oedema: skin.** This shows pitting oedema of the skin of the anterior tibial region in a patient with a nephrotic syndrome. In oedema there is an increased volume of extra-cellular and extravascular fluid, i.e. an excess of fluid within the tissue spaces. It is caused by conditions which interfere with the normal movement of blood, tissue fluid and lymph or which disturb the mechanism of fluid balance. These include lymphatic obstruction, increased vascular permeability, increased capillary pressure, decreased plasma protein, and sodium and water retention. **14.16 Digital gangrene.** This shows early gangrene of the top of the third ('ring') finger. The nail is bluish-black and the skin a dusky purplish-red. Gangrene is massive

necrosis of tissue to which there is added invasion by saprophytic organisms. Such a lesion is often called moist gangrene. Where the necrotic tissue is drier and much less heavily infected, the condition is one of dry gangrene. Ischaemic necrosis of the tip of an extremity may be due to thrombosis, embolism or vasospasm. This patient developed thrombosis of the digital arteries as a complication of intense peripheral vasoconstriction resulting from left ventricular failure which followed surgical repair of an atrial septal defect. **14.17 Pyogenic granuloma: skin.** The nature of granuloma pyogenicum is in dispute, some regarding it as a capillary haemangioma and others as an exuberant granulation tissue reaction to trauma and non-specific infection. Microscopically it consists of newly-formed capillaries, fibroblasts, and variable numbers of neutrophil polymorphs. This lesion was present on the skin of the abdomen of a 31-year-old man and it had recurred one month after removal. It forms a lobulated purplish-brown mass with an ulcerated tip. **14.18 Spider naevus.** In chronic liver disease, arteriovenous fistulas of the skin (vascular spider naevi) are often observed. They consist of a leash of tortuous venules radiating out from a central arteriole. Similar lesions have been described in the lungs and they may be the cause of the finger-clubbing and cyanosis that are found in some cirrhotic patients.

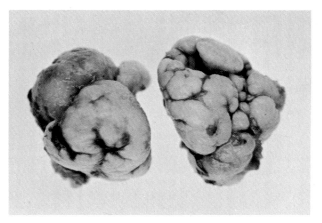

14.19 Seborrhoeic keratosis (basal cell papilloma)

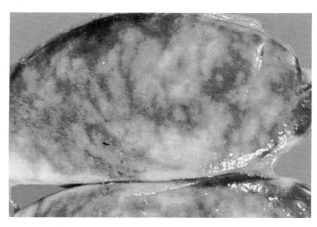

14.20 Histiocytoma cutis

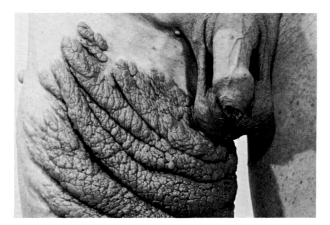

14.21 Neurofibromatosis

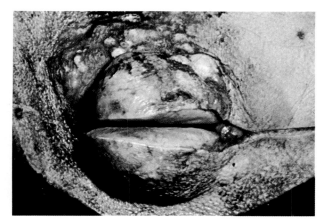

14.22 Dermatofibrosarcoma protuberans

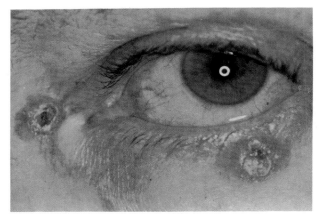

14.23 Basal cell carcinoma ('rodent ulcer')

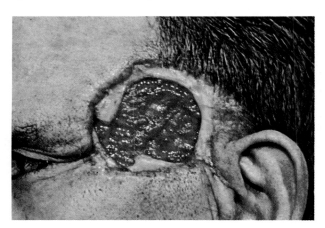

14.24 Basal cell carcinoma ('rodent ulcer')

14.19 Seborrhoeic keratosis (basal cell papilloma). This is one of the commonest skin tumours. Typically it is a sharply-defined papillomatous growth which is often covered by a 'greasy' crust. This shows one such mass which has been bisected. It is grey-brown and lobulated and measured 1.5 cm in diameter. The lesions are often multiple and may be pigmented. They may occur on any part of the body and are commoner in the elderly. **14.20 Histiocytoma cutis.** The lesion forms an oval mottled yellowish-brown mass (2 x 3 cm) underlying a stretched epidermis (top). It is a common skin tumour which is usually about 1 cm in diameter but may occasionally be up to 3 cm across. Microscopically it consists of fibroblasts, lipophages, blood vessels and a variable amount of haemosiderin. Some lesions contain a lot of haemosiderin and may be mistaken clinically for melanomas. The histogenesis is confused and sometimes the lesion is called sclerosing haemangioma or dermatofibroma. **14.21 Neurofibromatosis.** Neurofibromatosis (von Recklinghausen's disease of nerves) consists of multiple soft sessile or pedunculated tumours of the skin. In this man it takes the form of a large irregularly folded thickening of the thigh skin. The affected skin is wrinkled and dark brown from the presence of melanin. This is unusual, and the skin over a tumour is usually normal in colour. There are also a number of small non-pigmented nodular lesions. **14.22 Dermatofibrosarcoma protuberans.** An irregular nodular greyish-white polypoid tumour projects from the surface of the skin. This is a rare tumour, most frequently found in women. Classically it arises in the skin of the trunk around the hip or shoulder. Growth is slow and ulceration eventually develops. It is locally invasive and grows slowly over many years. Dissemination is rare. The absence of fat and haemosiderin and the tendency to ulcerate are the main differences from dermatofibroma. **14.23 and 14.24 Basal cell carcinoma ('rodent ulcer').** Basal cell carcinoma occurs predominantly in fair-skinned people in the part of the face bounded by the hairline, ears and upper lip. It grows slowly and invades locally. **14.23** A particularly characteristic site is the inner canthus of the eye and one of these two early lesions is situated over the inner canthus of the left eye. The other is on the lower lid. They are smooth elevated ulcerated papular growths with a rolled red border. **14.24** This is a more advanced lesion over the left temporal region. It is a large ulcer, with a bright red granular base and a smooth, white, rolled border. This is the cicatricial type of basal cell carcinoma, which is characterised by superficial peripheral spread with ulceration and subsequent central scarring. It occurs commonly on the forehead.

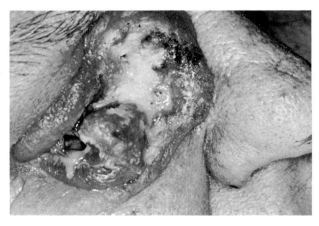

14.25 Squamous carcinoma

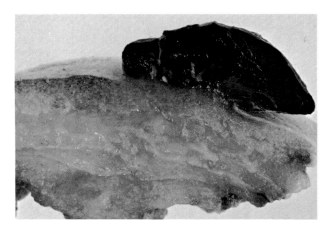

14.26 Malignant melanoma

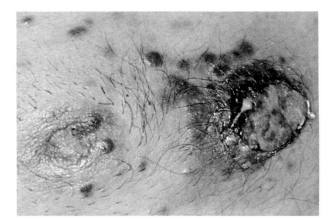

14.27 Malignant melanoma

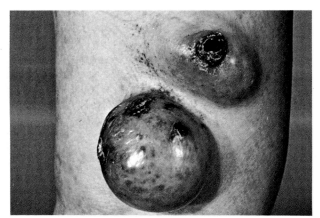

14.28 Malignant melanoma

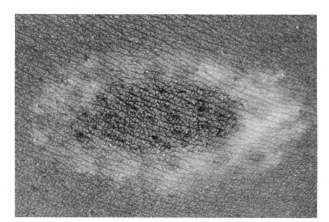

14.29 Halo naevus

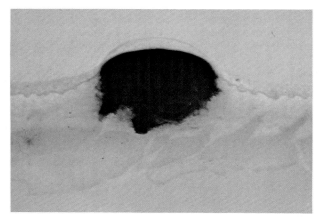

14.30 Blue naevus

14.25 Squamous carcinoma. Clinically, squamous carcinoma may be ulcerative or papillary, and this advanced lesion on the inner canthus of the right eye of an elderly woman has some of the features of both types. There is an exuberant growth of neoplastic tissue which forms a heaped-up mass as well as irregular areas of ulceration covered with a thick creamy-white necrotic slough. Squamous carcinoma is commoner on the skin of the face and hands, and in contrast to basal cell carcinoma it metastasises readily. The rate of growth is variable. Some grow rapidly and invade lymphatics early. **14.26-14.28 Malignant melanoma.** Malignant melanoma is the most malignant of all skin cancers. The lymph vessels in the vicinity of the primary growth are readily infiltrated and satellite deposits develop along the lymphatics draining the primary growth. Many melanomas arise in pre-existing pigmented naevi. When a naevus begins to darken, malignant transformation should be suspected. Ulceration, increase in size and bleeding are serious signs. **14.26** This deeply pigmented elevated tumour measuring 2 x 2 x 1 cm was situated on the skin of the back. Within the dermis, beneath and to the left of the tumour, there is a diffuse flat spreading brownish-coloured lesion. This appearance suggests that the melanoma arose in a previously benign intradermal naevus. **14.27** This illustrates local invasion. Many small satellite nodules have formed in the tissue around the ulcerated pigmented primary tumour which was situated on the chest. **14.28** This is the back of the knee. The larger spherical blue-black mass is the primary tumour. The ulcerated nodule above it is a metastatic satellite. **14.29 Halo naevus.** The halo naevus (Sutton's naevus) is formed by the progressive centrifugal extension of a zone of depigmentation around a naevus, the depigment-ation probably being provoked by subepidermal inflammation. In this case the patient is a negro and the halo of depigmentation (local vitiligo) around a flat bluish-black naevus is clearly visible. The same appearance is sometimes seen around small malignant melanomas. **14.30 Blue naevus.** This is a hemi-section of the naevus. It forms a black dome-shaped nodule with ill-defined margins within the dermis. The epidermis is thinned over it. Histologically it consisted of elongated melanocytes within the dermal connective tissue, with abundant melanin present. Blue naevi are rarely greater than 1 cm in diameter and are almost always benign, although lesions situated on the trunk or extremities are often mistaken clinically for malignant melanoma. The commonest sites are the extremities, face and perineal region. This one was on the thigh of a 14-year-old boy.

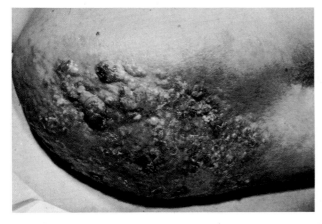

14.31 Carcinoma *en cuirasse*

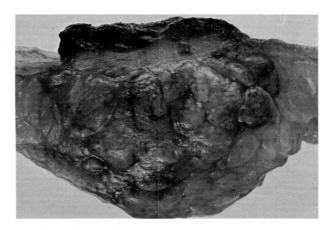

14.32 Secondary carcinoma

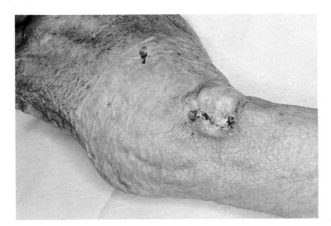

14.33 Secondary carcinoma

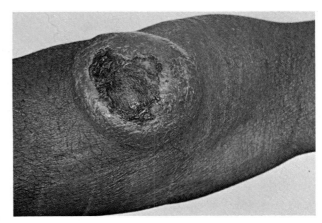

14.34 Lymphoma: skin

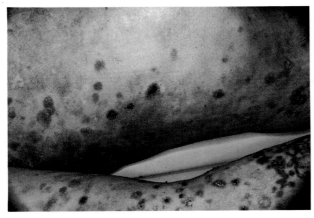

14.35 Mycosis fungoides

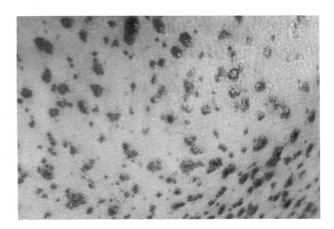

14.36 Letterer-Siwe disease

14.31 Carcinoma *en cuirasse*. In carcinoma of the breast, the skin may be involved by retrograde spread via the periductal lymphatics, lymphatics of Cooper's ligaments, or by direct continuity. The process of formation of multiple nodules of carcinoma in the skin of the breast and chest wall is known as cancer *en cuirasse*. This shows such a change on the infero-lateral aspect of a female breast in which there is a primary carcinoma. The skin is widely infiltrated by neoplastic nodules, many of which are ulcerated. **14.32 and 14.33 Secondary carcinoma.** The carcinomas most liable to produce skin metastases are those of breast, uterus, lung, gastrointestinal tract, pancreas, thyroid and prostate, in addition to melanomas, squamous carcinomas and lymphomas. **14.32** This shows, in cross-section, a raised ulcerated tumour which was removed from the skin of the chest wall in a 56-year-old man. The lesion is yellowish-brown and lobulated and there is extensive necrosis. Clinically it was diagnosed as a malignant melanoma but histology showed that it was metastatic squamous carcinoma and the primary was found in a bronchus. **14.33** This patient also had a carcinoma of bronchus. The wrist is swollen and deformed by the presence of a metastatic deposit in the radius which has invaded directly the skin over the radial aspect of the wrist, with formation of an irregular ulcerated pinkish-white nodule. **14.34 Lymphoma: skin.** A raised smooth spherical swelling with central ulceration is present on the forearm. In disseminated lymphomas, involvement of the skin is generally a late event but a

lymphoma may present in the skin as collection of nodules before there are signs of lymph node enlargement. Moreover, cases of follicular lymphoma, lymphosarcoma, histiocytic lymphoma and Hodgkin's disease have been reported as starting in skin. It is difficult however to assess whether such tumours have arisen in the skin or whether they are cutaneous manifestations of multicentric tumour. **14.35 Mycosis fungoides.** Multiple erythematous patches are present over the trunk and arm. Several plaques have a vesicular eczematous appearance, and others are circinate plaques with central ulceration. Mycosis fungoides is generally regarded as a malignant disease of the lympho-reticular cells of the dermis with three successive phases; the premycotic, the infiltrative, and the fungoid tumour stages. Though the lesions histologically resemble Hodgkin's disease or histiocytic lymphoma, the viscera are commonly spared, with only about 15% of the fatal cases showing involvement. **14.36 Letterer-Siwe disease.** The patient was an infant, and this shows the disseminated haemorrhagic maculo-papular cutaneous eruption that was present. Letterer-Siwe disease is an acute malignant disorder of the lympho reticular system, affecting infants and young children and currently related to the malignant histiocytosis of childhood, histiocytosis-X. Microscopically the dermal lesions contain accumulations of mono-cytoid cells, eosinophils and lymphocytes. The spleen, lymph nodes and liver are enlarged and there are similar lesions in the lungs and bone.

INDEX